Wards 101 pocket

Clinician's Survival Guide

Authors: Jed Abraham Katzel, M.D., Rosemary Garcia, M.D., Raluca Vucescu M.D.

Acknowledgements:
James Mazzara, M.D., Andrew Bohmart, M.D., Yolanda Brown, M.D., Abigail Chen, M.D., Ruchir Gupta, M.D., Saad Jazrawi, M.D., Linda Kirschenbaum, M.D., Ryan Knueppel, M.D., Stephen Kreiger, M.D., Reshma Mahtani, M.D., Jayson Mallie, M.D., Anatasios Manessis, M.D., Daniel Nichita, M.D., Salas Sabnis, M.D., Sonali Sethi, M.D., Margaret Smith, M.D., Ken Spaeth, M.D., Raghuraman Vidhun, M.D., Elizabeth Ward, M.D., Brian Wong, M.D., Fred Y. Wu, M.D., PhD.

Editors: Daniel Nichita, M.D., Rahul Ghugari, M.D.
Production: Alexander Storck
Publisher: Börm Bruckmeier Publishing, LLC, www.media4u.com

111½ Eucalyptus Drive, El Segundo, CA 90245
www.media4u.com
Third Edition

IMPORTANT NOTICE – PLEASE READ!
This book is based on information from sources believed to be reliable, and every effort has been made to make the book as complete and accurate as possible and to describe generally accepted practices based on information available as of the printing date, but its accuracy and completeness cannot be guaranteed. Despite the best efforts of authors, editors and publisher, the book may contain errors, and the reader should use the book only as a general guide and not as the ultimate source of information about the subject matter.
This book is not intended to reprint all of the information available to the author or publisher on the subject, but rather to simplify, complement and supplement other available sources. The reader is encouraged to read all available material and to consult the package insert and other references to learn as much as possible about the subject.
This book is sold without warranties of any kind, expressed or implied, and the publisher and authors disclaim any liability, loss or damage caused by the content of this book.
IF YOU DO NOT WISH TO BE BOUND BY THE FOREGOING CAUTIONS AND CONDITIONS , YOU MAY RETURN THIS BOOK TO THE PUBLISHER FOR A FULL REFUND.

Printed in China through Colorcraft Ltd., Hong Kong
ISBN 978-1-59103-266-3

Preface to the Third Edition

The demands exerted on all levels of medical practitioners from attendings, nurses, fellows, residents, interns and students continue to increase, while the speed of care delivery and medical progress reaches new heights. The challenge to provide excellent care is often at odds with time and cost limitations. This 3rd edition is dedicated to those individuals who take the extra time to sit at the bedside of their sickest patients and continue to recognize that they are our greatest responsibility and also our greatest teachers.

This edition would not be possible without the tremendous work of two chief residents from Kaiser, Santa Clara - now practicing attendings, Rosemary Garcia and Raluca Vucescu.

Just as with the first two editions, this is not intended to be an all-inclusive text. To the contrary, our intention is to include the minimum essential information that should be addressed during rounds. In the past, physicians (like my father) would carry a "little black book" in their pocket with clinical pearls. Even in this electronic information age, Wards 101 3rd edition is intended to be a modern version of that little black book.

I hope you and your patients benefit from this concise text.

Sincerely,

Jed A. Katzel

Coauthor preface and acknowledgments

Raluca Vucescu, M.D.
Internal Medicine Chief Resident 2010-2011 at Kaiser Santa Clara Hospital
Currently Internal Medicine Physician at Kaiser South San Francisco

As chief residents, the mindset is how can we teach our students and interns the relevant information in a clear and simple way - and Wards 101 is part of such an endeavor. During my chief resident year, I was very grateful for the opportunity to co-author the third edition of Wards 101 and I greatly enjoyed researching the clinical guidelines and literature for the latest updates.

We hope you will find this pocketbook helpful in every day learning, rounding and patient care, and as a teaching tool.

Acknowledgements: Jed Katzel, MD, Rosemary Garcia, MD, Fred Y Wu, MD, PhD

Coauthor preface and acknowledgments

Rosemary Garcia, M.D.
Internal Medicine Chief Resident 2010-2011 at Kaiser Santa Clara Hospital
Internal Medicine Physician at Kaiser San Diego

I am very grateful for having had the opportunity to work on researching new clinical updates for the third edition of this book. The endeavor to help succinctly organize and update this information was a great learning experience, and I hope the readers will continue to benefit from this reference book.

I would like to acknowledge and thank Dr. Jed Katzel who created this book series and extended the opportunity to co-author this book for this edition. I would also like to thank Dr. Raluca Vucescu, my Internal Medicine Co-Chief Resident at the time, as we both worked on suggestions for this edition.

To Liz, Jim, Marilyn

"Though a little one, the master-word looms large in meaning. It is the open sesame to every portal, the great equalizer in the world, the true philosopher's stone, which transmutes all the base metal of humanity into gold. The stupid man among you it will make bright, the bright man brilliant, and the brilliant student steady. With the magic word in your heart all things are possible, and without it all study is vanity and vexation. The miracles of life are with it; the blind see by touch, the deaf hear with eyes, the dumb speak with fingers...

...And the master word is **Work**, a little one, as I have said, but fraught with momentous sequences if you can but write it on the tablets of your hearts, and bind it upon your foreheads." -- William Osler

Additional titles in this series:

Acupuncture pocket
Anatomy pocket
Differential Diagnosis pocket
Drug pocket
Drug pocket plus
Canadian Drug pocket
ECG pocket
ECG Cases pocket
EMS pocket
Homeopathy pocket
Medical Abbreviations pocket
Medical Classifications pocket
Medical Spanish Dictionary pocket
Medical Spanish pocket
Medical Spanish pocket plus
Medical Translator pocket
Normal Values pocket
Nursing Dictionary pocket
Respiratory pocket

Börm Bruckmeier Publishing LLC on the Internet:
www.media4u.com

Contents

3 Endocrinology

4 Gastroenterology

Contents

9 Internal Medicine

10 Women's Health and Pregnancy

11 Nephrology

15 Pediatrics

16 Psychiatry

Contents

Algorithms

ACLS – Adult Cardiac Arrest

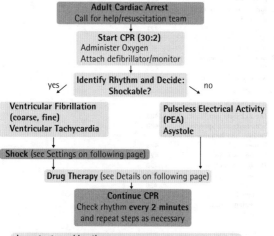

Adult Cardiac Arrest
Call for help/resuscitation team

↓

Start CPR (30:2)
Administer Oxygen
Attach defibrillator/monitor

↓

Identify Rhythm and Decide: Shockable?

yes ↙ ↘ no

yes:

Ventricular Fibrillation (coarse, fine)
Ventricular Tachycardia

↓

Shock (see Settings on following page)

↓

no:

Pulseless Electrical Activity (PEA)
Asystole

↓

Drug Therapy (see Details on following page)

↓

Continue CPR
Check rhythm **every 2 minutes**
and repeat steps as necessary

Important considerations:
- Ensure early IV access
- Minimize CPR interruptions
- Consider advanced airway (ET tube or supraglottic airway)
- Treat reversible causes

Adapted from the 2011 AHA/ESC Pocket Guidelines.

ACLS - Adult Cardiac Arrest: Doses and Details

CPR quality

- Push hard (≥ 2 inches [5 cm]) and fast (≥ 100/min) and allow complete chest recoil
- Minimize interruptions in compressions
- Avoid excessive ventilation
- Rotate compressor every 2 min
- If no advanced airway, 30:2 compression-ventilation ratio
- Quantitative waveform capnography
  - If $PETCO_2$ <10 mm Hg, attempt to improve CPR quality
- Intra-arterial pressure
  - If relaxation phase (diastolic) pressure <20 mm Hg, attempt to improve CPR quality

Reversible causes

- Hypovolemia
- Hypoxia
- Hydrogen ion (acidosis)
- Hypoglycemia
- Hypo-/Hyperkalemia
- Hypothermia
- Tension pneumothorax
- Tamponade, cardiac
- Toxins
- Thrombosis, pulmonary
- Thrombosis, coronary

Management

Shock energy for defebrillation	• **Biphasic:** Manufacturer recommendation (eg, initial dose of 120-200 J); if unknown, use maximum available. Second and subsequent doses should be equivalent, and higher doses may be considered • **Monophasic:** 360 J
Drug therapy	**Epinephrine IV/IO dose:** • 1 mg every 3-5 min.
	Vasopressin IV/IO dose: • 40 units can replace first or second dose of epinephrine
	Amiodarone IV/IO dose: • First dose: 300 mg bolus • Second dose: 150 mg
Advanced airway	• Endotracheal intubation or supraglottic advanced airway • Waveform capnography to confirm and monitor ET tube placement • 8-10 breaths per minute with continuous chest compressions
Return of spontaneous circulation (ROSC)	• Pulse and blood pressure • Abrupt sustained increase in $PETCO_2$ (typically ≥40 mm Hg) • Spontaneous arterial pressure waves with intra-arterial monitoring

ACLS – Adult Tachycardia

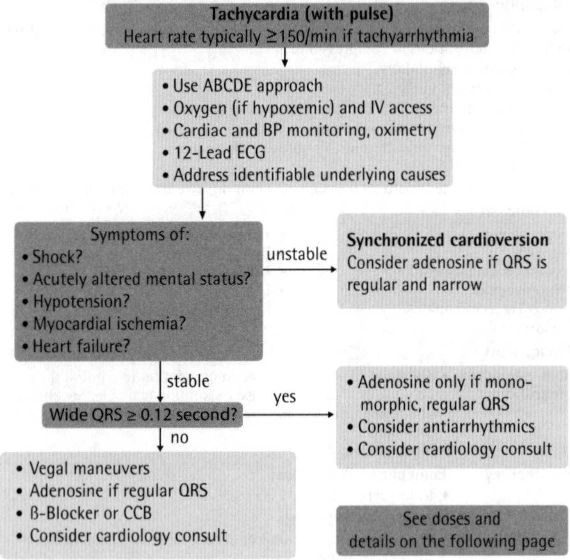

Adapted from the 2011 AHA/ESC Pocket Guidelines.

ACLS - Adult Tachycardia: Doses and Details	
Synchronized cardioversion	
Initial recommended doses	• Narrow regular: 50-100 J • Narrow irregular: 120-200 biphasic or 200 J monophasic • Wide regular: 100 J • Wide irregular: Defibrillation dose (NOT synchronized)
Adenosine IV dose	• First dose: 6 mg rapid IV push; follow with NS flush • Second dose: 12 mg if required
Antiarrhythmic infusions for stable Wide-QRS Tachycardia	
Procainamide IV dose	• 20-50 mg/min until arrhythmia suppressed, hypotension ensues, QRS duration increases >50%, or maximum dose 17 mg/kg given. • Maintenance infusion: 1-4 mg/min. Avoid if prolonged QT or CHF
Amiodarone IV dose	• First dose: 150 mg over 10 minutes. Repeat as needed if VT recurs • Maintenance infusion: 1 mg/min for first 6 hours
Sotalol IV dose	• 100 mg (1.5 mg/kg) over 5 minutes. • Avoid if prolonged QT.

ACLS-Adult Bradycardia

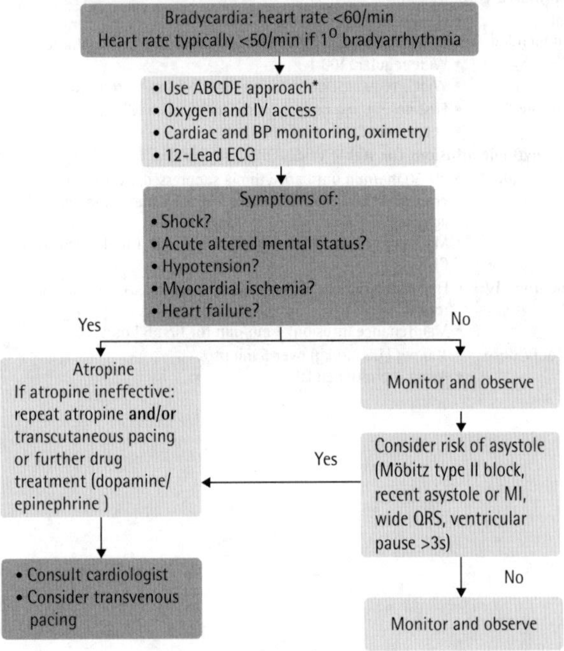
Bradycardia: heart rate <60/min
Heart rate typically <50/min if 1° bradyarrhythmia
• Use ABCDE approach*
• Oxygen and IV access
• Cardiac and BP monitoring, oximetry
• 12-Lead ECG
Symptoms of:
• Shock?
• Acute altered mental status?
• Hypotension?
• Myocardial ischemia?
• Heart failure?
Yes
No
Atropine
If atropine ineffective: repeat atropine and/or transcutaneous pacing or further drug treatment (dopamine/ epinephrine)
Monitor and observe
Yes
Consider risk of asystole (Möbitz type II block, recent asystole or MI, wide QRS, ventricular pause >3s)
No
• Consult cardiologist
• Consider transvenous pacing
Monitor and observe

Adapted from the 2011 AHA/ESC Pocket Guidelines.

ACLS - Adult Bradycardia: Doses and Details	
Drug therapy	
Atropine IV dose	• First dose: 0.5 mg bolus • Repeat every 3-5 minutes (max 3 mg)
Dopamine IV infusion	• 2-10 mcg/kg per minute
Epinephrine IV infusion	• 2-10 mcg per minute

PALS - Pediatric cardiac arrest

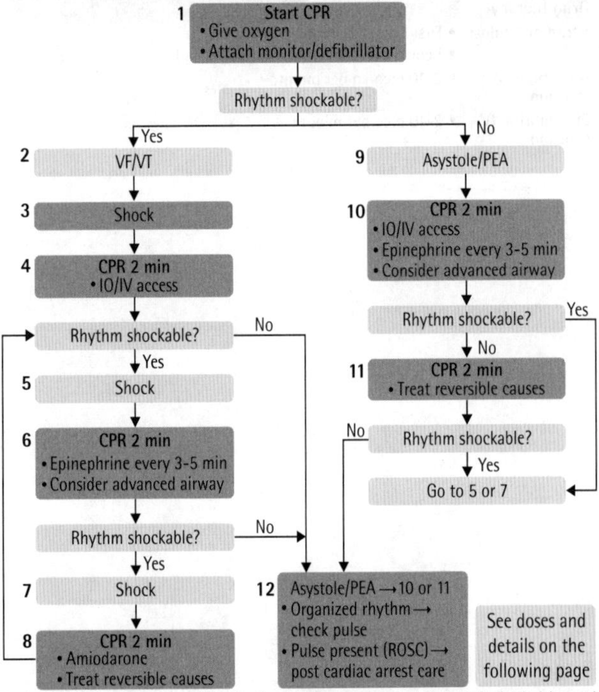

Monica E. Kleinman, Leon Chameides, Stephen M. Schexnayder, et al. Part 14: Pediatric Advanced Life Support: 2010 American Heart Association Guidelines for Cardiopulmonary Resuscitation and Emergency Cardiovascular Care. Circulation. 2010;122:S876-S908.

PALS - Pediatric Cardiac Arrest: Doses and Details

CPR quality

- Push hard (≥ 1/3 of anterior-posterior diameter of chest) and fast (at least 100/min) and allow complete chest recoil
- Minimize interruption in compressions
- Avoid excess ventilation
- Rotate compressor every 2 min
- If no advances airway, 15:2 compression-ventilation ratio. If advanced airway, 8-10 breaths per minute with continuous chest compression

Reversible causes

- Hypovolemia
- Hypoxia
- Hydrogen ion (acidosis)
- Hypoglycemia
- Hypo-/Hyperkalemia
- Hypothermia
- Tension pneumothorax
- Tamponade, cardiac
- Toxins
- Thrombosis, pulmonary
- Thrombosis, coronary

Management

Shock energy for defibrillation	First shock 2 J/kg, second shock 4 J/kg, subsequent shocks ≥ 4 J/kg, maximum 10 J/kg or adult dose
Drug therapy	**Epinephrine IV/IO dose:** • 0.01 mg/kg (0.1 mL/kg of 1:10,000 concentration). Repeat every 3-5 min. • If no IO/IV access, may give endotracheal dose: 0.1 mg/kg (0.1 mL/kg of 1:1000 concentration)
	Amiodarone IO/IV dose: • 5 mg/kg bolus during cardiac arrest. May repeat up to 2 times for refractory VF/pulseless VT
Advanced airway	• Endotracheal intubation or supraglottic advanced airway • Waveform capnography or capnometry to confirm and monitor ET tube placement • Once advanced airway in place give 8-10 breaths per minute
Return of spontaneous circulation (ROSC)	• Pulse and blood pressure • Spontaneous arterial pressure waves with intra-arterial monitoring

PALS - Pediatric Tachycardia

1 Identify and treat underlying cause

- Maintain patent airway; assist breathing as necessary
- Oxygen
- Cardiac monitor to identify rhythm; monitor blood pressure and oximetry
- IO/IV access
- 12-Lead ECG if available; don't delay therapy

2 Evaluate QRS duration

Narrow ($\leq$ 0.09 sec) → 3 | Wide (> 0.09 sec) → 9

3 Evaluate rhythm with 12-lead ECG or monitor → 4, 5

4 Probable sinus tachycardia

- Compatible history consistent with known cause
- P waves present/ normal
- Variable R-R; constant PR
- Infants: rate usually < 220/min
- Children: rate usually < 180/min

→ **6 Search for and treat cause**

5 Probable supra-venticular tachycardia

- Compatible history (vague, nonspecific); history of abrupt rate changes
- P waves absent/ abnormal
- HR not variable
- Infants: rate usually $\geq$ 220/min
- Children: rate usually $\geq$ 180/min

7 Consider vagal maneuvers (No delays) → 8

8 If IO/IV access present, give **adenosine**
OR
If IO/IV access not available, or if adenosine ineffective, synchronized cardioversion

9 Possible venticular tachycardia → 10

10 Cardiopulmonary compromise?

- Hypotension
- Acutely altered mental status
- Signs of shock

Yes → **11 Synchronized cardioversion**

No → **12 Consider adenosine if rhythm regular and QRS monomorphic** → 13

13 Expert consulatation advised

- **Amiodarone**
- **Procainamide**

See doses and details on the following page

Monica E. Kleinman, Leon Chameides, Stephen M. Schexnayder, et al. Part 14: Pediatric Advanced Life Support: 2010 American Heart Association Guidelines for Cardiopulmonary Resuscitation and Emergency Cardiovascular Care. Circulation. 2010;122:S876-S908.

PALS - Pediatric Tachycardia: Doses and Details

Synchronized cardioversion: Begin with 0.5-1 J/kg; if not effective, increase to 2 J/kg. Sedate if needed, but don't delay cardioversion.
Doses/details: Adenosine IO/IV dose: First dose: 0.1 mg/kg rapid bolus (maximum: 6 mg). Second dose: 0.2 mg/kg rapid bolus (maximum second dose 12 mg).
Amiodarone IO/IV dose: 5 mg/kg over 20-60 min , OR **Procainamide IO/IV dose:** 15 mg/kg over 30-60 min
Do not routinely administer amiodarone and procainamide together.

PALS - Pediatric Bradycardia

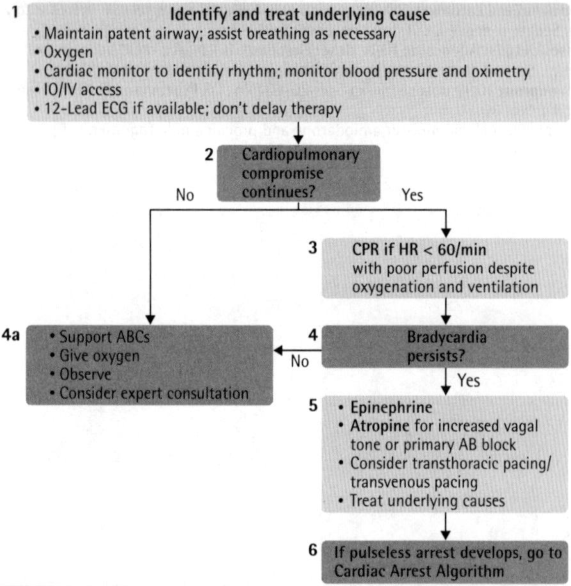
1
Identify and treat underlying cause
• Maintain patent airway; assist breathing as necessary
• Oxygen
• Cardiac monitor to identify rhythm; monitor blood pressure and oximetry
• IO/IV access
• 12-Lead ECG if available; don't delay therapy
2
Cardiopulmonary compromise continues?
No
Yes
3
CPR if HR < 60/min with poor perfusion despite oxygenation and ventilation
4a
• Support ABCs
• Give oxygen
• Observe
• Consider expert consultation
4
Bradycardia persists?
No
Yes
5
• Epinephrine
• Atropine for increased vagal tone or primary AB block
• Consider transthoracic pacing/ transvenous pacing
• Treat underlying causes
6
If pulseless arrest develops, go to Cardiac Arrest Algorithm

Cardiopulmonary compromise: Hypotension, acutely altered mental status, signs of shock

Doses/details: Epinephrine IO/IV dose: 0.01 mg/kg (0.1 mL/kg of 1:10,000 concentration). Repeat every 3-5 min. If IO/IV access not available but endotracheal (ET) tube in place, may give ET dose: 0.1 mg/kg (0.1mL/kg of 1:1000); **Atropine IO/IV dose:** 0.02 mg/kg. May repeat once. Minimum dose 0.1 mg and maximum single dose 0.5 mg.

Monica E. Kleinman, Leon Chameides, Stephen M. Schexnayder, et al. Part 14: Pediatric Advanced Life Support: 2010 American Heart Association Guidelines for Cardiopulmonary Resuscitation and Emergency Cardiovascular Care. Circulation. 2010;122:S876-S908.

Acute Coronary Syndrome

Presenting Complaints:
- Chest discomfort suggestive of ischemia
- Complaints may only be vague symptoms such as dyspnea, weakness, fatigue, or syncope in diabetics, the elderly, and women

Consider Differential Diagnoses:
- Anxiety
- Arrhythmia
- Pericarditis
- Aortic dissection
- Pulmonary embolism
- Pneumothorax
- Aortic stenosis
- Esophageal rupture
- Acute pancreatitis
- Perforated ulcer
- Myocarditis
- Tamponade

Suspected Acute Coronary Syndrome (ACS)

Initial Procedures:
- Secure and monitor ABCs, be prepared to defibrillate and give CPR
- Check vital signs, assess O_2 saturation
- Establish IV access
- Serial 12-lead ECGs
- Chem panel, cardiac markers, coags
- D-dimer if PE suspected
- Perform focused history and physical
- Chest X-ray unless emergent PCI
- Assess for fibrinolysis and check fibrinolytic contraindications

Initial STAT Therapy:
- Supplemental O_2 if needed to keep O_2 saturation > 90%
- Aspirin 162-325 mg chewed and swallowed; clopidogrel 300 mg if aspirin intolerant
- Nitroglycerin 0.4 mg SL q5min x3
- Morphine 5 mg IV (0.1 mg/kg)
- If pain persists start nitroglycerin drip at 20 mg/min

Assess Chest X-Ray:
Conditions to rule out:
- Widened mediastinum (> 8 cm) → poss aortic dissection
- Pneumomediastinum and left pleural effusion → Boerhaave syndrome
- Wedge-shaped infarct, elevated hemidiaphragm pulmonary embolism

Assess 12-Lead ECG

ST Elevation
- ≥ 0.1 mV in ≥ 2 contiguous leads
- Peaked T waves early and inverted T waves late or presumably new LBBB
- Most progress to **Q wave**

→ **STEMI**

Start Adjunctive Therapy:
- Clopidogrel or prasugrel[1]
- Anticoagulation[2]:
  UFH 60 U/kg bolus max 4000 U then 12 U/kg/h max 1000 U/h or enoxaparin 30 mg IV bolus, then 1 mg/kg SC q12h or fondaparinux 2.5 mg SC qd

Time from onset of symptoms < 12 hours?
- No → Admit to Cardiac Care Unit
- Yes → Perform Revascularization

Perform Revascularization:
- Primary PCI (door-to-balloon time < 90 min)
- Or thrombolytic therapy (door-to-drug time < 30 min)
- Or CABG

Continue adjunctive tx plus:
- ACE inhibitor or ARB if anterior MI, pulm edema, or LVEF < 40%, and no contraindications
- Statins (HMG CoA reductase inhibitors)
- Oral β-blockers, eg, metoprolol 100-200 mg/d PO div bid

No ST Elevation
- ST depression ≥ 0.1 mV in ≥ 2 contiguous leads
- Dynamic T wave inversions
- Most progress to **non-Q wave**

→ **Unstable Angina/ NSTEMI**

Start Adjunctive Therapy:
- Nitroglycerin
- GP IIb/IIIa inhibitors: eptifibatide or tirofiban[1]
- Clopidogrel or prasugrel[1]
- Anticoagulation as in STEMI

Admit to Cardiac Care Unit:
Continue or give β-blockers, ACEIs/ARBs, and statins
Assess high-risk criteria:
- Refractory chest pain
- Arrhythmias (v-tach)
- Recurrent/persistent ST deviation
- Heart failure signs

Yes → Diagnostic Angiography
No → LVEF < 40% on echo?
- Yes → Diagnostic Angiography
- No → High risk on stress test?
  - Yes → Diagnostic Angiography
  - No → Medical therapy only

Diagnostic Angiography:
- + → PCI or CABG within 48 hrs
- − → Medical therapy only

Medical therapy only:
- Aspirin 75-162 mg qd indefinitely
- Clopidogrel 75 mg PO qd x 1-12 mo
- Discontinue GP IIb/IIIa inhibitors and anticoagulants

No ST Elevation
- No ST depression
- Nonspecific ECG changes

→ **Unstable Angina Low/Intermediate Risk**

Recheck ECG, Troponin:
Development of high-risk ECG changes or troponin positive?
- Yes → Start Adjunctive Therapy (Unstable Angina/NSTEMI)
- No → Continue Monitoring

Continue Monitoring:
Continue monitoring in ED or chest pain unit:
- Serial ECGs
- Serial cardiac markers
- Consider stress test

High- or intermediate-risk criteria or troponin-positive?
- Yes → Admit to Cardiac Care Unit
- No →
  - No invasive diagnostic tests
  - Further evaluation per patient risk profile

- Continue telemetry monitoring
- Consider stress test
- Outpatient follow-up if low risk

Acute Coronary Syndrome - Footnotes

1. Consider 5 mg daily dose if patient weighs < 60 kg; prasugrel is indicated only in patients who are to be managed with PCI after the coronary anatomy has been defined; prasugrel can cause significant bleeding and should not be used in patients with active pathological bleeding or history of TIA or stroke, or in patients expected to undergo CABG; use of prasugrel is not recommended in patients older than 75 yrs.
2. Due to risk of heparin-induced thrombocytopenia, an anticoagulant other than UFH (eg, enoxaparin) should be used if anticoagulation persists beyond 48 hours; enoxaparin effects cannot be reversed by protamine.

ACLS Acute Stroke

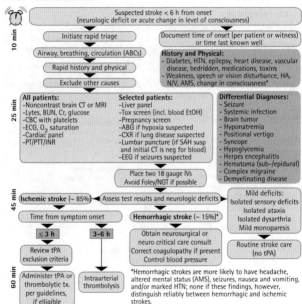

10 min

Suspected stroke < 6 h from onset (neurologic deficit or acute change in level of consciousness)

- Initiate rapid triage
- Airway, breathing, circulation (ABCs)
- Rapid history and physical
- Exclude other causes

Document time of onset (per patient or witness) or time last known well

History and Physical:
- Diabetes, HTN, epilepsy, heart disease, vascular disease, bedridden, medications, toxins
- Weakness, speech or vision disturbance, HA, N/V, AMS, change in consciousness*

25 min

All patients:
- -Noncontrast brain CT or MRI
- -Lytes, BUN, Cr, glucose
- -CBC with platelets
- -ECG, O_2 saturation
- -Cardiac panel
- -PT/PTT/INR

Selected patients:
- -Liver panel
- -Tox screen (incl. blood EtOH)
- -Pregnancy screen
- -ABG if hypoxia suspected
- -CXR if lung disease suspected
- -Lumbar puncture (if SAH susp and initial CT is neg for blood)
- -EEG if seizures suspected

Differential Diagnoses:
- Seizure
- Systemic infection
- Brain tumor
- Hyponatremia
- Positional vertigo
- Syncope
- Hypoglycemia
- Herpes encephalitis
- Hematoma (sub-/epidural)
- Complex migraine
- Demyelinating disease

Place two 18 gauge IVs
Avoid Foley/NGT if possible

45 min

Assess test results and neurologic deficits

Ischemic stroke (~ 85%) → Time from symptom onset
- ≤ 3 h → Review tPA exclusion criteria → (**60 min**) Administer tPA or thrombolytic tx. per guidelines, if elligible
- 3–6 h → Intraarterial thrombolysis

Hemorrhagic stroke (~ 15%)* → Obtain neurosurgical or neuro critical care consult; Correct coagulopathy if present; Control blood pressure

Mild deficits: Isolated sensory deficits; Isolated ataxia; Isolated dysarthria; Mild monoparesis → Routine stroke care (no tPA)

*Hemorrhagic strokes are more likely to have headache, altered mental status (AMS), seizures, nausea and vomiting, and/or marked HTN; none if these findings, however, distinguish reliably between hemorrhagic and ischemic strokes.

Status epilepticus

Status epilepticus

- Secure airway
- Give O_2
- Assess cardiac + respiratory function
- Secure IV access in large veins
- Collect blood for:
  glucose, CBCs, urea, electrolytes,
  liver enzymes, Ca, CK, AED levels
- Measure blood gases

Give lorazepam 4mg IV or diazepam 10mg IV/rectally

If status persists
- Repeat lorazepam 4mg IV **or**
  diazepam 10mg IV/rectally after max. 10min
- Determine etiology:
  - in hypoglycemia give 50ml 50% gluc. IV
  - in alcohol abuse give thiamine IV
  - give AED treatment orally/NG Tube

If status persists
Give fosphenytoin 18mg/kg IV (phenytoin equiv.) up to 150mg/min
or
phenytoin 18mg/kg IV, 50mg/min
both with ECG monitoring
(alternatively: valproic acid 900mg in 20-30min, max. 2400-3600mg/d)

If status persists
Phenobarbital up to 600mg IV (6min), max. 18-20mg/kg/d

If status persists
- General anesthesia
- ICU
- EEG monitoring

1 Fluids, Electrolytes, Acid-Base

1.1 General Concepts

1.1.1 Body water distribution

Total body water (TBW) = 60% of body weight (42L)		
Intracellular fluid (ICF) ~ 2/3 TBW (25L)	Extracellular fluid (ECF) ~1/3 TBW (17L)	
Note: In reality, the ICF volume is slightly less than 2/3 of TBW (25L), while the ECF volume is somewhat more than 1/3 of TBW (17L). The water distribution is markedly different in infants, with their TBW being about 75% of the body weight, and their ICF volume being about 1/2 of TBW.	Interstitial 3/4 ECF, 1/4 TBW (12L)	Plasma 1/4 ECF 1/12 TBW (5L)

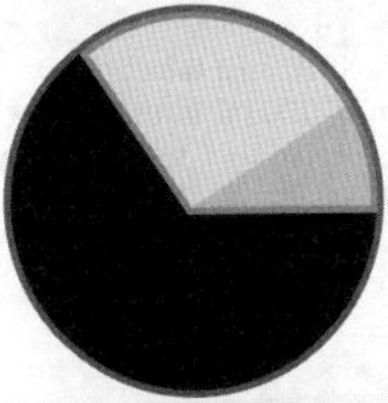

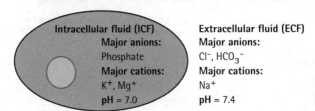

- Total body water (TBW) = 60% of body weight (eg, 42 L in a 70-kg person)
- Intracellular fluid (ICF) = 2/3 of TBW (25 L)
- Extracellular fluid (ECF) = 1/3 of TBW (17 L)
- Interstitial fluid = 3/4 ECF = 1/4 TBW (12 L)
- Plasma = 1/4 ECF = 1/12 TBW (5 L)

1.1.2 Electrolyte distribution and function

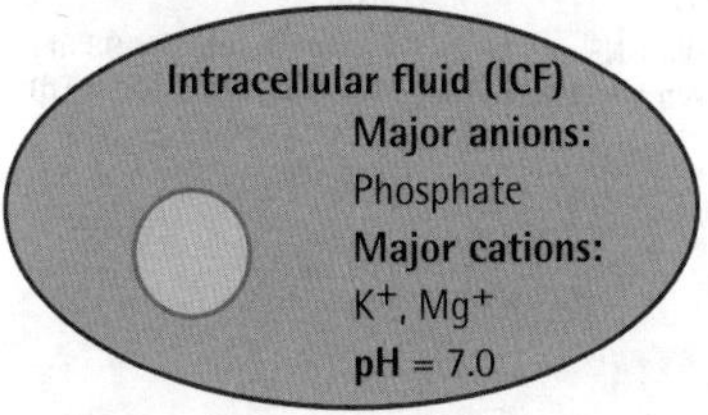

Extracellular fluid (ECF)
Major anions:
Cl^-, HCO_3^-
Major cations:
Na^+
pH = 7.4

1.1.3 Osmolality vs osmolarity

Osmolality (mOsm/Kg H_2O)	Milliosmoles per kg of water. The osmolality is the number of solute osmoles (number of particles that contribute to an osmotic pressure) in solution. For a fully dissociated salt, like NaCl, the osmolality of 1 mole of salt is 1 Osm of Na +1 Osm of Cl = 2 Osms.
Osmolarity (mOsm/L H_2O)	Milliosmoles per liter of water. At room temp., 1L = 1 kg water, therefore, this is equal to osmolality, but, since the density of water changes with temp., this measure is temp. dependent. However, for small solute concentrations, it can be assumed the two are equal.

1.2 Electrolyte Repletion

Electrolyte	Adult Dosing	Concentrations/Comments
Potassium		
K-Dur (Potassium chloride)	10, 20, or 40 mEq tablets Usual dosage: 1 tab PO q 4 h PRN	- Each 10 mEq tablet or 10 mEq/ 100 mL infusion is expected to ↑ serum [K^+] by 10 mg/dL - Use caution in patients with renal insufficiency
Potassium chloride	8, 10, 20, or 40 mEq in 100 mL NS over 1 h (recheck serum [K+] after 3–4 runs)	
Magnesium		
Magnesium gluconate	500 mg tablets Usual dosage: 500 mg PO TID x 1 day	- Each 500 mg tablet contains 27 mg elemental Mg^{2+} (2.2 mEq) - 1 gram IV contains 98 mg elemental Mg^{2+} (8.1 mEq) - PO use commonly causes diarrhea
Magnesium sulfate	1 g in 100 mL NS over 2 hours, given q 6 h	

Calcium		
Calcium carbonate	350, 500, 600, 750, 1000 mg tablets Usual dosage: 500 mg PO TID with food	- 1 gram PO contains 400 mg elemental calcium (20 mEq) - 1 gram IV contains 93 mg elemental calcium (4.7 mEq)
Calcium gluconate	1 g in 100 mL NS IV over 2 h q 6 h	
Phosphorus		
Potassium phosphate –Oral	1–2 packets PO QID; dissolve 1 packet in 75 mL of juice or water and take with food	- 1 packet contains 250 mg elemental phosphorus (8 mmol) - Use caution in patients with renal insufficiency - PO use commonly causes diarrhea
Potassium phosphate –IV	15 mmol in 250 mL NS over 6 h	

1.3 Fluid Management Basics

1.3.1 Assessing volume status

The first step in fluid management is determining the patient's total body fluid status. There are only three options:

1. **Hypovolemia** - Decreased total body fluid resulting in proportional decreases in intracellular and extracellular volume
2. **Euvolemia** - Normal volume status
3. **Hypervolemia** - Increased body fluid i

Clinical findings in expanded and contracted volume states	
Volume status	**Clinical findings**
Volume contraction	- Resting or orthostatic tachycardia - Hypotension - Absence of axillary sweat - Decreased skin turgor - Collapse of neck veins - Absence of peripheral edema and/or ascites
Volume expansion	- Presence of peripheral edema and/or ascites - Distended neck veins - Normal skin turgor - Normal axillary sweat - Signs of congestive heart failure
Volume expansion with intravascular depletion*	- Edema - Mental status changes - Decreased urine output (measured from catheter) - Increased urine specific gravity (>1.015) - Low urinary [Na] (<2 mEq/L) - Fractional excretion of sodium <0.2% - Increased Bun/Creatinine ratio >20:1 - Hemoconcentration (rise in hemoglobin)
* The intravascular space may be depleted even though the total body volume is expanded and the patient presents in an edematous state. The signs listed may give clues to the state of the intravascular compartment.	

1.3.2 Causes of edema formation

Congestive heart failure	Elevated intracapillary hydrostatic pressure at venous end of capillary caused by increased right heart pressure.
Hypoalbuminemic status	Decreased albumin production: - Cirrhosis - Starvation Increased albumin loss: - Nephritic states (proteinuria → loss of albumin in urine) Low albumin leads to decreased oncotic pressure

1.3.3 Three types of volume loss

	Plasma volume loss	Isotonic dehydration or ECF volume loss	Hypertonic dehydr. or free water loss
Example	Hemorrhage	Vomiting, diarrhea	Sweat, diabetes insip.
Na loss	Na loss = H_2O loss	Na loss = H_2O loss	H_2O loss > Na loss
Asymptomatic	800 ml	3500 ml (5% body wt)	10,500 ml
Tachycardia	800 - 1750 ml	7000 ml (10% body wt)	21,000 ml
Shock	>1750 ml	>7000 ml	>21, 000 ml

1.3.4 Systemic response to low effective circulating volume

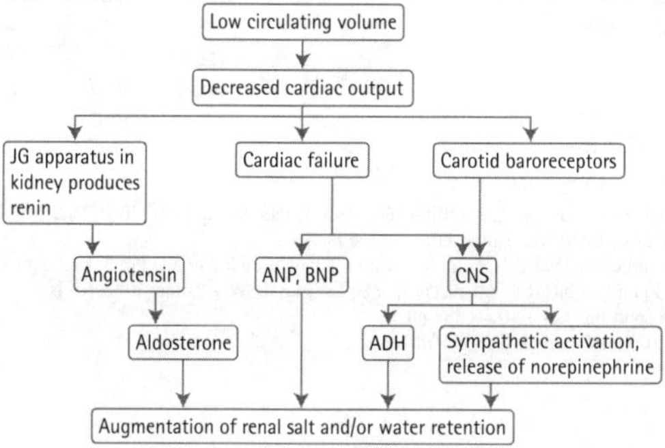

1.4 Fluid Replacement

1.4.1 Fluid types

Replacement fluids come in three general osmotic categories, based on their osmolarity relative to that of normal plasma (285 - 295 mOsm/L):

1. **Hypertonic:** Higher solute concentration than normal plasma
2. **Isotonic:** Roughly the same solute concentration as normal plasma
3. **Hypotonic:** Lesser solute concentration than normal plasma

Fluids are further categorized by the type of solutes they contain:

1. **Crystalloid solutions:** Saline solutions (eg, normal saline = 0.9% sodium chloride) D5NS, Lactated ringers etc.)
2. **Colloid solutions:** Aim to maintain oncotic pressure, eg, Hespan, albumin
3. **Blood:** Packed red blood cells (pRBC), whole blood

1.4.2 Crystalloid solutions

Solution	Na^+ mEq/L	Cl^- mEq/L	K^+ mEq/L	Ca^{2+} mEq/L	HCO_3^- mEq/L	Gluc mEq/L	Osm mOsm/Kg	kcal/L
NS	154	154					308	
1/2 NS	77	77					154	
1/4 NS	38.5	38.5					77	
D5 NS	154	154				252	560	205
D5 1/2 NS	77	77				252	406	205
D5 1/4 NS	38.5	38.5				252	330	205
D5W						252	252	205
D50W						2520	2520	2050
3% NS	513	513					1026	
5% NS	855	855					1710	
LR	147	156	4	9	28		310	

NS: Normal Saline 0.9% NaCl; **1/2NS:** 0.45% NaCl; **1/4NS:** 0.225% NaCl; **D5:** 5% Dextrose (50g/L); **D5W:** 5% Dextrose in Free Water; **LR:** Lactated Ringer's

Sodium bicarbonate ($NaHCO_3$) ampules (or amps) may be added to any fluids. Each amp of bicarb contains 50 mEq of bicarb in 50 mL (1000 mEq/L). Thus, D5W + 2 amps of bicarb is a slightly hypotonic solution (154 + 100 = 254 mEq).

Normal serum osmolality is 275-295 mOsm/L

1.4.3 Colloid solutions

Solution	Contents	Electrolytes (mEq/L)
Hespan	Hydroxyethyl starch	154 Na^+ and Cl^-
Plasminate	5% plasma protein factors	145 Na^+, 100 Cl^-, 0.25 K^+
Albumin*	5%, 10%, 25% human serum albumin (HSA) or recombinant human albumin (rHA)	130-160 Na^+ and Cl^- 1 K^+
*Albumin infusions are rarely used in order to preserve renal function during large volume-paracentesis, or with spontaneous bacterial peritonitis in cirrhotic patients with ascites		

1.4.4 Distribution of IV fluids in body compartments

Given that the intravascular space (IVS) is only 1/4 of the extracellular space (ECS), only a fraction of the infused crystalloids will stay in the vasculature. On the other hand, the protein or starch components of colloid solutions provide an oncotic force that keeps most of the administered volume in the IVS.

Solution	ICS distrib	ECS distrib	Plasma (IVS) distrib
NS (+/- D5)*	0 cc	1000 cc	250 cc
1/2 NS (+/- D5)	333 cc	667 cc	167 cc
1/4 NS (+/- D5)	500 cc	500 cc	125 cc
D5W	667 cc	333 cc	83 cc
3% NS	0 cc	1000 cc	250 cc
LR	100 cc	900 cc	225 cc
Colloids**	0 cc	1000 cc	1000 cc

ICS = Intracellular space, ECS = Extracellular space, IVS = Intravascular space
* Dextrose (d-glucose) is immediately absorbed by cells, therefore its presence does not alter the distribution of the fluid across the different body compartments. Dextrose in free water (D5W), for example, distributes very much like free water (2/3 ICF, 1/3 ECF).
Caution: Free water can NOT be given IV as it will cause RBC lysis!

1.4.5 Physiologic effects of various fluids

	Hypertonic fluid	H_2O	Isotonic (0.9%) NaCl
Plasma osmolality	↑	↓	↔
Plasma [Na]	↑	↓	↔
ECF volume	↑	↑ (transient)	↑

Urine [Na]	↑	↑ (transient)	↑
Urine osmolality	↑	↓	↔
ICF volume	↓	↑	↔
ECF volume	↑	↓	↑

1.4.6 Summary of rules for choosing replacement fluids

Purpose of infusion	Solutions
General hydration maintenance	1/2 NS or 1/4 NS (+/- D5), D5W
Intravascular volume replacement	NS, LR, colloid solutions* (Hespan, albumin)
Blood loss	Start with NS while awaiting blood from blood bank; not necessary to raise Hct >35

* Head-to-head studies have shown no mortality advantage to using colloid over crystalloid for fluid resuscitation. A multicenter trial randomly assigned nearly 7000 hypovolemic medical and surgical ICU patients to fluid resuscitation using either 4 percent albumin or normal saline. All-cause mortality at 28 days (the primary end point of the study), multiorgan failure, and the duration of hospitalization were similar in both groups. (AU Finfer S; Bellomo R; Boyce N; French J; Myburgh J; Norton R SO. A comparison of albumin and saline for fluid resuscitation in the intensive care unit. N Engl J Med 2004 May 27;350(22):2247-56)

1.4.7 Required volume of replacement fluids

The body needs a minimum level of maintenance hydration that depends on daily losses. In general, the I/Os of the average adult are as follows:

Daily intake	- Basal minimum: 30 ml/kg body weight	- Mean: 50 ml/kg body weight
Minimum obligate water output	- Urine: 500 ml - Skin: 500 ml	- Respiratory tract: 400 ml - Stool: 200 ml
Average normal daily losses*	- Renal: 1500 ml - Fecal: 100 ml - Insensible perspiration: 900 ml	- Perspiration: Additional 150 ml/d for each °C over 37°C - Total: 2.7 L - 4.7 L per day
Conditions that increase daily losses	- Fever - Diarrhea - Extensive burns - Tachypnea	- Sweating - Surgical drains - Polyuria

* These figures are difficult to estimate. Checking the patient's weight on a daily basis using the same scale at the same time of the day is the best way to assess losses.

1.4.8 4-2-1 Rule for maintenance fluids

100–50–20/4–2–1 Rule for Estimating Maintenance Fluids*	
First 10 kg body weight	100 mL/kg/24 h or 4 mL/kg/h
Second 10 kg body weight	50 mL/kg/24 h or 2 mL/kg/h
Each additional kg body weight	20 mL/kg/24 h or 1 mL/kg/h

Example: What is the daily and hourly infusion maintenance rate for a 22-kg child?
(10 x 100) + (10 x 50) + (2 x 20) = 1540 mL/24 h or (10 x 4) + (10 x 2) + (2 x 1) = 62 mL/h

Rough approximation of maintenance fluid rate in mL/h*

Rate (ml/h) = Body weight (kg) + 40
Example: If pt is 50 kg, rate = 50 + 40 = 90 ml/h
This order may be written as 1/2NS at 90 ml/h x 24 hours

Additional considerations

- If fluid loss exceeds a patient's oral intake, maintenance fluids should be started.
- Volume-depleted patients require additional fluids along with maintenance fluids (ie, a fluid bolus + maintenance fluids).
- **In cases of severe volume loss such as hypovolemic shock (due to hemorrhage, for example), rapid plasma volume replacement is key!**

***The values shown assume normal renal function, no CHF, and no edema. The rule applies to pediatric patients, but not for infants <14 days old.**

1.4.9 Fluid replacement in burn patients

Patients with extensive burns lose significantly higher volumes of body fluids due to the destruction of capillaries in the affected tissues. Therefore, the regular rules of volume replacement do not apply in the initial recovery phase. Instead, the Parkland formula and the 'Rule of 9s' is used to calculate required replacement volumes based on percent of body surface area are affected.

Rule of 9s	
Body area affected	**Total body surface area (TBSA)**
Each upper limb	9%
Each lower limb	18%
Anterior trunk	18%
Posterior trunk	18%
Head and neck	9%
Perineum and genitalia	1%

Parkland Formula
Volume of crystalloid / 24 h (ml) = TBSA (%) x weight (kg) x 4
Ex: 70 kg pt with 3rd-degree burn over back and left arm: Vol = (18 + 9) x 70 x 4 = 7560 ml/24h

Different protocols exist for the rate of replacement during the first 24 hours. An example replacement schedule is outlined in the table below:

Fluid Replacement Schedule in Burn Patients	
Time period during the first 24 hours	**% of total volume**
1 - 4 hours	25%
5 - 8 hours	25%
9 - 12 hours	12.5%
13 - 16 hours	12.5%
16 - 20 hours	12.5%
20 - 24 hours	12.5%

After the initial 24-36 hours, as the capillaries begin to regain integrity, the patient is usually switched to colloid (D5W or 5% albumin) at 0.5 ml/kg/TBSA%.

American Burn Association Burn Injury Severity Grading System			
Burn Type	**Minor**	**Moderate**	**Major**
Criteria	<10% TBSA burn in adults <5% TBSA burn in young or old <2% full-thickness burn	10 - 20% TBSA burn in adults 5 - 10% TBSA burn in young or old 2 - 5% full-thickness burn High-voltage injury Suspected inhalation injury Circumferential burn Medical problem predisposing to infection (eg, diabetes mellitus, sickle cell disease)	>20% TBSA burn in adults >10% TBSA burn in young or old >5% full-thickness burn High-voltage burn Known inhalation injury Any significant burn to face, eyes, ears, genitalia, or joints Significant associated injuries (fracture or other major trauma)
Disposition	Outpatient	Admit to hospital	Refer to burn center

TBSA: Total body surface area; burn: partial- or full-thickness; young or old: <10 or >50 years old; adults: > 10 or < 50 years old; adapted from: American Burn Association, J Burn Care Rehabil 1990; 11:98 and Hartford, CE, Total Burn Care, Philadelphia, WB Saunders, 1996

1.5 Electrolyte Abnormalities

1.5.1 Hypernatremia

Def: Serum $Na^+ > 145$ mEq/L.
Symptoms: Often asymptomatic, but can present with hypertension, rales, tachycardia, oliguria, lethargy, irritability, tremors, or flushed skin.
Differentiation: See diagram

Therapy
When to treat: Serum $Na^+ > 145$ mEq/L
Goal: ↓ Na^+ by < 0.5 mEq/L per hour and by not more than 12 mEq/L per 24 hrs
Treatment: IV or PO hypotonic fluids. Usually ~120ml of free water per hr and correction of underlying disorder Step 1: Calculate free water deficit = Desired Na^+ / [Total body water x (1- serum Na^+)] Step 2: Infusion rate (ml/hr) = [Required Na^+ (mmol) x 1000] / [Administered Na^+ (mmol/L) x Time (hours)]
Refer to the Conversions and Formulas section (→ 446) and the electrolyte solution section (→ 34) for information on these formulas and the Na^+ content in IVF saline solutions
Warning: Rapid decrease of Na may lead to cerebral contraction with associated neurologic sequelae including seizures

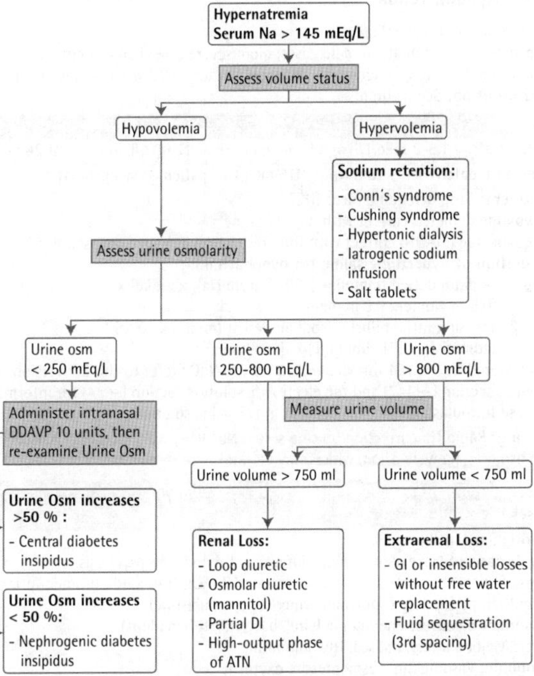
Hypernatremia
Serum Na > 145 mEq/L
Assess volume status
Hypovolemia
Hypervolemia
Sodium retention:
- Conn's syndrome
- Cushing syndrome
- Hypertonic dialysis
- Iatrogenic sodium infusion
- Salt tablets
Assess urine osmolarity
Urine osm < 250 mEq/L
Urine osm 250-800 mEq/L
Urine osm > 800 mEq/L
Administer intranasal DDAVP 10 units, then re-examine Urine Osm
Measure urine volume
Urine volume > 750 ml
Urine volume < 750 ml
Urine Osm increases >50 %:
- Central diabetes insipidus
Urine Osm increases < 50 %:
- Nephrogenic diabetes insipidus
Renal Loss:
- Loop diuretic
- Osmolar diuretic (mannitol)
- Partial DI
- High-output phase of ATN
Extrarenal Loss:
- GI or insensible losses without free water replacement
- Fluid sequestration (3rd spacing)

1.5.2 Hyponatremia

Def: Serum $Na^+ < 135$ mEq/L.
Symptoms: Asymptomatic in mild cases; more severe cases can present with hypotension, headache, tachycardia, lethargy, seizures, N/V, dry mucous membranes.
Differentiation: See diagram

Therapy
Goal: ↑ Na^+ by 1.5-2 mEq/L/h and by no more than 12 mEq/L in the first 24 hrs.
When to treat: When serum $Na^+ < 115$ mEq/L or patient is symptomatic.
Treatment: Stop offending meds (HCTZ). - If volume depleted correct with normal saline - If euvolemic (SIADH) correct with fluid restriction or hypertonic saline **Calculation of hypertonic saline for hyponatremia:** <u>Step 1</u>: Sodium deficit (mmol) = (120 -[serum Na]) x wt(kg) x (0.5 in women; 0.6 in men) <u>Step 2</u>: Infusion rate (ml/hr) = [sodium deficit (mmol) x 1000] / [administered Na (mmol/L) x time (hours)] Administered Na^+ is 154 for NS and 513 for 3% NaCl; refer to the Conversions and Formulas section (→ 447) and the electrolyte solution section (→ 34) for information on these formulas and the Na^+ content in IVF saline solutions.
Warning: Rapid Na correction (raising serum Na^+ level > 20 mEq/day) is associated with osmotic demyelination, which may be fatal.

SIADH (Syndrome of Inappropriate ADH secretion)
Causes
Tumors: Small cell lung cancer **CNS diseases:** Stroke, hemorrhage, infection, trauma, and psychosis **Drugs:** Typical antipsychotics, antidepressants (MAOI, TCA, SSRI), bromocriptine, chemotherapy (cyclophosphamide, vincristine, vinblastine) **Pulmonary diseases:** Pneumonia (viral, bacterial, tuberculous) **Other:** Major surgery, nausea, HIV, idiopathic **Iatrogenic:** Vasopressin, desmopressin, oxytocin
Treatment
Acute: Water restriction (1 L/day), hypertonic saline or NaCl tablets, loop diuretics **Chronic:** Water restriction, high-salt and high-protein diet, loop diuretics, or **demeclocycline**

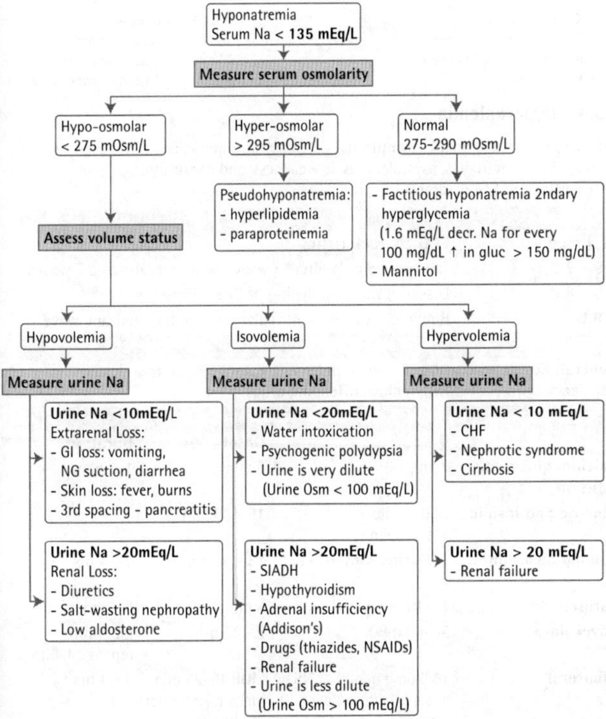
Hyponatremia
Serum Na < 135 mEq/L
Measure serum osmolarity
Hypo-osmolar
< 275 mOsm/L
Hyper-osmolar
> 295 mOsm/L
Normal
275-290 mOsm/L
Pseudohyponatremia:
- hyperlipidemia
- paraproteinemia
- Factitious hyponatremia 2ndary hyperglycemia (1.6 mEq/L decr. Na for every 100 mg/dL ↑ in gluc > 150 mg/dL)
- Mannitol
Assess volume status
Hypovolemia
Isovolemia
Hypervolemia
Measure urine Na
Measure urine Na
Measure urine Na
Urine Na <10mEq/L
Extrarenal Loss:
- GI loss: vomiting, NG suction, diarrhea
- Skin loss: fever, burns
- 3rd spacing - pancreatitis
Urine Na >20mEq/L
Renal Loss:
- Diuretics
- Salt-wasting nephropathy
- Low aldosterone
Urine Na <20mEq/L
- Water intoxication
- Psychogenic polydypsia
- Urine is very dilute (Urine Osm < 100 mEq/L)
Urine Na >20mEq/L
- SIADH
- Hypothyroidism
- Adrenal insufficiency (Addison's)
- Drugs (thiazides, NSAIDs)
- Renal failure
- Urine is less dilute (Urine Osm > 100 mEq/L)
Urine Na < 10 mEq/L
- CHF
- Nephrotic syndrome
- Cirrhosis
Urine Na > 20 mEq/L
- Renal failure

1.5.3 Factors affecting ICF-ECF potassium shifts

Drive K^+ out of cells:

Acidosis	Tissue necrosis
Beta blockers	Periodic paralysis
Hemolysis	

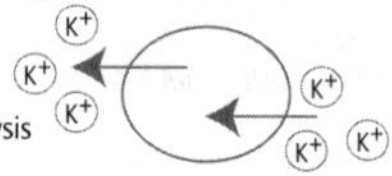

Drive K^+ into cells:

Insulin	Catecholamines
Alkalosis	Succinylcholine
Aldosterone	Periodic hypokalemia

1.5.4 Hyperkalemia

Def: Serum $K^+ > 5.0$ mEq/L. **Symptoms:** Often asymptomatic, but can present with bradycardia, arrhythmias, asystole, muscle weakness, and confusion.
Differentiation: See diagram

ECG Changes	
[K^+] mEq/L	**ECG characteristics**
6.5 - 7.5	Tall, peaked or "tented" T waves with narrow-based T waves
7.5 - 8.0	Loss of P waves, widening of QRS complexes
> 8.0	Biphasic QRSs, idioventricular rhythm, terminal sine wave

Therapy

General: Restrict exogenous K^+, treat underlying causes (eg, ex. treat insulin deficiency, correct acidosis), remove offending drugs.

Treatment for K^+ > 6, or ECG changes, or symptomatic	Dose	Onset	Duration
Calcium gluconate infusion	2 amps IV	5 min	1 - 2 hrs
Glucose and insulin	D50 1 amp + 10U insulin IV	15 - 30 min	1 - 4 hrs
Sodium bicarbonate	1-2 amps IV over 5-10 min	15 - 60 min	1 - 4 hrs
Furosemide	10-40 mg IV	5 min	IV 2 hrs
Kayexalate	30-60 g PO	2 - 12 hrs	Indefinite, repeat q4-6hrs
Albuterol	10-20mg in 4ml of NS by nasal inhalation over 10 min, or 0.5mg by IV infus.	MDI: 10-25 min (nebs take longer) IV: 30 min	3 - 4 hrs
Dialysis	-	Variable	Variable

Repeat ECG and serum K^+ measurements after treatment

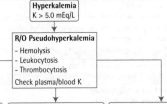

Hyperkalemia
K > 5.0 mEq/L

R/O Pseudohyperkalemia
- Hemolysis
- Leukocytosis
- Thrombocytosis

Check plasma/blood K

Excess K intake
(Urine spot K > 50 mEq/L)
- K supplements
- K penicillin
- Stored blood
- Salt substitutes

Translocation from ICF to ECF
- Acidosis
- Severe catabolism
- Rhabdomyolysis
- Tissue necrosis
- Insulin deficiency
- Mineralocorticoid deficiency (adrenal insufficiency, hyporeninemia, hypoaldosteronism)
- Periodic paralysis
- Aldosterone antagonists
- Digitalis toxicity
- Succinylcholine
- b-blockers
- Catecholamine deficiency states
- Hyperosmolarity

Decreased excretory deficiency
(Urine spot K < 50 mEq/L)
- Renal failure
- Oliguria
- Renal tubular disease
- K-sparing diuretics
- Hypoaldosteronism
- Cyclosporine
- ACE inhibitors
- NSAIDS

THERAPY GENERAL
- Treat underlying cause
- Restrict exogenous K

Remove offending drugs

K > 6
- Check ECG
- CaGluconate 2 amps. I/V
- D50 1 amp./10U insulin I/V
- $NaHCO_3$ 1-2 amps. I/V over 5-10
- Kayexalate 30-60 gm PO
- Lasix
- Dialysis
- Repeat K
- b agonist inhaled

1.5.5 Hypokalemia

Def: Serum $K^+ < 3.6$ mEq/L.
Symptoms: Often asymptomatic, but can include muscle weakness, fatigue, hypotension, headache, dizziness, and myocardial irritability.
Differentiation: See diagram

ECG changes
T wave flat, ST depression, U waves (may merge into TU waves)
Therapy
Find and **correct underlying cause** **Replace magnesium deficit first** Most deficits can be corrected with oral potassium chloride (K-Dur): - **K-Dur** 10-40 mEq PO 2-3x/day **Severe hypokalemia [K+] <2.5 mEq/L or symptomatic** (arrhythmias, marked muscle weakness): - Start with **potassium chloride IV:** 10 mEq in 100 ml NS over 1 hour along with PO supplementation. IV potassium may be painful.

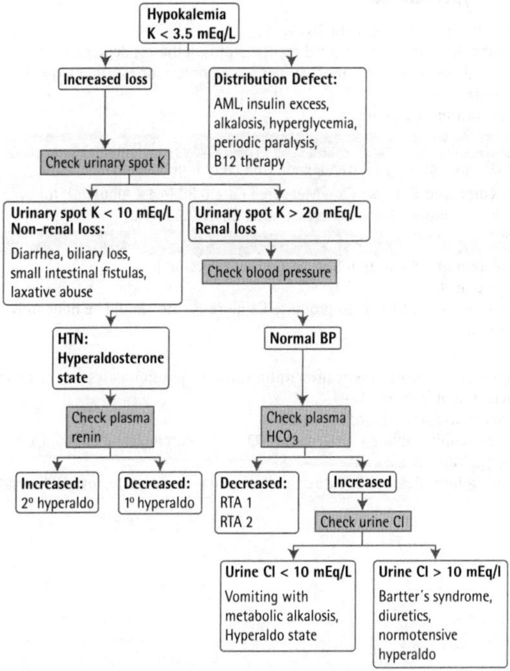
Hypokalemia
K < 3.5 mEq/L
Increased loss
Distribution Defect:
AML, insulin excess, alkalosis, hyperglycemia, periodic paralysis, B12 therapy
Check urinary spot K
Urinary spot K < 10 mEq/L
Non-renal loss:
Diarrhea, biliary loss, small intestinal fistulas, laxative abuse
Urinary spot K > 20 mEq/L
Renal loss
Check blood pressure
HTN:
Hyperaldosterone state
Normal BP
Check plasma renin
Check plasma HCO3
Increased:
2° hyperaldo
Decreased:
1° hyperaldo
Decreased:
RTA 1
RTA 2
Increased
Check urine Cl
Urine Cl < 10 mEq/L
Vomiting with metabolic alkalosis, Hyperaldo state
Urine Cl > 10 mEq/l
Bartter's syndrome, diuretics, normotensive hyperaldo

1.5.6 Hypercalcemia

Def: Serum $Ca^+ > 2.5$ mEq/L or 10 mg/dl.
Symptoms: N/V, headache, altered mental status, lethargy, depression, constipation, muscle/joint pains, polyuria, renal stones (mnemonic: stones, groans, psychiatric overtones).
Differentiation: See diagram

ECG changes
Short QT interval, long PR (rare), wide QRS (very high levels)
Verify corrected Ca: Corr Ca = Measured Ca + 0.8 * (4.4 - Albumin); for every 1 g/dl reduction in serum albumin, increase total Ca by 0.8 mg/dl.
Therapy
- Correction of dehydration (infuse 2-6L, as necessary) - Saline diuresis - Loop diuretics (if CHF) & to promote Ca diuresis. This should be done only AFTER hydration.
Treat causes: **Malignancy** - Anti-osteolytic prescription with bisphosphonates and calcitonin - **Calcitonin**: 8 U IM q6-12h - **Pamidronate**: 60-90 mg/d (1 dose) **Glucocorticoids**: Inhibit 1-OH Vitamin D3 for hematological malignancy, breast CA, granulomatous diseases - **Renal failure:** Restrict Ca intake, oral PO_4, low Ca dialysate, low Al dialysate

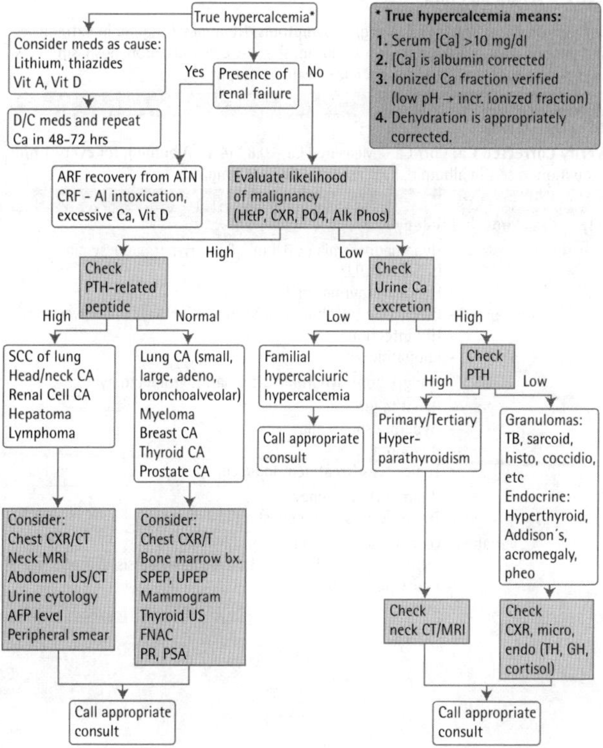
True hypercalcemia*
* True hypercalcemia means:
1. Serum [Ca] >10 mg/dl
2. [Ca] is albumin corrected
3. Ionized Ca fraction verified (low pH → incr. ionized fraction)
4. Dehydration is appropriately corrected.
Consider meds as cause: Lithium, thiazides Vit A, Vit D
D/C meds and repeat Ca in 48-72 hrs
Presence of renal failure
Yes
No
ARF recovery from ATN CRF - Al intoxication, excessive Ca, Vit D
Evaluate likelihood of malignancy (H&P, CXR, PO4, Alk Phos)
High
Low
Check PTH-related peptide
High
Normal
SCC of lung Head/neck CA Renal Cell CA Hepatoma Lymphoma
Lung CA (small, large, adeno, bronchoalveolar) Myeloma Breast CA Thyroid CA Prostate CA
Consider: Chest CXR/CT Neck MRI Abdomen US/CT Urine cytology AFP level Peripheral smear
Consider: Chest CXR/T Bone marrow bx. SPEP, UPEP Mammogram Thyroid US FNAC PR, PSA
Call appropriate consult
Check Urine Ca excretion
Low
High
Familial hypercalciuric hypercalcemia
Call appropriate consult
Check PTH
High
Low
Primary/Tertiary Hyper-parathyroidism
Granulomas: TB, sarcoid, histo, coccidio, etc Endocrine: Hyperthyroid, Addison´s, acromegaly, pheo
Check neck CT/MRI
Check CXR, micro, endo (TH, GH, cortisol)
Call appropriate consult

1.5.7 Hypocalcemia

Def: Serum Ca^{2+}< 2.0 mEq/L, 8 mg/dl. **Symptoms**: Numbness/tingling in extremities and perioral area (+ Chvostek, Trousseau signs), muscle cramps, bronchospasm/ laryngospasm, tetany, seizures, decreased cardiac output.

ECG Changes
Long QT interval
Verify Corrected Ca: Corr Ca = Measured Ca + 0.8 * (4.4 - Albumin); for every 1 g/dl reduction in serum albumin, increase total Ca by 0.8 mg/dl.

Differentiation		
PTH	**Phos**	**Etiology**
↓	↑	- Hypomagnesemia (< 0.8 mEq/L) or Hypermagnesemia (> 5.0 mEq/L) - Hypoparathyroidism - PTH action (alcoholism, diarrhea, diuretics, aminoglycosides) - HIV infection - Idiopathic
↓	↓	- Hungry bone syndrome after parathyroidectomy
↑	↑	- Renal failure - Hyperphosphatemia - Rhabdomyolysis - Tumor lysis (treatment induced)
↑	↓	- Vitamin D deficiency - Tumor lysis (spontaneous)
↑	variable	- Osteoblastic metastasis - Infiltrative dx of PTH gland (hemochromatosis, Wilson's, mets) - Acute pancreatitis - Sepsis

Therapy		
Before starting Ca treatment:		
- Check ionized Ca^{2+} or correct for albumin. - Prior to intervention, check creatine, PO_4, albumin, PTH, 25-OH-VitD. - Always replete magnesium before Ca^{2+} or K^+. - Stop potentially offending drugs: Bisphosphonates, calcitonin, loop diuretics, etc.		
Corrected Ca^{2+}	**Severity**	**Treatment**
> 7-8 mg/dl	Mild asymptomatic, ↓ Ca^{2+}	↑ dietary Ca^{2+} intake by 1000 mg/day
< 7 mg/dl (usually)	Symptomatic hypocalcemia	**Aggressive: Calcium Gluconate** 1-2 amps IV in 50-100mL D5W. Followed by gtt of 10 amps Calcium gluconate in 1L D5W at 50 mL/hr **Maintenance:** Calcium gluconate 1g in 100 ml NS over 2h, q6h
↓ Ca^{2+}, ↑ uric acid, ↑ Phos, ARF	Tumor lysis	IV fluids, pretreatment with allopurinol, consider early hemodialysis

1.5.8 Hypermagnesemia

Def: Serum Mg^{2+} > 2.1 mEq/L. **Symptoms:** Deep tendon reflex reduction (early sign at > 4 mEq/L), muscle weakness, respiratory depression (> 10 mEq/L), hypotension, cardiotoxicity (bradycardia, heart block, arrest) at > 14 mEq/L, hypocalcemia, impaired clotting. **Differentiation:** See diagram

ECG Changes	
Nonspecific	
Therapy	
Calcium Gluconate	**Calcium Gluconate** 100-300 mg IV in 150 ml D5W over 10 min → antagonizes Mg^{2+} effects
Glucose + Insulin	10 U IV and 50 mL D50W bolus or 500 mL D10W over 1 h → increases Mg^{2+} absorption into cells

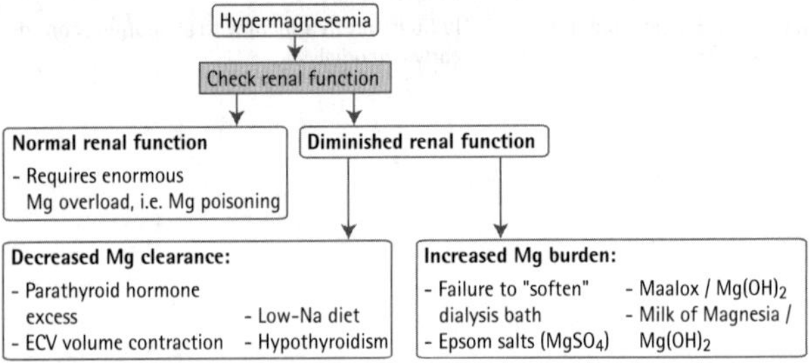

1.5.9 Hypomagnesemia

Def: Serum Mg^{2+} < 1.3 mEq/L. **Symptoms**: Usually asymptomatic until < 1.2 mEq/L, deep tendon reflex hyperactivity, mental status changes, muscle cramps, tremors, muscular fibrillations (+Chvostek, Trousseau signs), N/V, lethargy
Differentiation: See diagram

ECG Changes	
ST depression, altered T waves, PR prolongation, low voltage, wide QRS (severe)	
Therapy	
Mild cases (>1.2 mEq/L)	**Mg gluconate** 500mg PO TID (peds: 10-20mg/kg PO TID/QID, max 400mg/d); reduce dose by half in renal impairment
Symptomatic or < 1.2 mEq/L	**$MgSO_4$** 1g in 100ml NS IV over 1 hr
Severe with seizures or Torsades de Pointes	**$MgSO_4$** 2g IV over 10 min
Caution: Mg gluconate may cause diarrhea. Rapid infusion of Mg can be life-threatening, not to exceed 67 mEq over 8 hrs	

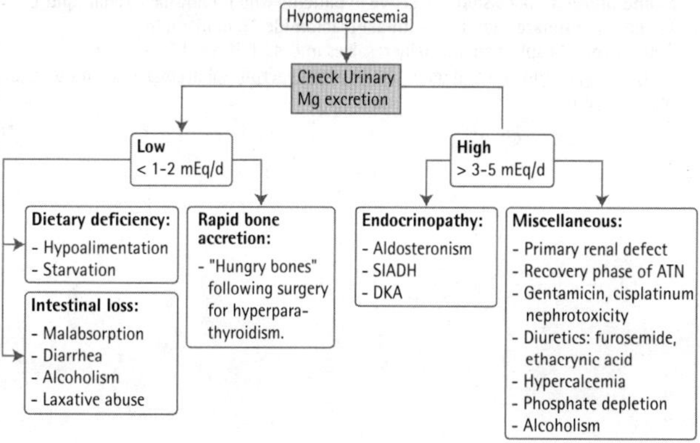

1.5.10 Hyperphosphatemia

Def: Serum phosphate > 4.5 mg/dl
Symptoms: Same as those attributable to hypocalcemia (tetany, paresthesias, etc).
Severe: tissue ischemia and calciphylaxis.
Chronic: contributes to renal osteodystrophy
Differentiation: See diagram

ECG Changes
Nonspecific

Therapy

- Dietary restriction to 600-900 mg/day.
- Oral phosphate binders including **Ca carbonate** 500mg PO daily with meals and **Sevelamer**

Phosphate level	Sevelamer dose
6 - 7.5 mg/dl	800 mg PO tid
7.5 - 9 mg/dl	1200 - 1600 mg PO tid
> 9 mg/dl	1600 mg PO tid

- **Saline diuresis** may also be effective in patients who do not have renal failure.
- Increase phosphate excretion with **acetazolamide** 15 mg/kg q3h.
- Acute hyperphosphatemia usually resolves in 6-12 h if renal function is intact.
- Dialysis may be indicated in renal failure with hyperphosphatemia and symptomatic hypocalcemia.

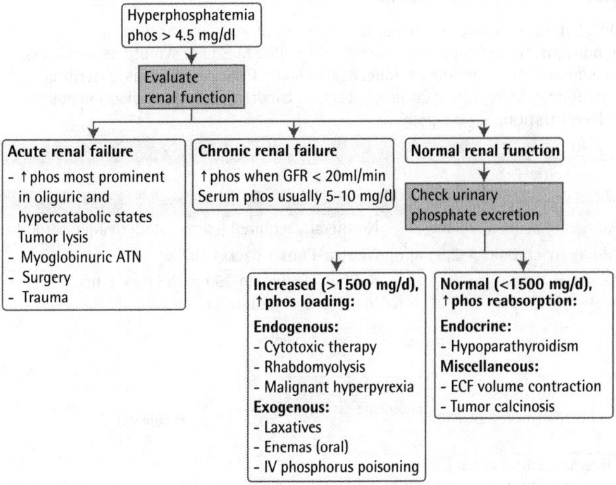
Hyperphosphatemia
phos > 4.5 mg/dl
Evaluate renal function
Acute renal failure
- ↑ phos most prominent in oliguric and hypercatabolic states
Tumor lysis
- Myoglobinuric ATN
- Surgery
- Trauma
Chronic renal failure
↑ phos when GFR < 20ml/min
Serum phos usually 5-10 mg/dl
Normal renal function
Check urinary phosphate excretion
Increased (>1500 mg/d), ↑ phos loading:
Endogenous:
- Cytotoxic therapy
- Rhabdomyolysis
- Malignant hyperpyrexia
Exogenous:
- Laxatives
- Enemas (oral)
- IV phosphorus poisoning
Normal (<1500 mg/d), ↑ phos reabsorption:
Endocrine:
- Hypoparathyroidism
Miscellaneous:
- ECF volume contraction
- Tumor calcinosis

1.5.11 Hypophosphatemia

Def: Serum phosphate < 3.5 mg/dl.
Symptoms: Become apparent at levels < 1 mg/dl. Muscular symptoms: weakness, rhabdomyolysis, respiratory failure, heart failure; CNS: paresthesias, dysarthria, confusion, seizure, coma; Chronic: rickets in children and osteomalacia in adults.
Differentiation: See diagram

ECG Changes	
Nonspecific	
Therapy	
Moderate acute 1-2.5 mg/dl	No therapy required (correct underlying disorder)
Moderate chronic 1-2.5 mg/dl	**Neutra-Phos** 1 packet TID
Severe < 1 mg/dl	**K-Phos** 15mmol in 250 ml NS over 6 hrs (may cause hypotension)

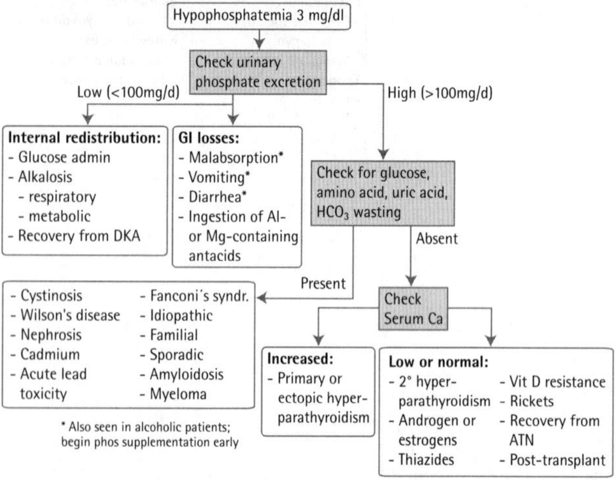

1.6 Acid-Base Disorders

1.6.1 Acid-base abnormalities chart

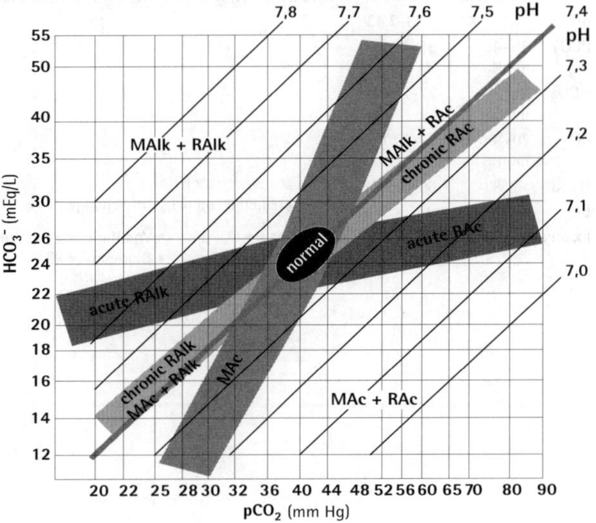

MAc = metabolic acidosis
MAlk = metabolic alkalosis
RAc = respiratory acidosis
RAlk = respiratory alkalosis

1.6.2 Acid-base disorders basics

	Normal Range		Simple Acid-Base Disorders			
	Arterial	Venous	Met acid	Resp acid	Met alk	Resp alk
pH	7.35-7.44	7.33–7.43	↓	↓	↑	↑
PCO_2	35-45 mmHg	36–48 mm Hg	↓	⇑	↑	⇓
HCO_3^-	21-27 mmol/L	22–29 mEq/ L	⇓	↑	⇑	↓
PO_2	70-100 mmHg	37–47 mm Hg	⇑/⇓ = primary change ↑/↓ = predicted compensatory change			
O_2 sat	>95%	60%–85%				
BE	-2 to 3					
Examples			• Diarrhea • CRF	• COPD • Resp depress.	• Vomiting • Diuretics	• Hypervent. • PE

Algorithm for Determining Acid-base Status				
1. Check pH (ABG) and metabolic panel, serum lactate	pH < 7.36 = Acidosis pH > 7.44 = Alkalosis			
2. Determine the 1° disorder	(Using the table in the previous section) Remember: The body **never** overcompensates			
3. Check compensation	**Disorder**	**1° disturbance**	**Compensation**	**Predicated Compensation**
	Metabolic acidosis	↓$[HCO_3^-]$	↓PCO_2	1 mEq/L ↓ HCO_3^- ⇒ 1.3 mmHg ↓PCO_2
	Metabolic alkalosis	↑$[HCO_3^-]$	↑PCO_2	1 mEq/L ↑ HCO_3^- ⇒ 0.7 mmHg ↑ PCO_2
	Acute resp. acidosis	↑PCO_2	↑$[HCO_3^-]$	1 mmHg ↑ PCO_2 ⇒ 0.1 mEq/L ↑ HCO_3^-
	Chron resp acidosis	↑PCO_2	↑$[HCO_3^-]$	1 mmHg ↑ PCO_2 ⇒ 0.4 mEq/L↑ HCO_3^-
	Acute resp. alkalosis	↓PCO_2	↓$[HCO_3^-]$	1 mmHg ↓ PCO_2 ⇒ 0.2 mEq/L↓ HCO_3^-
	Chronic resp. alkalosis	↓PCO_2	↓$[HCO_3^-]$	1 mmHg ↓ PCO_2 ⇒ 0.5 mEq/L↓ HCO_3^-
4. Check anion gap(AG)	$[Na^+] - [Cl^- + HCO_3^-]$ (Normal = 8-11)			
5. Check delta ratio (delta ratio = ↑AG/↓ bicarbonate)	< 1		1-2	> 2
	Hyperchloremic normal anion gap acidosis; consider combined high anion gap and normal anion gap acidosis		Uncomplicated high anion gap acidosis	Combined AG acidosis and metabolic alkalosis or pre-existing compensated respiratory acidosis
6. Clinical correlation	Correlate findings with history and physical examination.			

1.6.3 Primary respiratory acidosis algorithm

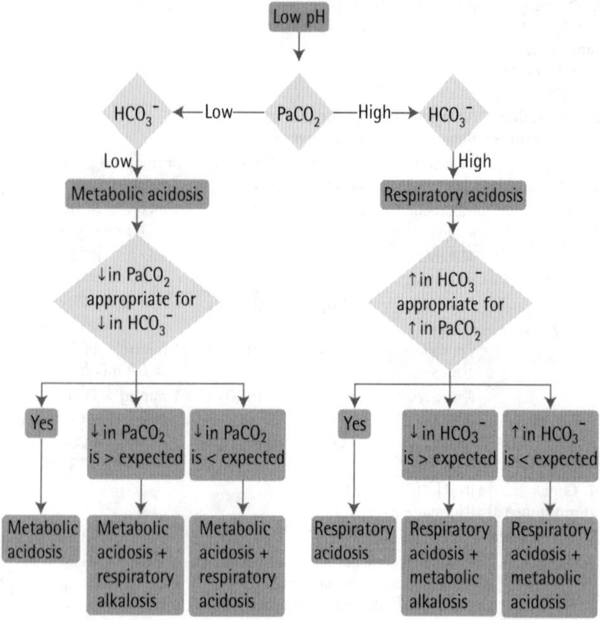

1.6.4 Primary respiratory alkalosis algorithm

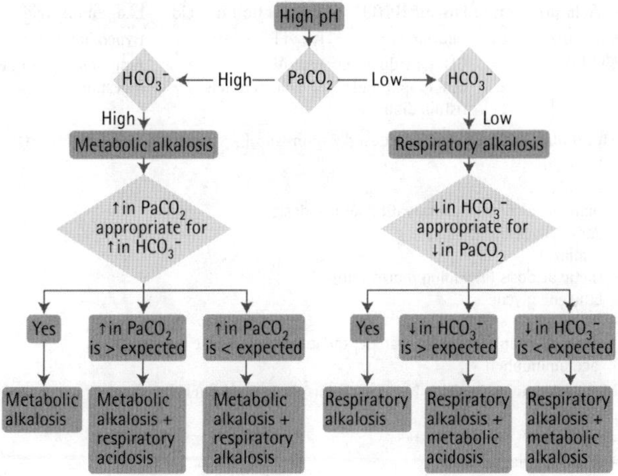

1.6.5 Metabolic acidosis

↑ Acid production	Loss of $HCO3^-$	↓ Excretion of acid	Exogenous acid
Use MUDPILES to identify the cause	Dilutional	Type I RTA-distal	Hyperalimentation
	GI losses: diarrhea, ileal loop, tube/ fistula drainage	Type IV RTA (↓ aldosterone)s	Ammonium chloride ingestion

Metabolic Acidosis With Increased Anion Gap (≥ 12 mEq/L) (MUDPILES + O)

- Methanol
- Uremia
- Diabetic, alcoholic, or starvation ketoacidosis
- Paraldehyde (rare)
- Isoniazid
- Lactic acidosis (including metformin)
- Ethylene glycol
- Salicylates
- Other: Carbon monoxide, cyanide, theophylline, toluene (glue sniffing), acetaminophen

Metabolic Acidosis With Normal Anion Gap (8–11 mEq/L)

- Diarrhea
- Dilutional
- Renal tubular acidosis
- Hyperalimentation
- Ammonium chloride or other acids

Elevated Osmolar Gap[1] (> 10 mOsm/L)

- The osmolar gap should be checked in patients with oNa+ or possible toxin ingestion.
- Some causes of metabolic acidosis also have an increased osmolar gap, for example
- Ethanol
- Methanol
- Ethylene glycol
- Isopropanol
- Sorbitol, mannitol
- IV contrast dye

[1]The osmolar gap is the difference between the measured and calculated osmolarity. The calculated osmolarity is 2[Na+] + [glucose]/18 + [BUN]/2.8.

1.6.6 Renal tubular acidosis

	Type I (Distal)	Type II (Proximal)	Type IV (↓ renin / aldosterone) *
Defect	Inability to excrete H^+ ions in the distal tubule	HCO_3^- lost in the proximal tubule	Defective NH_4 excretion
Urine pH	> 5.5	< 5.5	< 5.5
Serum [K+]	Low	Low	High
Fanconi's syndrome	-	+	-
Nephrolithiasis	+	-	-
Treatment	Bicarbonate tablets, 3-5 mEq/kg/d	Hydrochlorothiazide and Na^+ restriction	Lasix, Florinef, Kayexalate
Example	Amphotericin	Acetazolamide	Diabetes

1.6.7 Metabolic alkalosis

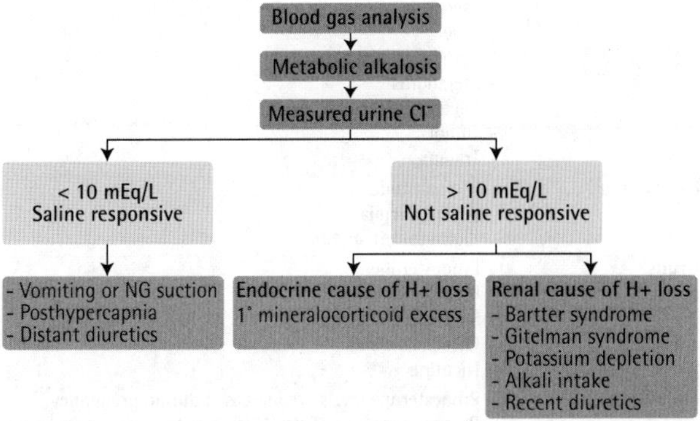

1.6.8 Respiratory acidosis (hypoventilation)

Pulmonary	Neuromuscular disease	CNS Depression
- Emphysema - Severe asthma - Chronic bronchitis - Obstructive sleep apnea	- Amyotrophic lateral sclerosis - Diaphragm paralysis - Severe kyphoscoliosis - Guillain-Barre syndrome - Myasthenia gravis - Muscular dystrophy	- Drugs: Narcotics, barbiturates, benzos, other CNS depressants - Neurologic disorders: Encephalitis, brainstem disease, trauma - Primary alveolar hypoventilation

1.6.9 Respiratory alkalosis

Disorder category	Causes
Central nervous system	- Pain - Hyperventilation syndrome - Anxiety - Psychosis - Fever - Cerebrovascular accident - Meningitis - Encephalitis - Tumor - Trauma
Hypoxemia	- High altitude - Severe anemia - Right-to-left shunts
Drugs	- Progesterone - Methylxanthines - Salicylates - Catecholamines - Nicotine
Endocrine	- Progesterone levels are increased during pregnancy. Progesterone causes stimulation of the respiratory center, which can lead to respiratory alkalosis. - Hyperthyroidism

Stimulation of chest receptors	- Pneumothorax/hemothorax - Pneumonia - Pulmonary edema - Pulmonary embolism - Aspiration - Interstitial lung disease
Miscellaneous	- Sepsis - Hepatic failure - Mechanical ventilation - Heat exhaustion - Recovery phase of metabolic acidosis

1.7 5 Board-Style Questions

1) The release of antidiuretic hormone is caused by all of the following factors except:
   a) Dehydration
   b) Hypovolemia
   c) Caffeine
   d) Nicotine

2) What are the three effects of aldosterone on Na^+, H^+, and K^+ in the late distal tubule and collecting duct?

3) All of the following conditions lead to edema formation EXCEPT:
   a) An increase in plasma oncotic pressure
   b) Lymphatic obstruction
   c) Capillary damage
   d) Arteriolar vasodilation
   e) Venous constriction

4) A patient has a $[Na^+]$ of 155 mEq/L with a urine osmolality of 50 mOsm/kg of water. This can be explained by such conditions as (more than one answer is possible):
   a) Lack of antidiuretic hormone
   b) Volume expansion with isotonic saline
   c) Nephrogenic diabetes insipidus
   d) Excessive water ingestion

5) Aldosterone secretion can be increased by an autonomous adrenal adenoma or in the presence of volume depletion. What will plasma renin activity be in these two conditions?

2 Cardiology

2.1 ECG Interpretation

Systematic approach:

1. Rate
2. Rhythm
3. P waves: P axis, RAE, LAE
4. PR interval
5. QRS: Width, axis, Q waves, hypertrophy
6. ST segment
7. T waves
8. QT segment

1. Rate
Use heart rate scale or count the number of QRS complexes on a 10 sec strip and multiply by six
60-100 bpm= normal
<60 bpm= bradycardia
>100 bpm= tachycardia
2. Rhythm
Check for normal sinus rhythm, with a P wave before each QRS, and a QRS after each P. Check P wave axis for sinus P waves (see next box).
3. P Waves
Axis - normal: Upright Ps in I and II, down-going in aVR
LAE - P wave ≥ 3mm **wide** and/or predominantly **downward** deflection in V_1
RAE - P wave ≥ 3mm **tall** and/or predominantly **upward** deflection in V_1
4. PR Interval
≤0.2 sec: normal
>0.2 sec: 1st-degree heart block is present
Changing PR interval: MAT, wandering atrial pacemaker, 2nd-degree heart block Mobitz type I (Wenckebach), or 3rd-degree heart block
5. QRS
Width
≤0.12 sec: normal
>0.12 sec for consistency wide complex (**Causes:** BBB, intraventricular conduction delay, Wolff- Parkinson-White, hyperkalemia, type I anti-arrhythmic drug, or pacemaker)

Axis	
Normal: -30^0 to $+90^0$	
-30^0 to -90^0 is LAD: Inferior wall MI, left anterior hemiblock	
$+120^0$ to $+180^0$ is RAD: Left posterior hemiblock, right ventricular hypertrophy, lateral wall infarct, lead reversal, dextrocardia	
$>180^0$ is extreme right (bizarre) axis: Same differential as RAD	
Q waves	
Pathologic Q waves are >0.04 sec in width and 1/3 of the height of the R wave.	
Hypertrophy	
Sokolow-Lyon criteria (most commonly used): $S_{V1} + R_{V5/V6}$ >35 mm or R_{aVL} >11 mm	
Cornell criteria: $R_{aVL} + S_{V3}$ >28 mm in males, >20 mm in females	
6. ST Segment	
ST segment is usually isoelectric with T-P interval	
>1 mm elevations are pathologic and represent: Acute ST elevation MI, variant angina, ventricular aneurysm, RV infarct (if seen in V1), or Brugada syndrome.	
>1 mm depressions are pathologic and represent: Ischemia, digoxin effect, LVH with strain, or BBB.	
Diffuse (multiple leads) ST segment elevation may be caused by acute pericarditis or early repolarization.	
7. T Waves	
Normally upright in I, II, V3-V6. They can be variable in III and aVL	
Peaked T waves are > 5 mm in limb leads or >10 mm in precordial leads are associated with hyperkalemia and infarction.	
8. QT Interval	
QT normally < ½ of R-R interval. QTc = QT/(R-R) < 0.44 sec	
Prolonged QTc > 0.45 sec has multiple causes, including: Congenital, metabolic (hypokalemia, hypocalcemia, hypomagnesemia, hypothyroidism), bradyarrhythmias; Medications: antiarrhythmics, antibiotics (fluoroquinolones), antihistamines, psychotropics (SSRIs, TCAs, risperidone)	

2.2 Important Differential Diagnoses

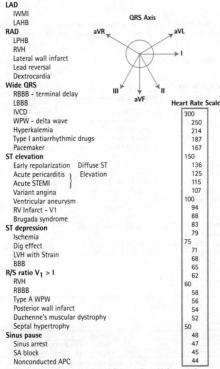

LAD
- IWMI
- LAHB

RAD
- LPHB
- RVH
- Lateral wall infarct
- Lead reversal
- Dextrocardia

Wide QRS
- RBBB - terminal delay
- LBBB
- IVCD
- WPW - delta wave
- Hyperkalemia
- Type I antiarrhythmic drugs
- Pacemaker

ST elevation
- Early repolarization
- Acute pericarditis
- Acute STEMI
- Variant angina
- Ventricular aneurysm
- RV Infarct - V1
- Brugada syndrome

(Early repolarization, Acute pericarditis, Acute STEMI: Diffuse ST Elevation)

ST depression
- Ischemia
- Dig effect
- LVH with Strain
- BBB

R/S ratio $V_1 > 1$
- RVH
- RBBB
- Type A WPW
- Posterior wall infarct
- Duchenne's muscular dystrophy
- Septal hypertrophy

Sinus pause
- Sinus arrest
- SA block
- Nonconducted APC

QRS Axis

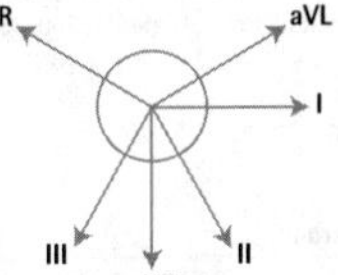

Heart Rate Scale

300
250
214
187
167
150
136
125
115
107
100
94
88
83
79
75
71
68
65
62
60
58
56
54
52
50
48
47
45
44

Narrow Complex Tachycardia

Regular

Sinus tachycardia rate: 100-160

PSVT (SNRT, AT, AVNRT, AVN reciprocal tach) vent rate: 180-220

Flutter with fixed conduction, atrial rate: 250-350 vent rate: 150, 300

Irregular

Afib

Flutter variable conduction

MAT

Wide Complex Tachycardia

SVT with aberrancy	Ventricular tachycardia	SVT and BBB
Rate 150-250 - intermittent	Rate 150-250	Rate 150-250 persistent
RBBB config predominates	RBBB or LBBB config	RBBB or LBBB
Triphasic rSR' in V1	Mono, biphasic R-V1	
Normal axis	LAD, extreme right axis	QRS >0.12
QRS < 0.14	QRS >0.14	
Initial deflection in V1 same as	Concordant precordial leads	
nonaberrant beat	QS V6, rS in V6	
qI, V6 normal septal	Pause following burst	
activation w/ RBBB config	Fusion beats (hybrid) 5%	
VR >250 consider	Capture beats -early,	
accessory pathway	narrow QRS	
	AV dissociation	

Abnormal P Axis Lead reversal, dextrocardia, ectopic rhythm

AV dissociation

Block CHB = 3° block upper PM rate > lower PM rate

Interference upper PM rate < lower PM rate

LAHB LAD, qRI, rSIII, axis -45° to -60°

LPHB RAD, rSI, qRIII, Axis +120°

PE SI, QIII, inverted T's V1-V4

RVH RAD >100°, R>S in V1

QT Prolongation <1/2 of R-R or QTc=QT/Sqrt(R-R) < 0.44 (genetic, electrolytes, antiarrhythmics, antibiotics, antipsychotics)

Uwave LVH, hypo K^+

LVH criteria

Sokolow-Lyon	Cornell
S V1 + R in V5 or V6 > 35mm	R aVL + S V3 > 28mm males
R aVL > 11mm	R aVL + S V3 > 20mm females

Used with permission: Mazzara J, Katzel J. Electrocardiographic Interpretation
Systematic Approach. © 2007

2.3 Ischemia Localization from ECG Changes

Leads with ischemic changes	Myocardium involved	Artery involved
II, III, aVF	Inferior	RCA
V1 ~ V2	Anteroseptal	LAD
V3 ~ V5	Anterior	LAD
V5 ~ V6	Apical or lateral	LAD or PDA or marginal branch
I, aVL	High lateral	Marginal branch or diagonal
V1 ~ V2 (Reciprocal)	Posterior	RCA
V3R ~ V4R	Right ventricular	RCA

Note: Obtain right-sided ECG when you have a patient with inferior wall infarction

Coronary Circulation (Normal Type)

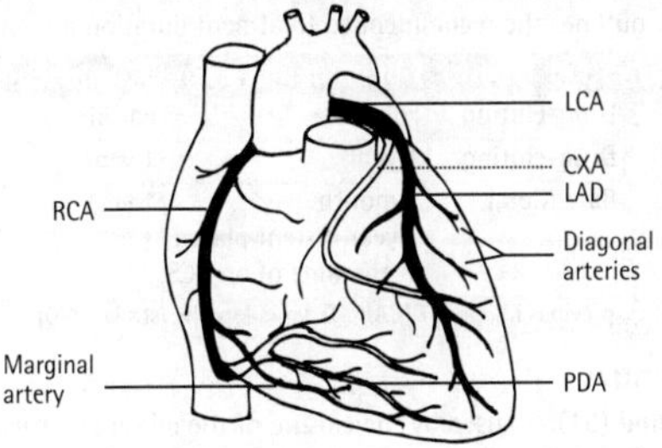

Coronary Circulation (Normal type)

LCA Left coronary artery
CXA Circumflex artery (branch of LCA)
LAD Left anterior descending (branch of LCA)
RCA Right coronary artery
PDA Posterior descending artery (branch of RCA)

2.4 Angina Classification

Class	Description
0	Asymptomatic
I	Angina with strenuous exercise
II	Angina with moderate exercise
III	Angina with mild exertion - Walking 1-2 level blocks at normal pace - Climbing 1 flight of stairs at normal pace
IV	Angina at any level of physical exertion

Source: Adapted from Canadian Cardiovascular Society (CCS) Angina Classification

2.5 Post-Angioplasty Care

Patients who receive stents require **Plavix 75mg PO once daily** on discharge in addition to lifelong Aspirin.

The table below outlines the recommended treatment duration intervals for Plavix:

Risk	Stent Type	Minimum duration	Recommended duration
High risk*	Drug-eluting	For life	For life
Average risk	Drug-eluting	1 year	1 year
Average risk	Bare Metal	1 month 1 year if stent placed at the time of an ACS	1 year

* High risk: diabetics, previous MI, prior PTCA/CAD, vasculopathy (stroke, PVD)

2.6 Murmurs

First Heart Sound (S1): Caused by the closure of the mitral and tricuspid valves.

Loud S1	Soft S1
Mitral stenosis	Mitral regurgitation
Short PR interval	Long PR interval
Tachycardia	LBBB, ↑ LVEDP (AS, AI)
Thyrotoxicosis	Immobile mitral valve

Second Heart Sound (S2): Caused by the closure of the aortic and pulmonic valves.

Wide splitting	Narrow or paradoxical	Fixed
MR, VSD	AS	ASD
RBBB	HCM	
RV volume overload (L→R shunt)	Severe HTN	
RV pressure overload (PS, PAH)	Acute MI	

Third Heart Sound (S3):
- Best heard at the apex with the bell of the stethoscope
- Abnormal for age > 40 yrs
- Suggests an enlarged ventricular chamber
- Associated with: MR, TR, and CHF

Fourth Heart Sound (S4):
- Best heard at the apex with the bell of the stethoscope
- Suggests decreased ventricular compliance
- Associated with: LVH, HTN, AS, HCM, PAH, MI, acute MR, and PS

Innocent vs. Pathologic Murmurs	
Innocent murmurs	**Pathologic murmurs**
Peak or end in the first half of systole	Diastolic murmur
Less than III/IV in intensity	New or very loud > III/IV
Loudest at LLSB without radiation	Abnormally split S2
Intensity decreases with Valsalva	Intensity increases with Valsalva
Patient younger than 45 yrs	Patient older than 45 yrs

Murmur Differentials	
Systolic	AS, PS, high flow states (anemia, pregnancy, adolescence), ASD, MVP, HCM
Holosystolic	MR, TR, VSD
Diastolic	AR, PR, MS, TS, ASD
Continuous	PDA, coarctation of aorta, AV fistula, mammary souffle (in pregnancy)

2.7 Valvular Disease

Disease	Classic murmur	Common cause	Surgery indications
Aortic stenosis (AS)	- Midsystolic crescendo-decrescendo murmur at RUSB that radiates to carotids and apex	- Rheumatic valve - Congenital bicuspid - Calcific valve	When symptomatic with or if severe AS: - Valve area < 0.6 cm^2 - Mean gradient > 60mmHg - Aortic jet velocity > 5 m/sec
Aortic regurgitation (AR)	3 murmurs: 1) Blowing early diastolic 2) Austin Flint: apical diastolic rumble 3) Midsystolic flow murmur	- Rheumatic disease - Connective tissue disorder - Rheumatologic (RA, SLE) - Endocarditis - Syphilis - Chronic volume overload	Symptoms at rest Symptoms during stress test Asymptomatic pts with: - LV end-diastolic diameter >75mm - LV end-systolic diameter >55 mm - EF <50%
Mitral stenosis (MS)	- Mid-diastolic apical rumble and opening snap: use bell	- Rheumatic disease - Congenital - Vegetation - Calcific	- Surgery when symptoms arise: valvuloplasty or MVR
Mitral regurgitation (MR)	- Holosytolic apical blowing murmur that radiates to axilla	- Rheumatic disease - MVP - Endocarditis - Mitral annular calcification - Papillary muscle rupture (post MI) - Marfan's syndrome	- Surgery for severe MR even if asymptomatic if EF <55% or LV end-systolic dimension ≥40mm
Mitral valve prolapse (MVP)	- Midsystolic click followed by late-systolic murmur that increases with Valsalva and also increases with handgrip	Most common congenital valvular disease in adults	May lead to MR
Hypertrophic cardio-myopathy (HCM)	- Systolic murmur at apex - Increases with Valsalva and decreases with handgrip	Congenital	Severe symptoms (NYHA class III or IV) or recurrent syncope despite pharmacological therapy; consider AICD placement

2.8 Endocarditis

2.8.1 Duke criteria

Pathologic criteria	Culture or histology directly from valve, after surgery or autopsy
Clinical criteria (2 major criteria, or 1 major + 3 minor criteria, or 5 minor criteria)	
Major criteria	Positive blood cultures x 2 of typical organisms Positive echo or presence of new regurgitant murmur
Minor criteria	- Presence of predisposing heart condition (IV drug abuse or valve abnormality) - Fever > 38°C - Embolic disease - Immunologic phenomena (glomerulonephritis, Osler nodes) - Positive blood culture x 1 or rare organism cultured

2.8.2 Risk stratification

Cardiac Conditions Associated With the Highest Risk for Endocarditis for Which Prophylaxis With Dental Procedures is Reasonable
• Prosthetic cardiac valve or prosthetic material used for cardiac valve repair
• Previous IE
• Congenital heart disease (CHD) – Unrepaired cyanotic CHD, including palliative shunts and conduits – Completely repaired congenital heart defect with prosthetic material or device, whether placed by surgery or by catheter intervention, during the first six months after the procedure – Repaired CHD with residual defects at the site or adjacent to the site of a prosthetic patch or prosthetic device (which inhibit endothelialization)
• Cardiac transplant recipients who develop cardiac valvulopathy
Source: Wilson W, Taubert KA, Gewitz M, et al. Lockhart, Larry M. Prevention of Infective Endocarditis: Guidelines From the American Heart Association: A Guideline From the American Heart Association Rheumatic Fever, Endocarditis, and Kawasaki Disease Committee, Council on Cardiovascular Disease in the Young, and the Council on Clinical Cardiology, Council on Cardiovascular Surgery and Anesthesia, and the Quality of Care and Outcomes Research Interdisciplinary Working Group. *Circulation* 2007;116;1736-1754

2.8.3 Prophylaxis

Procedures Requiring Prophylaxis in Patients with High Risk Conditions	
Dental	All dental procedures that involve manipulation of either gingival tissue or periapical region of teeth or perforation of the oral mucosa
Respiratory Tract	Procedures of the respiratory tract that involve incision or biopsy of the respiratory mucosa
GI and GU	Procedures in patients with ongoing GI or GU tract infections
Skin/Muscle/Bone	Procedures on infected skin, or musculoskeletal tissue
Pregnancy	Optional in women with high risk conditions at the time of delivery
Cardiac Surgery	ALL patients undergoing surgery to place prosthetic heart valves or prosthetic intravascular or intracardiac materials
Source: Wilson W, Taubert KA, Gewitz M, et al. Lockhart, Larry M. Prevention of Infective Endocarditis: Guidelines From the American Heart Association: A Guideline From the American Heart Association Rheumatic Fever, Endocarditis, and Kawasaki Disease Committee, Council on Cardiovascular Disease in the Young, and the Council on Clinical Cardiology, Council on Cardiovascular Surgery and Anesthesia, and the Quality of Care and Outcomes Research Interdisciplinary Working Group. *Circulation* 2007;116;1736-1754	

Prophylaxis Regimens		
Situation	**Adult**	**Children**
Dental Procedure - Administer single dose 30-60 minutes before procedure		
Oral	Amoxicillin 2 grams (g)	Amoxicillin 50 mg/kg
Can not tolerate PO	Ampicillin 2g IM/IV	Ampicillin 50 mg/kg IM/IV
PCN allergy	Cephalexin 2g or Clindamycin 600 mg or Azithromycin 500 mg or Clarithromycin 500mg	Clindamycin 20 mg/kg or Azithromycin 15 mg/kg
PCN allergy and can not tolerate PO	Cephazolin or Ceftriaxone (1g iv) or Clindamycin 600 mg IM/IV	Cephazolin or Ceftriaxone 50 mg/kg or Clindamycin 20 mg/kg IM/IV
GI or GU Procedure- Provide enterococcal coverage		
	Amoxicillin 2g PO or Ampicillin 2g IM/IV or Vancomycin 1g IV	Amoxicillin 50 mg/kg or Ampicillin 50 mg/kg IM/IV or Vancomycin 15 mg/kg
Skin and Musculoskeletal Tissue- Identical to Dental Procedures		
Source: Wilson W, Taubert KA, Gewitz M, et al. Lockhart, Larry M. Prevention of Infective Endocarditis* (see above)		

2.9 Rheumatic Heart Disease

Jones Criteria *	
Major criteria	- Carditis - Polyarthritis - Chorea - Erythema marginatum - Subcutaneous nodules
Minor criteria	- Fever - Arthralgia - Previous rheumatic fever or rheumatic heart disease
Evidence of recent strep infection	- Elevated antistreptolysin O or other streptococcal antibodies - Positive throat culture for Group A beta-hemolytic streptococci - Positive rapid direct Group A strep antigen test - Recent scarlet fever

* Diagnosis of rheumatic heart disease can be established by **2 major criteria or 1 major + 2 minor criteria** in addition to evidence of recent streptococcal infection

2.10 Chest Pain

Protocol for Chest Pain Management in the Emergency Department

- ABCs first
- MONA (Morphine, O_2, Nitrates until pain free, ASA 162-325 mg)
- 12-lead ECG
- IV access and labs sent (CBC, SMA-7, cardiac enzymes, INR)

If ACS is suspected by labs or ECG -**BATMAN** jumps into action. Cath lab is put on notice

B – Beta blocker
A – Aspirin
T – Thrombolytics (consider if cath lab is not available)
M – Morphine
A – Antiplatelet (heparin or IIb/IIIa agents)
N – Nitrates

Nine Critical Causes of Chest Pain	
Cause of pain	**Necessary initial steps**
Myocardial infarction, ischemia	EKG, cardiac enzymes
Pulmonary embolus	CT angiography
Pneumothorax	CXR
Tension pneumothorax	CXR
Aortic dissection	B/L pulses and BP, CT or TEE, call surgery
Ruptured AAA	CT, call surgery
Myocarditis/pericarditis	ECG (diffuse changes), H&P
Perforating peptic ulcer	CXR or water-soluble contrast study
Esophageal rupture	CXR or water-soluble contrast esophagram

2.11 Cardiovascular Health

2.11.1 Blood pressure: JNC VII classification for adults

BP Classification	SBP (mmHg)	DBP (mmHg)
Normal	< 120	and < 80
Pre-hypertension	120 - 139	or 80 - 89
Stage I HTN	140 - 159	or 90 - 99
Stage II HTN	> 160	or > 100

2.11.2 Cardiovascular risk factors

Major risk factors

- Hypertension
- Age (men > 55, women > 65)
- Diabetes mellitus
- Elevated LDL (or total) cholesterol, or low HDL cholesterol
- Estimated GFR < 60 ml/min
- Family history of premature cardiovascular disease (men < 55, women < 65)
- Microalbuminuria
- Obesity (BMI > 30)
- Physical inactivity
- Tobacco usage, particularly cigarettes

2.11.3 HTN target organ damage

- **Heart - LVH:** Angina/prior MI, prior coronary revascularization, heart failure
- **Brain:** H/O stroke or transient ischemic attack (TIA), dementia
- **Chronic kidney disease (CKD)**
- Peripheral arterial disease
- Retinopathy

2.11.4 Cholesterol classification and guidelines

ATP III Classification of LDL, Total, and HDL Cholesterol (mg/dl)	
LDL cholesterol	
< 100	Optimal
100-129	Near optimal/above optimal
130-159	Borderline high
160-189	High
> 190	Very high
Total cholesterol	
< 200	Desirable
200-239	Borderline high
> 240	High
HDL cholesterol	
< 40	Low
> 60	High

Major risk factors (exclusive of LDL cholesterol) that modify LDL goals

- Cigarette smoking
- Hypertension (BP > 140/90 mmHg or on hypertensive medications)
- Low HDL cholesterol (< 40 mg/dl)
- Family history of premature CHD (< 55 in males, < 65 in females, 1st-degree relative)
- Age (men > 45, women > 55)

Risk categories that modify LDL cholesterol goals	
Risk category	**LDL goal (mg/dl)**
0–1 risk factors	< 160
Multiple (2+) risk factors	< 130
CHD or CHD risk equivalents	< 100

Guidelines for Achieving LDL Goals by Therapeutic Lifestyle Changes (TLC) vs. Pharmacotherapy in Different Risk Categories			
Risk category	**LDL goal (mg/dl)**	**Start TLC**	**Consider starting pharmacotherapy**
0 - 1 risk factors*	< 160	≥ 160	≥190 160-189: Drug optional
2+ risk factors (10-yr risk ≥ 20%)	< 130	≥ 130	10-yr risk 10-20%: >130 10-yr risk < 10%: ≥160
CHD or CHD risk equivalents (10-yr risk > 20%)	< 100	≥100	≥ 130 100-129: Drug optional**

* Virtually all people with 0-1 risk factor have a 10-year risk < 10%, thus a 10-year risk assessment is not necessary for people in this category

** Some sources recommend use of LDL-lowering drugs in this category if LDL < 100mg/dL cannot be achieved through lifestyle changes alone. Others prefer use of TG- and HDL-modifying

2.11.5 Metabolic syndrome

Clinical Criteria Defining Metabolic Syndrome in Adults	
Waist circumference	**Men:** > 102 cm (40 in) **Women:** > 88 cm (35 in)
Blood pressure	> 130 mmHg systolic and/or >85 mmHg diastolic
Fasting glucose	> 110 mg/dl (6.1 mmol/L)
Triglycerides	> 150 mg/dl or 1.69 mmol/L
HDL cholesterol	**Men:** < 40 mg/dl **Women:** < 50 mg/dl

2.12 Drugs Affecting Lipoprotein Metabolism

Drug Class	Effects	Side Effects	Contra-indications	Clinical Trial Results
HMG CoA Reductase inibitors (statins)	LDL: ↓ 18-63% HDL: ↑ 5-15% TG: ↓ 7-30%	- Myopathy - ↑ liver enzymes - Rhabdomyolysis (rare)	**Absolute:** Active or chronic liver disease **Relative:** Concurrent use of certain drugs	Reduced major coronary events, CHD death, coronary procedure need, stroke, total mortality
Bile acid sequestrants	LDL: ↓ 15-30% HDL: ↑ 3-5% TG: No change	- GI distress - Constipation - ↑ absorption of other drugs	**Absolute:** dys-beta-lipoproteinemia TG > 400 mg/dl **Relative:** TG > 200 mg/dl	Reduced major coronary events and CHD deaths
Nicotinic acid	LDL: ↓ 5-25% HDL: ↑ 15-35% TG: ↓ 20-50%	- Flushing - Hyperglycemia - Hyperuricemia (gout) - Upper GI distress - Hepatotoxicity	**Absolute:** Chronic liver disease Severe gout **Relative:** Diabetes Hyperuricemia Peptic ulcer disease	Reduced major coronary events and possibly total mortality
Fibric acids	LDL: ↓ 5-20% HLD: ↑ 10-20% TG: ↓ 20-50%	- Dyspepsia - Gallstones - Myopathy - Unexplained non-CHD deaths in WHO study	**Absolute:** Severe renal disease Severe hepatic disease	Reduced major coronary events

2.13 Hypertensive Emergency

2.13.1 Definitions of terms

Term	Definition	Steps
Hypertensive urgency	- SBP >180mmHg - DBP >120mmHg - NO evidence of end-organ damage - NOT considered an emergency	- DO NOT undertake aggressive BP reduction steps - Rapid BP reduction increases risk of cerebral, renal, and cardiac hypoperfusion - BP should be controlled over 1-2 days
Hypertensive emergency (accelerated hypertension)	- High BP (>180/120) WITH evidence of end-organ damage (neurologic, cardiac, renal)	- IMMEDIATE BP control required

2.13.2 Possible causes

- Progression of chronic hypertension
- Renal or renovascular disease (renal artery stenosis)
- Drugs (cocaine, methamphetamines)
- Drug withdrawal (β-blocker withdrawal)
- Eclampsia (pregnancy)
- Endocrine (pheochromocytoma, hyperthyroidism, Cushing's)
- CNS (tumor, SAH)
- Trauma (particularly head trauma)

2.13.3 Pharmacologic treatment

Drug	Dose	Mechanism	Onset	Duration	Notes
nitro-prusside	0.25-10µg/kg/min IV infusion	Veno and arterial dilation	2-3 s	1-2 min	Never give longer than 10 min - causes cyanide accumulation
labetalol	IV bolus: 10-80mg q10min IV infusion: 0.5-2.0 mg/min	Combined beta + alpha adrenergic blocker	1-2 min	10-30 min	Safe in CAD pts; safe in pregnancy; contraindicated in: asthma, bradycardia
nitro-glycerin	init: 5 µg/min, increase up to 100 µg/min	Veno and arterial dilation	2-5 min	5-10 min	Headache is common, SE, reflex tachycardia
nicar-dipine	init: 5 mg/h, may be increased up to 15 mg/h	Dihydro-pyridine Ca^{2+} channel blocker	10-15 min	10-30 min (short-acting formula-tion)	Avoid in heart failure + coronary ischemia
hydra-lazine	10-20 mg q 20-30 min	Arterial vasodilator	5-20 min	1-4 hours	Use with caution in pulmonary hypertension; may cause hypotension

2.14 Atrial Fibrillation (AF)

2.14.1 Classification

Atrial Fibrillation (AF) Classification	
Recurrent	2 or more episodes of AF
Paroxysmal	Self-terminating, lasts 7 days or less and typically <24 hours
Persistent	Lasts longer than 7 days
Permanent	Cardioversion has failed or has not been attempted
Long-standing	Lasts longer than 1 year
Lone	Age <60 years without clinical or echo evidence of cardiopulmonary disease, including HTN
Nonvalvular	No rheumatic mitral valve disease, prosthetic valve or valve repair

2.14.2 Evaluation and workup

AF Evaluation and Workup	
Minimum evaluation	
1) History and physical examination to define presence and nature of symptoms, frequency, duration, precipitating factors, and modes of termination of AF; response to any pharmacological agents; and presence of underlying heart disease or other reversible conditions (eg, hyperthyroidism or alcohol consumption) 2) Electrocardiogram 3) Transthoracic echocardiogram 4) Blood tests: thyroid, renal, and hepatic function	
Workup	
Physical	HTN, murmurs (valve disease), cardiomegaly, edema, thyromegaly
ECG	Rate, rhythm, A/V hypertrophy, block, MI, preexcitation, RR, QRS, QTc intervals
Labs	TSH, free T4, electrolytes, CBC, cardiac markers, D-dimer
Imaging	Chest x-ray to assess cardiomegaly, pulmonary edema; transthoracic echo to rule out thrombus and assess valve defects, hypertrophy; transesophageal echo (TEE) to r/o left atrial appendage thrombus; chest CT or V/Q scan to rule out PE if clinically indicated
Stress tests	6-minute walk, exercise, stress test
Holter monitor	Characterize arrhythmia
EP study	Characterize arrhythmia, evaluate for AF ablation

2.14.3 Pharmacological management

Pharmacological Management Guidelines for Patients with AF	
General Principles - 3 main components:	
Rate control*	Administration of β-blockers, CCBs or cardiac glycosides to reduce ventricular rate and prevent hemodynamic instability
Rhythm control	Administration of antiarrhythmic drugs (AADs) or electrical cardioversion to return the heart to normal sinus rhythm
Anticoagulation	Anticoagulant or antiplatelet agents are considered for each patient. CHADS2 score is used to assess risk of stroke.
Newly Discovered AF	
Paroxysmal AF	• Therapy is not needed unless severe symptoms of hypertension, heart failure, angina pectoris, etc • Anticoagulate as necessary
Persistent AF	• Rate control and anticoagulation as necessary • Consider AAD therapy or cardioversion
Recurrent Paroxysmal AF	
Minimal or no symptoms	• Anticoagulation and rate control as necessary
Disabling symptoms	• Anticoagulation and rate control as necessary • AAD therapy • AF ablation if AAD therapy fails
Recurrent Persistent or Permanent AF	
Recurrent persistent	**Minimal or no symptoms:** • Anticoagulation and rate control as necessary **Disabling symptoms:** • Anticoagulation and rate control • AAD therapy • Electrical cardioversion • Continue anticoagulation and therapy to maintain sinus rhythm • Consider ablation for severely symptomatic recurrent AF after
Permanent	Anticoagulation and rate control as necessary

*The AFFIRM trial (N Engl J Med. 2002;347(23):1825) demonstrated an almost significant trend toward a decrease in all-cause mortality with rate control (21.3% vs 23.8%, HR 0.87, 95% CI 0.75-1.01). There was no difference between the two groups in the incidence of cardiac death, arrhythmic death, or deaths due to ischemic or hemorrhagic stroke. The RACE trial (N Engl J Med. 2002;347(23):1834.) showed an almost significant trend toward a lower incidence of adverse events with rate control (17.2% vs 22.6% with rhythm control, HR 0.73, 90% CI 0.53-1.01). There was no difference in cardiovascular mortality (6.8% vs 7%).

Adapted from the 2006 ACC/AHA/ESC Guidelines on AF and 2011 ACCF/AHA/HRS Focused Updates.

2.14.4 Management of newly discovered AF

Management of Patients with Newly Discovered AF

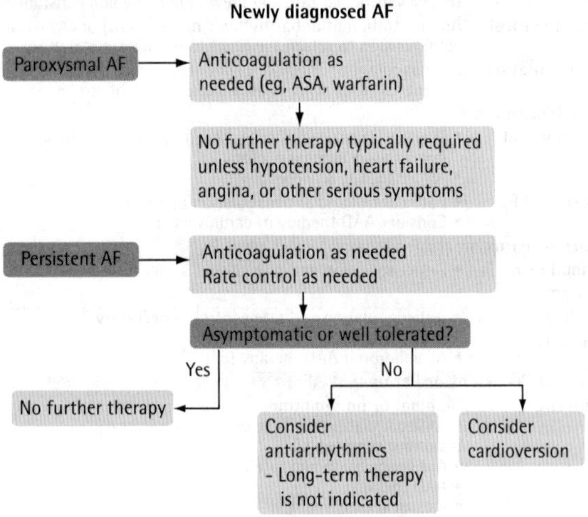

Adapted from the 2011 AHA/ESC Pocket Guidelines.

2.14.5 Pharmacological heart rate control in AF

Pharmacologic Heart-Rate Control in Atrial Fibrillation			
Drug	**Control of Acute Episode**	**Control of Sustained AF**	**Comments**
Calcium Channel Blockers			
Diltiazem	0.25 mg/kg over 2 min Maintenance infusion of 5–15 mg/hr	Oral controlled-released formulation 120–360 mg daily in divided doses;	Long-term control may be better with the addition of digoxin
Verapamil	0.075 to 0.15 mg/kg over 2 min	Slow-release formulation 120 –360 mg daily in divided doses	Causes elevation in digoxin levels. May be more negatively inotropic than diltiazem
Beta-Blockers			
Metoprolol	2.5 to 5 mg IV bolus over 2 min up to 3 doses	PO 25-100 mg twice a day	Useful if there is concomitant coronary artery disease
Esmolol	500 mcg/kg IV over 1 min, then 60-200 mcg/kg/min (increase rate to desired response in 50 mcg/kg/min increments q 4 min)	Not indicated	-
Propranolol	0.15 mg/kg IV	80 to 240 mg daily in divided doses, orally	-

Cardiac Glycosides			
Digoxin	0.25 mg every 2 h, up to 1.5 mg 0.125 to 0.375 mg daily IV or orally	0.125–0.375 mg daily	Use in patients who have HF. Renally excreted. Slow onset even if given IV, with less effective control than other agents, although may be synergistic with them. Poor efficacy for exertional heart rate control
Amiodarone	150 mg over 10 min then 0.5 to 1.0 mg/min	200 mg daily	Second-line therapy used when the other drugs failed
Adapted from the 2006 ACC/AHA/ESC Guidelines on AF and 2011 ACCF/AHA/HRS Focused Updates.			

2.14.6 Rate control vs rhythm control in AF

Rate Control vs Rhythm Control for AF	
Rate control is superior to conversion in:	
- Age > 65 - CAD - HTN	- Female gender - No CHF
Note: The bigger the size of the left atrium, the smaller the chance that the patient will remain in sinus rhythm	
AFFIRM Trial: Wyse DG, et al. Atrial Fibrillation Follow-up Investigation of Rhythm Management (AFFIRM) Investigators. A comparison of rate control and rhythm control in patients with atrial fibrillation. N Engl J Med. 2002 Dec 5;347(23):1825-33.	

2.14.7 Anticoagulation in nonvalvular AF

Guidelines for Anticoagulation for Nonvalvular AF		
For evaluation of risk factors use the CHADS2 score		
CHADS2 = CHF(1) , HTN (1), Age>75 (1), DM (1), Stroke/TIA (2) The CHADS2 score is calculated by adding the points shown in parenthesis if the patient has a history of the respective item.		
Total CHADS2 score	Yearly risk of stroke	Treatment
0	0.5% to 1.7%	ASA or no therapy
1	2%	Warfarin (INR 2-3) more effective than ASA
2+	4% to 10%	Warfarin (INR 2-3) or dabigatran or rivaroxaban

2.14.8 Invasive therapies in AF

Invasive Therapies in AF		
AV node ablation	Performed for rate control; requires pacemaker implantation.	
Left atrial appendage ligation	• The majority of thrombi in nonvalvular atrial fibrillation occur in the left atrial appendage. • Performed while undergoing other cardiac surgery.	
MAZE procedure	Interrupts potential reentry pathways by surgical incision of the myocardium in a specific pattern.	
	Success rate	Up to 70%-90% of patients at 10 years post-MAZE.
	Complications	Injury to conduction pathway requiring permanent pacing.

Ablation	• Map, isolate, and "burn" atrial fibrillation foci in the pulmonary veins and posterior left atrium using various energy sources. • Endovascular endocardial and minimally invasive epicardial approaches are available. • Quality of life favors ablation over medical therapy.	
	Success rate	Approx. 85% among paroxysmal atrial fibrillation patients and 68% among permanent atrial fibrillation patients at 10 months post-ablation.
	Complications	• Pericarditis, valve injury, recurrence of atrial fibrillation, mortality, heart failure, thromboembolism. • The incidence of major complications such as tamponade, atrioesophageal fistula, or pulmonary vein stenosis is <1%.
Source: Anthony Bavry MD and Calvin Y. Choi MD (U. of Florida). Atrial Fibrillation pocketcard Set. Borm Bruckmeier Publishing.		

2.15 Heart Failure

2.15.1 NYHA heart failure classification

New York Heart Association (NYHA) Heart Failure Classification	
Class I	No limitation of physical activity
Class II	Slight limitation of physical activity
Class III	Marked limitation of physical activity
Class IV	Symptoms at rest

2.15.2 History and physical examination

Symptoms	Comments
Exertional dyspnea	LHF > RHF; Dysfunctional LV cannot sustain sufficient CO; progresses to dyspnea at rest in advanced HF stage
Orthopnea	LHF > RHF; recumbency increases blood return to heart leading to pulm. congestion due to LV dysfunction; rapid onset/recovery, often associated with dry cough; pts use pillows to maintain upper body elevated
PND	Bronchospasm, with severe anxiety, feeling of suffocation; may mimic asthma attack clinically; slow recovery (30 min or more)
Fatigue, muscle weakness	Heaviness in the limbs; common in advanced HF
Nocturia	Recumbency increases blood flow and renal perfusion; may progress to oliguria in severe LHF
Psychiatric	Low CO → poor cerebral perfusion → confusion, memory impairment, psychosis, headache, delirium
GI	RHF: Often leads to venous hypertension and accompanying congestive hepatomegaly, ascites, RUQ abd. pain, anorexia, bloating, constipation; in severe HF (RHF or LHF) poor bowel perfusion leads to pain, distention, bloody stools
Physical Findings	
General	Pts appear dyspneic, easily fatigued, may appear cyanotic or jaundiced, swollen, are generally well nourished but may appear cachectic in terminal HF
HEENT	Possible eye pulsations in severe HF with tricuspid regurgitation, jaundice, flushed facial appearance with malar rash.
Skin	Cyanotic, cold, diaphoretic, clammy, secondary to increased adrenergic stimulation
Pulmonary	Rales over bases, wheezing, blood-tinged sputum
Cardiovascular	Weak rapid pulse, S3 gallop, loud P2, pulsus alternans, possible JVD (RHF) and + Kussmaul sign, peripheral edema, possible cardiomegaly
Abdominal	Ascites, increased abdominal girth, hepatomegaly, RUQ pain, + hepatojugular reflex (RHF)
Neuropsychiatric	Impaired CO → increased adrenergic stimulation → anxiety, clamminess, pallor; psych: confusion, delirium, psychosis
Extremities	Peripheral edema evident if significant water retention (>5L)

2.15.3 Heart failure workup

Test	Findings
SMA7	- Watch for hypokalemia in diuretics use (hyperkalemia if K-sparing diuretics or low GFR) - Hyponatremia (dilutional) - Low HCO3 (acidosis due to hypoxia) - High BUN/Cr in severe HF (low GFR)
LFTs	- High AST (> x10 normal), ALT, alk phos, LDH, bili (> 15-20 mg/dL), low albumin
Coagulation	- Elevated PT in longstanding chronic HF (hepatic dysfunction)
BNP	- > 100 pg/mL → 95% specific, 98% sensitive for HF; normal ranges increase with age; correlates well with PCWP press. and clinical outcomes - **Note:** Found to be the single most important predictor of short-term outcome in CHF
ABG	- Hypoxia; hypocapnia in initial stages → hypercapnia in advanced HF with severe pulmonary edema. - **Consider** intubation if marked hypercapnia + resp. acidosis
ECG	- Look for signs of MI (ST segment changes, flipped Ts, Q waves), LVH (SV2 + RV5 > 35mm), MAT or A-fib (atrial enlargement)
Chest X-ray	- Look for cardiomegaly, butterfly pattern infiltrates (pulm. edema), loss of clear pulm. vasculature patterns, hazy hilar area, Kerley-B lines (thickened interlobular septa due to fluid in interlobular space) - Typical findings can take up to 12 hrs to develop from onset of acute HF episode
Echocardiography	- Best method for LV function assessment - Consider transesophageal echo in obese or ventilated pts - **Look** for wall thickness or motion abnormalities, valvular abnormalities, chamber diameter increase
Radionuclide Multiple Gated Acquisition Scan (MUGA)	- Very reliable in determining global heart function and LV ejection fraction - Not useful in assessment of valvular or pericardial disease

2.15.4 Heart failure treatment

Any patient with documented heart failure requires treatment prior to discharge as outlined below:

ACE inhibitors / angiotensin receptor blockers (ARB)	• ACE inhibitors are 1st line, if contraindicated: document clearly • Titrate to maximum tolerated dose • If ACEIs are contraindicated, use ARBs: - **losartan** (Cozaar) 25-100 mg Po daily - **valsartan** (Diovan) 40mg PO twice daily, titrate up to 160mg PO twice daily - **candesartan** (Atacand) 16mg PO qday to max of 32mg PO qday
Beta Blockers	Sample β-blockers: - **carvedilol** (Coreg) start 3.125mg PO twice daily, titrate to max tolerated dose of 25mg PO twice daily - **Toprol XL** 25mg PO once daily, titrate to max tolerated dose of 200mg PO once daily - **metoprolol** 25mg PO twice daily, titrated up to 100mg PO twice daily - Atenolol - Not FDA indicated for HF therapy
Diuretics	- **furosemide** (Lasix) - Titrate to achieve euvolemic state - **spironolactone** - Class II and III CHF and EF < 30%, 25mg PO once daily In African Americans with EF <40%, add hydralazine and a nitrate (Isordil)
Drugs used for control of in-hospital acute CHF	
- IV nitroglycerin - Dobutamine - Dopamine - IV milrinone	

2.15.5 Congestive heart failure (CHF) overview

	Systolic Dysfunction	Diastolic Dysfunction
LVEDP	↑	↑
LVEF	↓	Normal

Echo Findings		
Chambers	Dilated	Normal
Hypertrophy	-	-/+
Contractility	↓	Normal
Treatment	ACEIs (ARBs if ACEI not tolerated), -Blockers, Hydralazine + nitrates (in black patients with class III/IV HF), aldosterone antagonists (post MI, severe HF), Diuretics, Digoxin	β-Blockers, Verapamil, ACEIs., Diuretics, Nitrates - no clear benefit for any specific medication. Goal is to control BP, HR, treat volume overload
LVEDP=Left ventricular end diastolic press; LVEF=Left ventricular ejection fraction; BNP levels correlate with severity of CHF		

2.16 Syncope

Cardiogenic	**Arrhythmias**
	- AV block with bradycardia - Sinus pauses/bradycardia (vagal stimulation, sick sinus syndrome, overdose on negative chronotropic drug: β–blockers, calcium channel blockers) - Ventricular tachycardia due to structural heart disease
	Not caused by < arrhythmias
	- Hypertrophic cardiomyopathy - Aortic stenosis
Non-cardiogenic	**Reflex mechanisms**
	Vasovagal syncope Micturition Cough
	Orthostatic hypotension
	- Fluid depletion - Dysautonomias - Drugs: sympathetic blockers
Neurologic	- Seizure - Stroke

Psychogenic	- Hysterical - Panic/anxiety
Drug-induced	- Alcohol, drugs
Unknown	- Approx 50% are of unknown etiology

2.17 Aortic Aneurysms

Aneurysm Location	Indications for Surgery
Abdominal aortic aneurysm	> 5.5 cm, or growth > 0.5 cm in 6 months
Ascending aortic aneurysm	> 5 cm, or growth > 1 cm per year
Descending aortic aneurysm	> 6 cm

Note: Use ultrasound to diagnose, angiogram prior to surgery
Follow patients with ultrasonography

Dissecting Aortic Aneurysm Classification

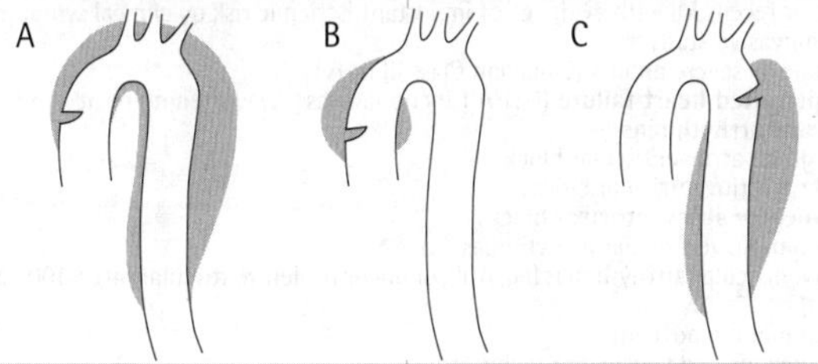

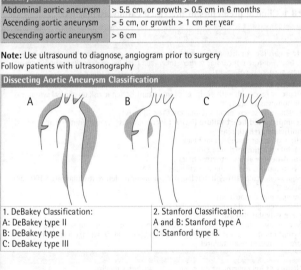

1. DeBakey Classification:	2. Stanford Classification:
A: DeBakey type II B: DeBakey type I C: DeBakey type III	A and B: Stanford type A C: Stanford type B.

2.18 Perioperative Cardiovascular Evaluation

The recommendations outlined in this section are based on the most recent evidence-based guidelines released by the American College of Cardiology and American Heart Association in 2007 and updated in 2009. These guidelines apply only to **noncardiac procedures**.

Source: Fleisher LAet al. 2009 ACC/AHA Focused Update on Perioperative Beta Blockade Incorporated Into the ACC/AHA 2007 Guidelines on Perioperative Cardiovascular Evaluation and Care for Noncardiac Surgery. Circulation 2009;120:e169

2.18.1 Clinical predictors of increased cardiovascular risk

Clinical Predictors of Increased Perioperative Cardiovascular Risk (Myocardial Infarction, Heart Failure, Death)	
Active cardiac conditions for which the patient should undergo evaluation and treatment before noncardiac surgery (may lead to delay or cancellation of surgery, unless surgery is emergent)	
Unstable coronary syndromes - Acute or recent MI with evidence of important ischemic risk by clinical symptoms or noninvasive study - Unstable or severe angina (Canadian Class III or IV) **Decompensated heart failure** (NYHA functional class IV, worsening or new-onset) **Significant arrhythmias** - High-grade atrioventricular block - Mobitz II atrioventricular block - Third-degree atrioventricular block - Symptomatic ventricular arrhythmias - Supraventricular arrrhythmias (eg, Afib, or uncontrolled ventricular rate >100 bpm at rest) - Symptomatic bradycardia - Newly recognized ventricular tachycardia **Severe valvular disease** - Severe aortic stenosis (gradient > 40 mmHg, area < 1.0 cm^2, or symptomatic) - Symptomatic mitral stenosis (progressive dyspnea on exertion, exertional presyncope, or heart failure)	
Clinical Risk Factors	
- History of ischemic heart disease - History of compensated or prior HF - History of cerebrovascular disease	- Diabetes mellitus - Renal insufficiency (SeCr >2 mg/dL)
*The American College of Cardiology National Database Library defines recent MI as greater than 7 days but less than or equal to 1 month (30 days); acute MI is within 7 days; may include "stable" angina in patients who are unusually sedentary.	

2.18.2 Assessing functional capacity

The patient's capacity for activity is also used as an important clinical predictor of post-op recovery. This functional capacity is measured in metabolic equivalents (METS). 1 MET represents resting O_2 consumption (VO_2) and is approximately 3.5 ml O_2/kg/min for a 40-year-old male. The MET requirements of various human activities have been described and are outlined in the diagram below (adapted from the Duke Activity Status Index, and the AHA Exercise Standards).

1 MET ↓	Can you take care of yourself? Eat, dress, or use the toilet? Walk indoors around the house? Walk a block or two on level ground at 2 to 3 mph or 3.2 to 4.8 km per h?	4 METs ↓	Climb a flight of stairs or walk up a hill? Walk on level ground at 4mph or 6.4 km per hour? Run a short distance? Do heavy work around the house like scrubbing floors or lifting or moving heavy furniture? Participate in moderate recreational activities like golf, bowling, dancing, doubles tennis, or throwing a baseball or football?
4 METs	Do light work around the house like dusting or washing dishes?	Greater than 10 METs	Participate in strenuous sports like swimming, singles tennis, football, basketball, or skiing?

Sample METS table

Activity	Description	METS
Cycling	Leisurely (< 10 mph)	4
	Moderate (12-13.9 mph)	8
Conditioning exercise	General light to moderate effort	4.5
	Vigorous effort (push-ups, pull-ups, sit-ups)	8.0
	Circuit training, ski machine	8.0 - 9.5
Dancing	Aerobic, general moderate intensity	6.0
Home activities	Carpet/floor sweeping	2.5
	Cleaning house, general	3.5

Lawn and garden	Chopping wood	6.0
	Lawn mowing (power push mower)	4.5
	Lawn raking	4.0
	Shoveling snow	6.0
Occupation	Standing, moderate effort	3.5
	Construction	5.5
	Farming, carrying heavy loads, lifting	8.0
Running	5 mph (12-minute mile)	8.0
	6 mph (10-minute mile)	10.0
	7.5 mph (8-minute mile)	12.5
	Up the stairs	15.0
Sports	Baseball	5.0
	Basketball, football, hockey	8.0
	Golf (power cart - carrying clubs)	3.5–5.5
	Racquetball	10.0
	Soccer	10.0
	Tennis (doubles - singles)	6.0–8.0
Walking	2.5 - 4.0 mph (light - brisk pace)	3.0 - 4.0
	Hiking, cross-country	6.0
	Up stairs, climbing ladder	8.0
Water activities	Canoeing, rowing (2 - 6 mph)	3.0–7.0
	Sailing	3.0
	Water skiing	6.0
	Swimming (leisurely - vigorous)	6.0–10.0
Winter activities	Ice skating	5.5–9.0
	Skiing, cross-country light pace, flat surface	7.0
	Skiing, cross-country uphill, max effort	16.5
	Skiing, downhill light-moderate effort	5.0
	Skiing, downhill, vigorous effort, racing	8.0
	Snow shoeing	8.0

2.18.3 Risk stratification for noncardiac procedures

In addition to the patient's general cardiovascular condition, as assessed by pathologic clinical predictors and functional capacity, the risk inherent in each procedure is also an important consideration in the perioperative assessment. The table below outlines the relative risks of a number of noncardiac procedures.

Cardiac Risk* Stratification for Noncardiac Surgical Procedures
High (Reported cardiac risk often greater than 5%)
- Aortic and other major vascular surgery - Peripheral vascular surgery
Intermediate (Reported cardiac risk generally less than 5%)
- Carotid endarterectomy - Head and neck surgery - Intraperitoneal and intrathoracic surgery - Orthopedic surgery - Prostate surgery
Low (Reported cardiac risk generally less than 1%)**
- Endoscopic procedures - Superficial procedures - Cataract surgery - Breast surgery - Ambulatory surgery
*Combined incidence of cardiac death and nonfatal myocardial infarction **Do not generally require further preoperative cardiac testing

2.18.4 Perioperative cardiac evaluation algorithm

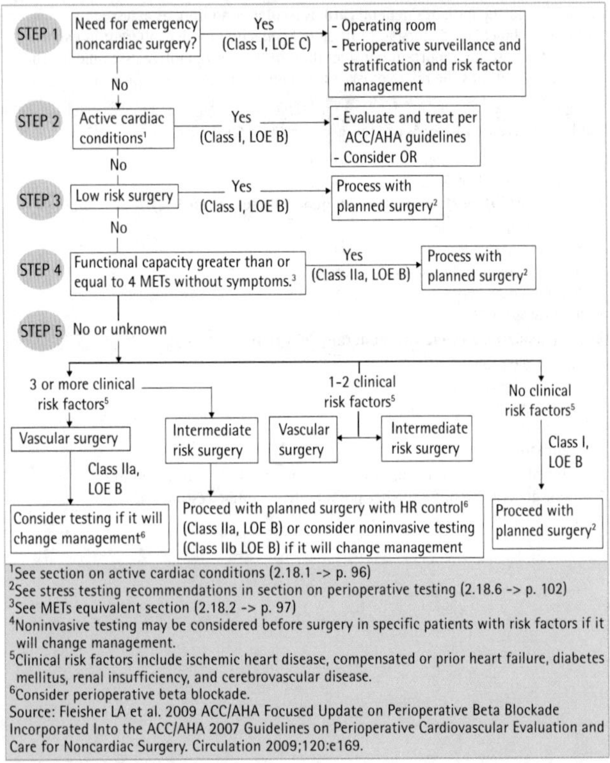

[1]See section on active cardiac conditions (2.18.1 -> p. 96)
[2]See stress testing recommendations in section on perioperative testing (2.18.6 -> p. 102)
[3]See METs equivalent section (2.18.2 -> p. 97)
[4]Noninvasive testing may be considered before surgery in specific patients with risk factors if it will change management.
[5]Clinical risk factors include ischemic heart disease, compensated or prior heart failure, diabetes mellitus, renal insufficiency, and cerebrovascular disease.
[6]Consider perioperative beta blockade.
Source: Fleisher LA et al. 2009 ACC/AHA Focused Update on Perioperative Beta Blockade Incorporated Into the ACC/AHA 2007 Guidelines on Perioperative Cardiovascular Evaluation and Care for Noncardiac Surgery. Circulation 2009;120:e169.

2.18.5 Exercise testing in patients with CAD

Patients with proven or suspected CAD who demonstrate an ischemic response in an ECG-monitored stress test, fall into the risk categories outlined below.

Prognostic Gradient of Ischemic Responses During an ECG-Monitored Exercise Test in Patients with suspected or proven CAD
High risk
Ischemia induced by low-level exercise (less than 4 METs or heart rate less than 100 bpm, or less than 70% age-predicted) manifested by one or more of the following: - Horizontal or down-sloping ST depression greater than 0.1 mV - ST segment elevation greater than 0.1 mV in noninfarct lead - Five or more abnormal leads - Persistent ischemic response longer than 1-3 min after exertion - Typical angina
Intermediate risk
Ischemia induced by moderate-level exercise 4 to 6 METs or heart rate 100 to 130 bpm [70 to 85% age-predicted] manifested by one or more of the following: - Horizontal or downsloping ST depression greater than 0.1 mV - Persistent ischemic response longer than 1 to 3 min after exertion - Three to four abnormal leads
Low risk
No ischemia or ischemia induced at high-level exertion (greater than 7 METs or heart rate greater than 130 bpm, greater than 85% age-predicted) manifested by: - Horizontal or downsloping ST depression greater than 0.1 mV - One or two abnormal leads
Inadequate test
Inability to reach adequate target workload or heart rate response for age without an ischemic response. For patients undergoing noncardiac surgery, the inability to exercise to at least the intermediate-risk level without ischemia should be considered an inadequate test.
Workload and heart rate estimates for risk severity require adjustment for patient age. Maximum target heart rates for 40- and 80-year-old subjects on no cardioactive medication are 180 and 140 bpm.

2.18.6 Evidence-based guidelines for the perioperative testing of surgical patients undergoing non-cardiac procedures

The 2007 ACC/AHA Practice Guidelines make recommendations on the appropriateness of perioperative testing in patients undergoing noncardiac surgical procedures. These guidelines are based on the evidence-based classification developed by reviewing relevant research articles.

ACC/AHA Evidence-based Classification System	
Class I	Recommendation that the procedure/therapy is useful and effective, based on Level A evidence from multiple randomized clinical trials or meta-analyses. Benefit >>> Risk. The procedure/treatment SHOULD be performed/administered.
Class II	Conditions for which there is conflicting evidence and/or a divergence of opinion about the usefulness/efficacy of performing the procedure/therapy.
IIa	Additional studies with focused objectives needed. IT IS REASONABLE to perform procedure/administer treatment.
IIb	Additional studies with brad objectives needed; additional registry data would be helpful. Procedure/treatment MAY BE CONSIDERED.
Class III	Risk > Benefit. Procedure/treatment should NOT be perfomed/ administered SINCE IT IS NOT HELPFUL AND MAY BE HARMFUL.

Recommendations for Preop ECG Evaluation		
Class I		- For patients with at least 1 clinical risk factor who are undergoing vascular surgical procedures - For patients with known CAD, PAD or cerebrovascular disease who are undergoing intermediate-risk surgeries
Class II	**IIa**	Patients with no clinical risk factors undergoing vascular surgery
	IIb	Patients with at least 1 clinical risk factor undergoing intermediate risk surgery
Class III		Not indicated in asymptomatic subjects undergoing low-risk operative procedures

Recommendations for Preoperative Noninvasive Evaluation of Left Ventricular Function		
Class II	IIa	Patients with current or prior HF with worsening dyspnea or change in clinical status, if test not done within 12 months patients with dyspnea of unknown origin
	IIb	Reassessment of LV function in clinically stable patients with previously documented cardiomyopathy is not well established
Class III		Not recommended as a routine perioperative test of LV function

Recommendations for Exercise or Pharmacological Preop Stress Testing		
Class I		Patients with active cardiac conditions (Unstable Angina, MI within 30 days, decompensated HF, significant arrhythmias, severe valvular disease) should be evaluated and treated per respective guidelines prior to the noncardiac surgery
Class II	IIa	In patients with 3 or more clinical risk factors and poor functional capacity (<4 METs)undergoing vascular surgery -if it will change management
	IIb	Patients with at least 1-2 clinical risk factors and poor functional capacity (<4 METs)undergoing intermediate-risk or vascular surgery - if it will change management
Class III		Not indicated for patients with no clinical risk factors undergoing intermediate-risk noncardiac surgery or for patients undergoing low-risk surgery

Recommendations for Preoperative Coronary Revascularization		
Class I		- Patients with stable angina who have significant left main coronary artery stenosis or 3-vessel disease or 2-vessel disease with significant proximal LAD stenosis and either EF< 50% or demonstrable ischemia on noninvasive testing - Patients with high-risk UA or NSTEMI, or with acute STEMI
Class II	IIa	1. In patients in whom PCI is appropriate for mitigation of cardiac symptoms and who need elective noncardiac surgery in the subsequent 12 months, a strategy of balloon angioplasty or bare-metal stent placement followed by 4 to 6 weeks of dual-antiplatelet therapy is probably indicated 2. In patients who have received a drug eluting stent and who must undergo urgent surgery that mandates the discontinuation of Plavix, it is reasonable to continue Asa if possible and restart the Plavix as soon as possible
	IIb	The usefulness of preoperative coronary revascularization is not well established in high-risk ischemic patients or for low-risk ischemic patients with an abnormal dobutamine stress echo
Class III		1. Routine prophylactic coronary revascularization is not recommended in patients with stable CAD before noncardiac surgery 2. Elective noncardiac surgery is not recommended within 4-6 weeks of bare metal stent implantation or within 1 year of DES if the Asa + Plavix will have to be discontinued perioperatively 3. Elective noncardiac surgery is not recommended within 4 weeks of balloon angioplasty

Recommendations for Perioperative Medical Therapy		
Class I		1. Beta blockers* - should be continued in patients taking this medication for treatment of conditions with ACC/AHA Class I guideline indications for the drugs 2. Statin: - should be continued for patients currently taking statin and scheduled for noncardiac surgery
Class II	IIa	Beta blockers titrated to HR and BP: - patients undergoing vascular surgery who are at high cardiac risk from CAD or the presence of >1 clinical risk factor, or the finding of cardiac ischemia on preop testing - patients with CAD or > 1 clinical risk factor undergoing intermediate-risk surgery Statin: - for patients undergoing vascular surgery statin use is reasonable
	IIb	Beta blockers: Their usefulness is uncertain for: - patients undergoing intermediate-risk procedure or vascular surgery with a single clinical risk factor in the absence of CAD - patients undergoing vascular surgery with no clinical risk factors who are not currently taking beta-blockers Statins - may be considered for patients with at least 1 clinical risk factor who are undergoing intermediate-risk procedures
Class III		Beta blockers: - should not be given to patients undergoing surgery who have absolute contraindication to beta blockade. - routine administration of high-dose beta blockers in the absence of dose titration is not useful and may be harmful to patients not currently in beta blockers undergoing noncardiac surgery

*Beta blockers should ideally be initiated > 1 week prior to the surgery and titrated during the preop and periop to achieve HR 55-65 and BP control, avoiding hypotension and bradycardia.

2.19 5 Board-Style Questions

1) What drug should be avoided in treating cocaine-induced chest pain?
2) A patient is found to have an acute inferior wall MI along with hypotension. Closer inspection of the rhythm strip on the ECG reveals a 2nd-degree heart block, Mobitz Type II. What should be considered immediately for this patient?
3) Patient with a history of "severe" aortic stenosis according to the medical record now presents to the hospital with chest pain. The ECG shows new inverted T waves when compared with the old ones in the chart. What is best next step in this patient's management?
4) During cardiac catheterization the following is noted: Left ventricular end-diastolic pressure = 10 mmHg, and pulmonary artery wedge pressure = 60 mmHg. What is the most likely cause of this finding?
5) Your patient has a history of mitral valve prolapse. She has no murmur, and the most recent echo shows thickened leaflets. She is scheduled to undergo a dental extraction in one month. What should you do for the patient?

3 Endocrinology

The Central Dogma of Endocrinology

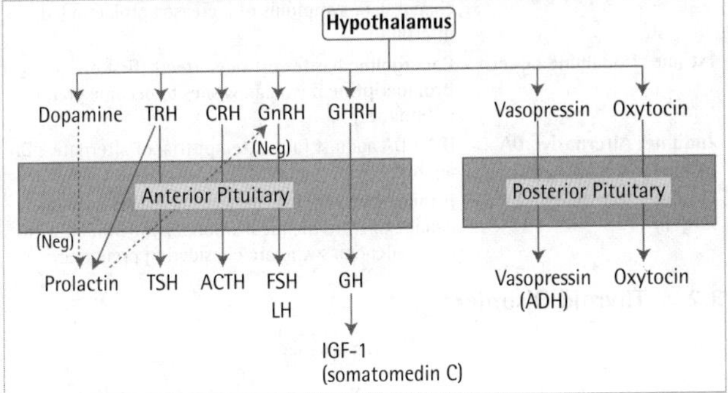

3.1 Pituitary Disorders

3.1.1 Ten causes for hyperprolactinemia

Physiologic	- Pregnancy - Nipple stimulation - Stress
Pathologic	- Prolactinomas - Decreased dopaminergic inhibition of prolactin secretion - Tumors or infiltrative disease of the hypothalamus - Decreased clearance of prolactin - Hypothyroidism - Chronic renal failure - Idiopathic
Drugs	- Most commonly: Haloperidol, phenothiazines, risperidone, olanzapine, clomipramine, cimetidine, metoclopramide, verapamil, morphine, codeine, methyldopa, estrogens

3.1.2 Treatment of prolactinoma

Indications for treatment	- Presence of neurologic deficits (including vision changes), or symptoms of increased prolactin (eg, infertility)
1st line: Dopamine agonist	- **Cabergoline** has fewest side effects (first drug) - **Bromocriptine** if woman wishes to become pregnant (alternative)
2nd line: Alternative DA agonist	- If 1st DA agonist fails, attempt trial of alternative DA agonist
3rd line: Transphenoidal surgery	- If there is no response to dopamine agonist, patient cannot tolerate the medication, or for women with giant adenomas who are considering pregnancy

3.2 Thyroid Disorders

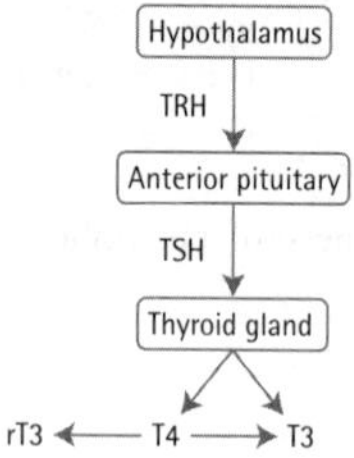

3.2.1 Hyperthyroidism (elevated T3/T4)

TSH level	Condition	Causes
Normal or high	- Secondary hyperthyroidism	- TSH-producing tumor
Low	- Primary hyperthyroidism: Check radioactive iodine (RAI)	- ↑ RAI: Diffuse homogenous = Graves disease - Heterogeneous ↑ RAI = multinodular goiter - Focal ↑ RAI = toxic adenoma - ↓ RAI uptake = subacute thyroiditis, factitious thyrotoxicosis

3.2.2 Thyroid storm - emergency!

Signs	Treatment
- Tachycardia - Congestive heart failure - Hyperpyrexia to 104-106° F - Agitation, delirium, psychosis - Stupor, coma - Severe nausea, vomiting, or diarrhea - Hepatic failure with jaundice	1) Propranolol (beta-blocker; controls symptoms of increased adrenergic tone) 2) Methimazole (thionamide) (blocks new hormone synthesis) or PTU 3) Iodine solution (blocks release of thyroid hormone) 4) Hydrocortisone, glucocorticoids (reduces T4-to-T3 conversion and possibly treats autoimmune processes in Graves disease

3.2.3 Hypothyroidism (low T3, T4)

TSH	Condition	Causes
High	- Primary hypothyroidism	- Hashimoto's thyroiditis - Neck radiation - Post-RAI or post-surgery - Iodine deficiency - Subacute thyroiditis - Lymphocytic - Drugs (lithium, amiodarone)
Normal or low	- Secondary hypothyroidism: Check MRI and measure other hormones	- Pituitary lesion - Hypothalamic lesion

3.2.4 Myxedema coma

Myxedema coma is an Emergency! (mortality rate of 30%-40%)	
Signs	**Interventions**
- Altered mental status - Hypothermia - Bradycardia - Hyponatremia - Hypoglycemia - Hypotension - Hypoventilation - Precipitating illness	- Draw serum T4, TSH and cortisol - Give **thyroxine** 200-400 µg (0.2-0.4 mg) IV followed by daily doses of 50-100 µg and **triiodothyronine** 5-20 µg IV followed by 2.5 -10 µg every 8 hours - Stress-dose steroids: Hydrocortisone 100mg IV q 8-12h - Convert to PO dose of thyroxine whenever possible (PO = IV/0.75) - Supportive measures as needed - Mechanical ventilation - Fluids and pressors - Passive rewarming

3.3 Diabetes

3.3.1 Diagnostic criteria

Test	Prediabetes	Diabetes
Hemoglobin A1C	5.7%-6.4%	**≥6.5%**
Fasting Plasma Glucose (FPG)	100–125 mg/dL 5.6–6.9 mmol/L (IFG)	**≥126 mg/dL** **≥7.0 mmol/L**
Oral Glucose Tolerance Test (OGTT)*	140–199 mg/dL 7.8–11.0 mmol/L (IGT)	**≥200 mg/dL** **≥11.1 mmol/L**
Random Plasma Glucose**	-	**≥200 mg/dL** **≥11.1 mmol/L**

IFG = impaired fasting glucose, IGT = impaired glucose tolerance
*OGTT is peformed by measuring plasma glucose levels at 2 hours after ingestion of standard 75 g dose of glucose.
**The diagnosis of diabetes may be made if the blood glucose level exceeds the indicated values In a patient with classic symptoms of hyperglycemia or hyperglycemic crisis.
Adapted from the American Diabetes Association. Standards of Medical Care in Diabetes - 2012. Diabetes Care. 2012 Jan;35 Suppl 1:S11-S63.

3.3.2 Treatment goals

Test	Frequency	Goals/Comments
Hemoglobin A1C	3-6 months	≤7%
Fasting glucose	-	70-130 gm/dL
2 hr postprandial glucose	-	<180 mg/dL
Blood pressure	3 months	<130/80
Lipid panel	Annually	LDL <100 mg/dL (maybe <70) HDL >40 mg/dL in men and >50 in women, TG <150 mg/dL
Eye examination	Annually	Retinal exam
Foot examination with microfilament	Annually	Every visit if peripheral vascular disease or neuropathy is present
Urine for microalbumin	Annually	If microalbuminuria is present, then begin ACE inhibitor or ARB (slows progression to macroalbuminuria)
Medication	**Indication**	
Aspirin	If cardiovascular disease is present	
ACE inhibitor	Pts with HTN, micro or macroalbuminuria or renal insufficiency	
β-blocker	For 2 years post-MI or undergoing major surgery	
Statin	In patients with cardiovascular disease or age >40 and ≥1 cardiovascular risk factor	
Vaccines	**Frequency**	
Influenza vaccine	Annually	
Pneumococcal vaccine	Once - revaccinate if age >64 y and previously immunized when age <65 y, and more than 5 years before	
Management	**Frequency**	
Smoking cessation counseling	Annually	
Education/Nutrition	Annually	
Source: Diabetes Care January 2010. vol. 33 no. Supplement 1 S4-S10.		

3.3.3 Classification of diabetes mellitus

Classification of Diabetes Mellitus (adapted from AACE 2007 and ADA 2011)	
Prediabetes	
• Definition of intermediate group of patients with IFG and/or IGT and/or HbA1c 5.7% - 6.4%, whose glucose levels are too high to be considered normal	
Type 1 Diabetes Mellitus	
• 5%–10% of all diabetics • Absolute deficiency in insulin secretion due to autoimmune, viral, or idiopathic destruction of pancreatic beta-cells	
Type 2 Diabetes Mellitus	
• 90%–95% of all diabetics • Complex metabolic disorder with insulin resistance, progressive decline in pancreatic insulin secretion, excessive hepatic glucose production, hyperglycemia; obesity is common	
Other Specific Types	
• Genetic defects of beta–cell function (MODY) • Genetic defects in insulin action • Endocrinopathies • Other genetic syndromes associated with diabetes (eg, Down syndrome)	• Diseases of the exocrine pancreas • Drug- or chemical-induced • Infections • Uncommon forms of immune-mediated DM
Gestational Diabetes Mellitus	
• Any degree of glucose intolerance with onset or first recognition during pregnancy	

3.3.4 Insulin pharmacokinetics

Insulin Pharmacokinetics (adapted from AACE, 2007)			
Insulin Formulation (Brand)	**Onset**	**Peak**	**Duration**
Rapid-acting			
Insulin aspart (Novolog)	5-15 min	30-90 min	<5 h
Insulin lispro (Humalog)	5-15 min	30-90 min	<5 h
Insulin glulisine (Apidra)	5-15 min	30-90 min	<5 h
Short-acting			
Regular (Humulin R, Novolin R)	30-60 min	2-3 h	5-8 h
Intermediate, basal			
NPH (Humulin N, Novolin N)[1]	2-4 h	4-10 h	10-16 h
Long-acting, basal			
Insulin glargine (Lantus)[2,3]	2-4 h	No peak	20-24 h
Insulin detemir (Levemir)[2,3]	3-8 h	No peak	5.7-23.2 h
Premixed insulins			
Lispro 75% protamine susp/25% inj (Humalog Mix 75/25)	5-15 min	Dual	10-16 h
Lispro 50% protamine susp/50% inj (Humalog Mix 50/50)	5-15 min	Dual	10-16 h
Aspart 70% protamine susp/30% inj (Novolog Mix 70/30)	5-15 min	Dual	10-16 h
70% NPH / 30% regular (Humulin 70/30, Novolin 70/30)	30-60 min	Dual	10-16 h

[1]NPH = neutral protamine Hagerdon (insulin isophane suspension)
[2]May require 2 daily injections in patients with T1DM
[3]Assumes 0.1-0.2 U/kg per injection. Onset and duration may vary significantly by injection site.

3.3.5 Oral antidiabetic drugs

Sulfonylureas – 1st Generation	
Tolazamide	**Use of these agents is not recommended unless the patient has established a history of taking them (NDEP) AE:** hypoglycemia, nausea, allergic skin reactions **CI:** T1DM, ketoacidosis, renal insufficiency, coma, severe infection, severe thyroid or liver disease, trauma or surgery; DKA or IDDM as sole therapy
ini 100–250 mg PO, maint 250–500 mg PO qd, max 1g/d; doses >500 mg/d: div bid	
Tolbutamide	
ini 1 g PO qd, maint 250 mg – 2 g PO qd, max 3 g/d	

Sulfonylureas - 2nd Generation	
Glimepiride	**AE**: hypoglycemia, nausea, GI distress, skin reactions, weight gain, drug interactions **CI**: as above; caution in renal/hepatic dysfunction or elderly
ini 1-2 mg PO qd, maint 1-4 mg PO qd, max 8 mg/d	
Glipizide	
ini 5 mg PO qd, maint 10-15 mg/d, max 40 mg/d; if >15 mg, div bid; XL: ini 5mg PO qd, maint 5-10 mg PO qd, max 20 mg/d	
Meglitinides	
Repaglinide	**AE:** hypoglycemia **CI:** DKA, T1DM, hypersensitivity
0.5-4 mg PO tid within 30 min before a meal; max 16 mg/d	
Alpha-Glucosidase Inhibitors	
Acarbose	**AE: (acarbose, miglitol)**: diarrhea, abdominal pain, flatulence; **CI: (acarbose)**: hypersensitivity to acarbose, DKA, inflammatory bowel diseases, colonic ulceration, partial obstruction **CI: (miglitol)**: DKA, chron. intestinal diseases characterized by marked digestive or absorptive DO, hypersensitivity to miglitol, inflammatory bowel disease or other conditions which may deteriorate with gas formation ↑, intestinal obstruction
ini 25 mg PO tid, ↑ to 50 mg PO tid, max 300 mg/d	
Miglitol	
ini 25 mg PO tid, ↑ to 50 mg PO tid after 4-8 wks, max 300 mg/d	
Biguanides	
Metformin	**AE:** lactic acidosis, N/V/D, flatulence, anorexia, complete blood count changes **CI:** T1DM, renal/hepatic/respiratory/cardiac insufficiency, Cr >136 µmol/L in men/>124 umol/L in women, CHF, severe infections, hypersens. to metformin, metabolic acid., concomit. use of iodinated contrast media, DKA, alcohol abuse
Ini 500 mg PO qd-bid or 850mg PO qd, ↑ by 500 mg q wk or 850 mg q 2 wks, max 2550mg/d extended release: ini 500mg PO qd, ↑ by 500mg/d qwk, max 2000 mg/d	

Thiazolidinediones	
Pioglitazone	**AE**: edema, weight gain, anemia. Comb. with metformin: anemia, hypo- and hyperglycemia, headache, diarrhea, abdominal pain, nausea, tiredness, edema; Comb. with sulfonylureas: anemia, thrombopenia, hypo- and hyperglycemia, weight gain, edema **CI**: acute heart failure, hepatic impairment, hypersensitivity to product ingredients
Monotherapy or in combination with sulfonylureas, metformin, or insulin: ini 15–30 mg PO qd, max 45 mg/d	
Rosiglitazone	
Monotherapy or in combination with metformin or sulfonylureas: ini 4 mg PO qd or 2 mg bid, ↑ after 8–12 wks to max 8 mg/d	
Dipeptidylpeptidase-4-Inhibitors (DPP-4)	
Sitagliptin	**AE**: (**sitagliptin**): HA, nasopharyngitis, upper respiratory tract infections, hypoglycemia, diarrhea, abdominal pain, nausea; **CI**: none; **AE**: (**saxagliptin**): upper respiratory tract infection, UTI, headache, peripheral edema, hypoglycemia, urticaria, facial edema **CI**: none
Monotherapy or in combination with metformin or thiazolidinediones: 100 mg PO qd	
Saxagliptin	
Monotherapy or in combination with metformin, sulfonylureas, or thiazolidinediones: 2.5 or 5 mg PO qd	
Amylin, Incretin Mimetics	
Exenatide	**AE: (pramlintide)**: N/V, headache, hypoglycemia, anorexia, fatigue, dizziness, pharyngitis, arthralgia, cough, injection site reaction; **CI: (exenatide)**: hypersensitivity to exenatide **CI: (pramlintide)**: hypersensitivity to pramlintide, confirmed gastroparesis, hypoglycemia, confusion
T2DM on metformin or sulfonylurea: 5 µg SQ bid 60 min before meals, ↑ prn after 1 mo to 10 µg bid	
Pramlintide	
T1DM: ini 15 µg SQ just before major meals, ↑ by 15 µg q3d to 30–60 µg, reduce rapid or short-acting insulin dose 50% **T2DM:** ini 60 µg SQ just before major meals, ↑ to 120 µg in 3–7 d if nausea tolerable; reduce rapid- or short-acting insulin dose 50%; after 1 mo to 10 µg bid	

Combinations	
Metformin + Glyburide	**AE: (met+gly)**: hypoglycemia, lactic acidosis (rare), GI adverse events; **AE: (met+rosi)**: diarrhea, anemia, upper resp. tract infections, headache, fatigue; **AE: (rosi+glim)**: headache, dizziness, heart failure, edema, changes in vision, sinusitis, N/V, diarrhea, abdominal pain, liver toxicity, hypoglycemia, upper respiratory infection, allergic skin reactions, UTI; **AE: (pio+glim)**: headache, dizziness, changes in vision, heart failure, edema, N/V, diarrhea, abdominal pain, UTI, liver toxicity, weight gain, hypoglycemia, upper respiratory infection **CI: (met+gly)**: renal disease, congestive heart fail., hypersens. to metformin or glyburide, acute/chronic metabolic acidosis, DKA **CI: (met+rosi)**: renal disease, congest. heart fail., acute/chronic metab. acidosis **CI: (rosi+glim)**: hypersens. to rosiglitazone, glimepiride, diabetic ketoacidosis, CHF (NYHA 3-4) active hepatic dysfunction, T1DM, metabolic acidosis, pregnancy, breastfeeding **CI: (pio+glim)**: hypersensitivity to pioglitazone or glimepiride, hepatic dysfunction, acute or chronic metabolic acidosis, diabetic ketoacidosis, T1DM
Ini 250+1.25mg PO qd or bid, ↑ prn by 250+1.25mg to max 2000+20mg	
Metformin + Pioglitazone	
500–850+15mg PO qd-bid, max 2550+45mg/d	
Metformin + Rosiglitazone	
Ini 500+1–2mg PO bid, max 2000+8mg/d	
Metformin + Glipizide	
Ini 250+2.5mg PO qd-bid, ↑ prn to max 2000+10mg	
Metformin + Sitagliptin	
500–1000+50mg PO qd-bid, max 2000+100mg/d	
Rosiglitazone + Glimepiride	
Ini 4 +1 mg or 4 + 2 mg PO qd, max 8 mg + 4 mg/d	
Pioglitazone + Glimepiride	
30+2–4mg PO qd	

3.3.6 Contraindications to metformin use

Metformin increases the risk of lactic acidosis and is contraindicated in the following conditions:

- Reduced creatinine clearance (creatinine >1.5 mg/dL men, >1.4mg/dL women)
- CHF exacerbation
- Acute illness (sepsis, shock)
- Impaired liver function
- EtOH abuse
- Acute or chronic metabolic acidosis with or without coma (including DKA)
- Any surgical procedure until renal function is verified
- Temporarily discontinue in patients undergoing radiologic studies with iodinated IV contrast

3.3.7 Metformin toxicity

Effect	Essential lab tests	Intervention
- Lactic acidosis	- ABG to determine acid-base status - BUN & creatinine to determine renal function - Serum lactate level to confirm lactic acidosis - Fingerstick glucose	- ABCs: mechanical ventilation is rarely necessary - Activated charcoal for acute ingestions - Supportive care including IVF - Hemodialysis for critically ill patients with severe metabolic acidosis (pH < 7.1) who fail to improve with supportive care or have renal insufficiency

3.3.8 Treatment of type 2 diabetes melitus

Management of Type 2 Diabetes Melitus (adapted from ADA 2012)

Healthy lifestyle: Health eating, weight control, increased physical activity

+

Initial drug monotherapy with METFORMIN

If need to reach individualized HbA1c target after 3 months, proceed to two-drug combination

⇓

2-Drug Combination: METFORMIN plus 1 of the following:

Side effects	Second antidiabetic				
	SU	TZD	DPP-4i	GLP-1ra	Insulin
Efficacy	+++	+++	++	+++	++++
Hypoglycemia risk	++	+	+	+	+++
Weight	+	+	+/-	-	+
Major side effects	hypo-glycemia	edema, HF, Fx's	rare	GI	hypo-glycemia
Cost	+	+++	+++	+++	variable

If need to reach individualized HbA1c target after 3 months, proceed to three-drug combination

⇓

3-Drug Combination: METFORMIN plus 2 of the following:

SU	TZD	DPP-4i	GLP-1ra	Insulin
+	+	+	+	+
TZD	SU	SU	SU	TZD
or DPP-4i	or DPP-4i	or TZD	or TZD	or DPP-4i
or GLP-1ra	or GLP-1ra	or Insulin	or Insulin	or GLP-1ra
or Insulin	or Insulin			

If combination therapy that includes basal insulin has failed to achieve HbA1c target after 3-6 months, proceed to a more complex insulin strategy, usually in combination with one or two non-insulin agents

⇓

INSULIN (multiple daily doses)

SU=sulfonylureas, TZD=thiazolidinediones, DPP-4i=dipeptidylpeptidase-4-Inhibitors, GLP-1ra=glucagon-like peptide-1 receptor agonist (incretin mimetic)
HF=heart failure, FX's=bone fractures, GI=gastrointestinal
Adapted from Inzucchi SE, et al. Management of Hyperglycemia in Type 2 Diabetes: A Patient-Centered Approach. Diabetes Care. 2012 Jun;35(6):1364-79. Epub 2012 Apr 19.

Insulin Strategies in Type 2 Diabetes (adapted from ADA 2012)

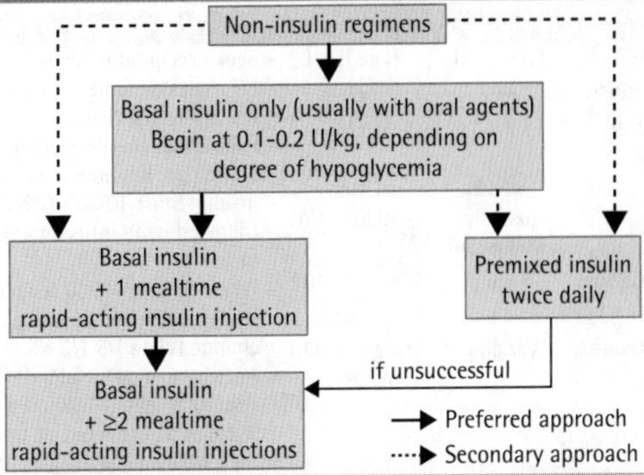

Additional Notes

- Basal insulin alone (0.1-0.2 U/kg), depending on the degree of hyperglycemia, is usually the optimal initial regimen; usually given with 1-2 noninsulin agents.
- In patients with higher HbA1c levels (≥9.0%) who are willing to take more than one injection, consider twice-daily premixed insulin or a more advanced basal plus mealtime insulin regimen (dashed arrow lines).
- When basal insulin has been titrated to an acceptable fasting glucose, but HbA1c remains above target, consider basal plus mealtime insulin, consisting of 1-3 injections of rapid-acting analogs.
- Consider progressing from basal to a twice-daily premixed insulin (dashed arrow line); if this is unsuccessful, move to basal plus mealtime insulin.
- Once a strategy is initiated, titration of the insulin dose is important, with dose adjustments made based on the prevailing glucose levels as reported by the patient. Noninsulin agents may be continued, although insulin secretagogues (sulfonylureas, meglitinides) are typically stopped once more complex regimens beyond basal insulin are utilized.
- Comprehensive education regarding self-monitoring of blood glucose, diet, exercise, and the avoidance of, and response to, hypoglycemia are critical in any patient on insulin therapy.

Adapted from Diabetes Care. 2012 Jun;35(6):1364-79. Epub 2012 Apr 19.

3.3.9 Treatment of DKA and NKH*

	DKA	NKH	Treatment
Cause	Type I > II	Type II > I	- Seek precipitating cause - IVF: Assess volume deficit and give 1L NS within the first hour - Follow labs closely every hr: Glucose, anion gap, K+, phos, pH, bicarbonate - Insulin: Start 10 unit IV bolus followed by IV infusion at 0.1 IU/kg/hr - When glucose < 250 reduce (not stop) insulin to 0.05 IU/kg/hr and change IVF to D5 1/2 NS - Anticipate a potassium deficit by adding at least 10-20 mEq of KCl to IV fluids at the onset of treatment, then follow closely. - Indications for bicarbonate: pH < 7.0 or severe hyperkalemia
Met. acidosis	+++	+/-	
Anion Gap >10	++	+/-	
Plasma Glucose	>250 (usually < 800 mg/dL)	Often > 1000 mg/dL	
Avg. fluid loss	3 - 6 L	Up to 8 - 10 L	
Ketones	++	Trace	
Serum Osm	Variable	Usually > 320 mOsm/kg	
Stupor/coma	+/-	Common	- Potentially fatal complications: Volume overload, hypoglycemia, cerebral edema from rapid correction of Na, hypo/hyperkalemia, hypophosphatemia, arterial thrombosis/CVA - Your attending will appreciate a flow sheet tracking all labs and interventions
Mortality	< 5%	15 %	
Best test to follow	Anion gap	Fluid deficit	

*DKA = Diabetic ketoacidosis; NKH = Non-ketotic hyperglycemia

3.4 Adrenal Disorders

3.4.1 Adrenal crisis

<table>
<tr><th>When to suspect adrenal crisis</th><th>Treatment</th></tr>
<tr><td>- Any patient with peripheral vascular collapse
- Unexplained severe hypoglycemia
- Recent withdrawal of steroids
- Hyperpigmentation
- Hyperkalemia with hyponatremia and volume depletion, eosinophilia</td><td rowspan="3">When suspicion is high, therapy should not be delayed for diagnostic tests. Adrenal crisis is a life-threatening emergency!

Emergent therapy:
- Fluid resuscitation with D5NS (0.9% saline with 5% dextrose)
- Dexamethasone 10mg IV (Dexamethasone does not interfere with a corticotrophin stimulation test, which should be performed concurrently to establish the diagnosis)
- Change to Hydrocortisone 50-100mg IV q 6-8h after stimulation test is done

Maintenance Therapy (after 1-3 days of IV therapy):
- Hydrocortisone 10 mg PO every morning and 5 mg every evening
- Fludrocortisone 0.1 mg PO daily, for mineralocorticoid replacement, along with liberal salt intake

Discharge Considerations:
- Medical alert bracelet/necklace
- Prefilled dexamethasone syringes that can be administered by the patient in case of crisis</td></tr>
<tr><th>Labs</th></tr>
<tr><td>1. Check basal ACTH, cortisol level:
-Low cortisol <10 µg/dL with high ACTH confirms primary adrenal insufficiency
2. Perform corticotrophin (Cosyntropin, Cortrosyn) stimulation test: Cosyntropin 250 µg, given IV, and plasma cortisol is measured 30 and 60 minutes later:
-Normal response (plasma cortisol > 18.5 µg/dL) rules out adrenal insufficiency, unless serum albumin is <2.5 mg/dL</td></tr>
</table>

3.4.2 Adrenal incidentaloma

Initial Work-Up	Indications for Surgical Resection
1) Measure blood pressure 2) Serum K^+ 3) 1 mg overnight dexamethasone suppression test and check 8 am serum cortisol 4) 24-hr urine for catecholamines, VMA, and plasma metanephrines	1) Functioning tumor on lab tests 2) Mass greater than 4 cm 3) Smaller than 4 cm but evidence of growth on repeat CT scan
If all tests are negative consider repeat CT scan in 3 months. Consider FNA if >4 cm or suspicious findings on CT (increased density, irregular borders, dense or vascular appearance)	

3.4.3 Pheochromocytoma

Clinical signs	Workup	Preparation for surgery
Triad: Headache, sweating, tachycardia (low risk)	24-hr urinary metanephrines + catecholamines; if positive, do adrenal CT or MRI	Preoperatively give alpha-adrenergic blockade with **phenoxybenzamine,** followed by **propranolol** to prevent severe elevations in blood pressure. Beta blockade is titrated to control the tachycardia Laparoscopic adrenalectomy can then be performed by an experienced endocrine surgeon
Paroxysmal or poorly controlled hypertension (low pre-test probability)	24-hr urinary metanephrines; if positive, do adrenal CT or MRI	
Adrenal incidentaloma	24-hr urinary fractionated metanephrines and catecholamines. If mass is suspicious for pheochromocytoma, then plasma free metanephrines should also be checked as well as CT or MRI	
Familial syndromes: MEN2, von Hippel-Lindau, or previous pheochromocytoma are at high risk.	Plasma-free metanephrines. If elevated then do CT or MRI and 24-hr urinary metanephrines	

3.4.4 MEN syndrome

Type I (Wermer's syndrome)	Type 2A (Sipple's syndrome)	Type 2B (Type III)
3 Ps: Pituitary adenoma (Prolactinoma most common) Parathyroid hyperplasia or tumor Pancreatoma	- Pheochromocytoma - Medullary thyroid cancer - Parathyroid hyperplasia or tumor	- Pheochromocytoma - Medullary thyroid cancer - Mucocutaneous neuromas, particularly of the GI tract

3.4.5 Systemic steroid equivalency table

Steroid	RGCP	RMCP	EHL	Indications: Dose
cortisone	0.8	0.8	0.5h	**Adults:** Adrenal insufficiency, inflamm. disease: 25-300 mg PO qd or 25-150 mg IM q12-24h **Peds:** Adrenal insufficiency: 0.5-0.75 mg/kg/d PO; Inflamm. disease: 2.5-10 mg/kg/d PO
hydrocortisone	1	2	1-2h	**Adults:** Adrenal insufficiency: 5-30 mg PO bid-qid; Inflamm. disease: 10-320 mg/d PO div tid-qid or 100-500 mg IV/IM q12h **Peds:** Adrenal insufficiency: 0.5-0.75 mg/kg/d PO div tid; Inflamm. disease: 2.5-10 mg/kg/d PO div tid-qid
prednisolone	4	1	2.6-3h	**Adults:** Inflamm. disease: 5-60 mg PO/IV/IM qd **Peds:** Inflamm. disease: 0.1-2 mg/kg/d PO/IV div qd-qid

Steroid	RGCP	RMCP	EHL	Indications: Dose
methyl-prednisolone	5	0	2-3h	**Adults:** Inflamm. disease: 10-250 mg IV/ IM q4h; 4-48 mg PO qd; 4-80 mg intraarticular (methylprednisolone acetate), may be repeated after 1-5 wks; Spinal cord injury: init 30 mg/ kg IV over 15 min, then 5.4 mg/kg/h IV for 23h; Lupus nephritis: 1g IV qd for 3d **Peds:** Inflamm. disease: 0.5-1.7 mg/kg/d PO/IV/IM div q6-12h; Spinal cord injury: see adults
triamcinolone	5	0	n/a	Inflamm. disease: 4-48 mg/d PO div qd-qid; 2.5-15 mg, max 40 mg intraarticular (triamcinolone acetonide)
fludrocortisone	10	125	3.5h	Adrenal insufficiency: 0.1-0.2 mg POqd; Salt-losing adrenogenital syndrome: 0.1- 0.2 mg PO qd
dexamethasone	30	0	3.3h	**Adults:** Inflamm. disease: 0.75-9 mg/d PO/ IM/IV div bid-qid; Cerebral edema: init 10mg IV, then 4 mg IM q6h or 2 mg PO bid-tid **Peds:** Inflamm. disease: 0.08-0.3 mg/kg/d PO/IM/IV div bid-qid; Cerebral edema: init 1.5 mg/kg IV, then 1.5 mg/kg/d IV div q4-6h; fetal lung maturation, maternal antepartum: 6 mg IM q12h x 4 doses

RGCP = relative glucocorticoid potency; RMCP = relative mineralocorticoid potency;
EHL = estimated half-life

3.5 5 Board-Style Questions

1) A patient is found to have both primary adrenal insufficiency and hypothyroidism. Which one should be treated first?

2) A 25-year-old woman presents to the ED with severe dizziness, weakness, nausea, and vomiting for 1 week. Blood pressure is 88/62 supine and 80/50 standing. The skin is well tanned, and there is markedly increased pigmentation of the gums and palmar creases.
   Labs: Hb 13%, Cr 1.2, BUN 340, Na 124, K 6.8, Glucose 61.
   What is the most likely underlying cause of this patient's condition?
   a) Pituitary apoplexy
   b) Acute adrenal hemorrhage
   c) Fulminant meningococcemia
   d) Autoimmune adrenalitis
   e) Tuberculosis

3) What hormone is responsible for hypercalcemia, often associated with sarcoid?

4) What is the best drug for treating thyrotoxicosis during pregnancy?

5) An 18-year-old man is found to have low LH, and FSH levels. He is also found to have hypogonadism and anosmia. What condition does this patient likely have, and how might it be treated?

4 Gastroenterology

4.1 GI Bleeds

4.1.1 Causes of GI bleeds

Upper GI bleeds	
Ulcers	Peptic ulcer disease (PUD)/acid-related disease (55% of cases): Gastric or duodenal ulcer disease, Zollinger-Ellison syndrome, gastroesophageal reflux disease (GERD); stress ulcers
Infectious	Helicobacter pylori, cytomegalovirus, herpes simplex virus
Drug-induced	Erosions, ulcers, or bleeding caused by aspirin, other NSAIDS, or pill-induced (tetracycline, quinidine, potassium chloride tablets), anticoagulation therapy
Trauma	Mallory-Weiss tear, foreign body ingestion.
Vascular lesions	Varices, angiomas, telangiectasia and ectasia, vascular malformation, Dieulafoy's lesion
Tumors - benign	Lipoma, leiomyoma
Tumors - malignant	Adenocarcinoma, metastatic tumor, lymphoma, Kaposi's sarcoma, carcinoid, melanoma
Miscellaneous	Hemobilia, hemosuccus pancreaticus (in pancreatitis pts), unknown cause
Lower GI bleeds	
Diverticular	Colonic diverticulosis (42% of cases)
Infectious	Pseudomembranous colitis (C. difficile), CMV colitis (HIV and immunosuppressed pts), other acute infectious colitis (bacterial)
Inflammatory	Ischemic bowel, inflammatory bowel disease (Crohn's disease, ulcerative colitis)
Vascular	Hemorrhoids, colonic angiodysplasia, arteriovenous malformation, radiation, post-polypectomy hemorrhage
Neoplastic	Benign polyps, colorectal adenocarcinoma, other malignancy

4.1.2 Steps to diagnosing suspected GI bleeds

Upper GI bleed
1. Check ABCs (Airway, Breathing, Circulation) 2. Vitals, physical exam with rectal 3. Gastric lavage 4. Begin intravenous proton pump inhibitor 5. Esophagogastroduodenoscopy (EGD) - May be diagnostic and therapeutic 6. If all studies are negative, then consider arteriography (interventional radiology) or surgery
Lower GI bleed
1. Check ABCs (Airway, Breathing, Circulation) 2. Vitals, physical exam with rectal 3. If patient has orthostatic hypotension* or maroon stools, consider gastric lavage and EGD 4. Colonoscopy - Urgent may be done unprepped; prepped is done 12 hrs post-bowel cleansing 5. Bleeding scan (diagnostic) or arteriogram (diagnostic and may be therapeutic) 6. Consider surgery
Occult GI bleed
1. Suspect occult bleed if stool is guaiac+ and patient has iron deficiency anemia 2. Perform EGD 3. Colonoscopy 4. Capsule endoscopy, therapeutic enteroscopy 5. If all studies are negative then begin iron replacement and observe closely
*Orthostatic hypotension: Drop in systolic BP >20 mm Hg or drop in diastolic BP >10 mm Hg, or rise in pulse rate of >15 beats/min when patient sits or stands suggests 10%-20% loss of circulatory volume. Clinical diagnosis may be made if patient feels dizzy when sitting or standing.

4.1.3 Approach to a patient with a GI bleed

Test	Findings	Next intervention
Check vitals	- Tachycardia, hypotension suggest >20% loss of circulatory volume	- Emergent IV fluids - Packed RBC transfusion - O-negative blood is universal donor
Orthostatic BP	- Drop in systolic BP >20 mm Hg, or drop in diastolic BP > 10 mmHg, or rise in pulse rate of >15 beats/min when patient sits or stands suggests 10%-20% loss of circulatory volume	- Emergent IV fluids - Packed RBC transfusion
Correct coagulopathy	- Review patient's recent use of anticoagulants and current PT/INR/PTT	- 2-4 units of FFP will reverse most coagulopathies as long as no inhibitor is present - Vitamin K 10mg SQ or IV effective for vitamin deficiency or warfarin therapy - Platelet transfusion if < 50,000/mm^3 - protamine rapidly reverses heparin
Ventilation	- Monitor for altered mental status, respiratory distress, or hematemesis	- Consider intubation for airway protection
Gastric lavage	- Presence of coffee grounds identifies upper GI bleeds	- Prepare patient for EGD
Rectal exam	- Digital rectal exam to verify presence of blood/occult bleeding; check for anal fissures, hemorrhoids	- Prepare patient for colonoscopy – should be performed on all patients with acute lower GI bleed from an unknown source

Test	Findings	Next intervention
Technetium-99m tagged RBC scanning	- Can identify GI bleeding rates as low as 0.1 mL/min. Is specific but only ~45% sensitive (when positive it accurately identifies the source of bleeding)	- Prepare patient for arteriography, or surgery
Arteriography	- May identify and permit embolization of source of bleeding if bleeding rate >0.5 mL/min. May localize angiodysplasia, bleeding diverticula, or tumor	- If embolectomy was not effective then prepare patient for surgery

4.1.4 Variceal hemorrhage

Octreotide infusion	50-100 µg bolus followed by infusion at 25-50 µg/hr
Vasopressin (alternative)	0.3 units/min IV, then increase by 0.3 units/min IV every 30 min until bleeding stops or maximum dose of 0.9 units/min is reached
Endoscopy	Possible variceal banding or ligation, sclerotherapy
TIPS	Transjugular intrahepatic portosystemic shunt

4.2 Liver Dysfunction

4.2.1 Approach to abnormal liver function tests

Causes	Tests
Search for common causes first - Medications - EtOH - Hepatitis B and C - Hemochromatosis screening - Evaluate for NAFLD (non-alcoholic fatty liver disease)	- Prescription, herbal, illicit drugs - AST/ALT >2:1 - HBsAg, HBsAb, HBcAb, HCV Ab - Caucasian pts: transferrin saturation (iron/TIBC), if >45%, check ferritin. If iron overload is present do genetic testing and liver biopsy - AST/ALT <1, obtain liver ultrasound
Exclude nonhepatic sources - Hypothyroidism - Celiac disease - Adrenal insufficiency	- TSH - History of diarrhea, iron deficiency - Serum tTG antibodies (tissue transglutaminase) and IgA - History of hyperpigmentation, ↓Na^+ ↑K^+
Less common hepatic causes - Wilson's disease - Alpha-1-antitrypsin deficiency - Autoimmune liver disease	- Serum ceruloplasmin, urinary copper - Alpha-1-antitrypsin level - SPEP for diffusely elevated IgG, ANA, and anti-smooth muscle antibodies
Consider liver biopsy	- If ALT and AST are persistently abnormal and cause remains obscure for 6 months

Pratt DS, Kaplan MM. Evaluation of abnormal liver-enzyme results in asymptomatic patients. *New England Journal of Medicine.* 2000;342(17):1266-1271.

4.2.2 Common drug causes of abnormal liver function tests

1. Tylenol	5. Augmentin	9. Amiodarone
2. NSAIDS	6. Tetracycline	10. Quinidine
3. Oral contraceptive pills	7. Sulfa drugs	11. Methotrexate
4. Erythromycin	8. Statins	12. Phenytoin

4.2.3 Discriminant function - steroid administration in alcoholic hepatitis

Discriminant Function (DF) = 4.6 x (PT - control PT) + serum bilirubin	
DF <32	DF ≥32
Do not administer steroids	High short-term mortality, administer steroids: Prednisone 40mg PO qdaily x 1 month

4.2.4 Modified MELD Score

Purpose	The Model End-Stage Liver Disease score is used for liver transplant candidate stratification and allocation of organs for liver transplantation. Predicts mortality associated with alcoholic hepatitis, hepatorenal syndrome, surgical procedures in chronic liver diseases, and TIPS.		
Formula	**MELD[1] = 10 x [0.957 x ln (SeCr) + 0.378 x ln (Bili) + 1.12 x ln (INR) + 0.643 x Cause_Factor]** Where: SeCr=Serum Creatinine, Bili=Serum Total Bilirubin, INR=International Normalized Ratio, Cause_Factor=0 if cirrhosis is caused by alcohol or cholestasis, and 1 if caused by something else (carcinoma, etc.); ln is the natural log ($\log_e$).		
Interpretation	Minimum score is 6, maxium score is 40. Hepatocellular carcinoma is assigned a minimum MELD score of 24.		
	MELD Score Prognostic Values[2]		
	Score	**% of Pts Hospitalized**	**3-Month Mortality**
	<= 9	4%	2%
	10-19	27%	5.6%
	20-29	76%	50%
	30-39	83%	N/A
	>=40	100%	N/A
Other considerations for liver transplant	Blood type, number of other patients for transplant in the local area and their MELD scores, number of livers available in the local area.		

1. Chalasani N, Kahi C, et al. Letter to the Editor: Model for End-Stage Liver Disease (MELD) for predicting mortality in patients with acute variceal bleeding. *Hepatology.* 2002; 35: 1282-1284.
2. Kamath PS, Wiesner RH, et al. A model to predict survival in patients with end-stage liver disease. *Hepatology.* 2001; 33: 464-470.

4.3 Hepatitis

4.3.1 Viral hepatitis serology

Hepatitis type	Test results					
Hepatitis A (HAV)						
Recent infection	IgM anti-HAV +					
Past infection	IgG anti-HAV +					
Hepatitis B (HBV)						
	DNA	**sAg**	**sAb**	**cAb**	**eAg**	**eAb**
Acute infection	+	+	-	IgM	+	-
Vertical transmission	+	+	-	IgG	+	-
Chronic acquired after childhood	+	-	-	IgG	+	-
Chronic inactive carrier	+/-	-	-	IgG	-	+
Resolved infection	-	+	+	IgG	-	+
Vaccinated	-	-	+	-	-	-
Hepatitis C (HCV)						
Acute infection	HCV RNA+, anti-HCV Ab+ in 8-10 weeks (tests may be negative)					
Past infection	anti-HCV Ab+, HCV RNA-					
Chronic infection	anti-HCV Ab+, HCV RNA+					
Hepatitis D (HDV)						
Acute (+HBV)	IgM anti-HDV+, HDV Ag+					
Chronic (+HBV)	IgG anti-HDV+					
Hepatitis E (HEV)						
	- No tests available - Suspected in patients who reside or travel to endemic areas (Asia, Africa, Middle East, Central America). - Epidemics, high fatality rate in pregnant women					

4.3.2 Extrahepatic manifestations of hepatitis

Hepatitis B	Hepatitis C
- Polyarthritis nodosa - Glomerulonephritis	- Essential mixed cryoglobulinemia - Monoclonal gammopathies - Lymphoma - Porphyria cutanea tarda - Thyroid disease - Glomerulonephritis - Ocular disease

4.3.3 Treatment of hepatitis B and C

	Hepatitis B	Hepatitis C
Treatment indications	- Abnormal LFTs - (>2x normal) with a high viral load - Evidence of fibrosis on biopsy	- Abnormal LFTs - Active inflammation on biopsy
Regimen	- **Interferon alpha** SQ for 16 weeks **OR** - Oral therapy with **lamivudine**[1], **adefovir**[2], or **telbivudine** for a prolonged period	**Pegylated interferon + ribavirin** - Genotype 1 & 4: Treat for 48 weeks - Genotype 2 & 3: Treat for 24 weeks*

[1] Lamivudine is a synthetic nucleoside analog. Typical dose is 100mg PO qdaily; In lamivudine-resistant patients, entecavir may be appropriate. Entecavir is a deoxyguanine nucleoside analog with a typical dose of 0.5 mg PO qday; in lamivudine-resistant chronic HBV use 1mg PO qday (renal dose adjustment is required for GFR < 50ml/min)

[2] Adefovir dipivoxil is a synthetic nucleotide analog; typical dose is 10mg PO qday (renal dose adjustment required for GFR < 50 ml/min)

*Source: Ghany MG, Strader DB, Thomas DL, Leonard B. Seeff LB. AASLD PRACTICE GUIDELINES - April 2009 Diagnosis, Management, and Treatment of Hepatitis C: An Update. Hepatology. 2009;49(4):1335-1374.

4.4 Jaundice

4.4.1 Differential diagnoses of jaundice

Lab abnormality	Etiology	Common cause	Additional tests
None	Pseudojaundice	- Eating carrots/beets	- Dietary history
↑ indirect bilirubin	↑ production	- Hemolysis - Transfusion - Hematoma resorption - Dyserythropoiesis	- Blood smear for schistocytes - Haptoglobin - Coombs test - CT abdomen and pelvis for hematoma
	↓ bilirubin uptake	- Congestive heart failure - Drugs (rifampin)	- ANP, echo - History
	↓ conjugation	- Gilbert's syndrome - Crigler-Najjar type I + II - Hyperthyroidism - Chronic hepatitis - Wilson's disease - Cirrhosis	- Hepatitis serology - Serum ceruloplasmin, slit lamp examination
↑ direct bilirubin	Hepatocellular injury	- Drug - Hypotension - Hypoxemia - Acute hepatitis - Wilson's disease - Budd-Chiari	- Doppler US for perfusion - Hepatitis serologies - Liver biopsy

↑ direct bilirubin	Intrahepatic cholestasis	- Alcoholic hepatitis - NASH - Primary biliary cirrhosis - Drugs - Sepsis (hypoperfusion) - Infiltrative disease: amyloid, lymphoma, TB - Pregnancy - Viral hepatitis	- History - Antimitochondrial antibodies - Ultrasound - +/- ERCP
	Extrahepatic cholestatis	- Choledocolithiasis - Tumors - Primary sclerosing cholangitis - AIDS cholangiopathy - Pancreatitis - Parasites: ascaris, flukes	- Ultrasound - Cholangiography
Note: Jaundice may occur when serum bilirubin levels > 2mg/dl.			
Source: Reisman Y, Gips CH, Lavelle SM, Wilson JH. Clinical presentation of (subclinical) jaundice - the Euricterus project in the Netherlands. United Dutch Hospitals and Euricterus Project Management Group. Hepatogastroenterology. 1996;43:1190.			

4.4.2 Congenital causes of jaundice

	Findings	Treatment
Gilbert's syndrome	- Common disorder (7% of the population) - Male predominance, autosomal recessive - Decreased amount of UDP-glucuronyl trasferase activity, slowed hepatic bilirubin uptake, and mild hemolysis. - Usually detected in teens or twenties - Asymptomatic except during starvation or stress - Bilirubin level is usually less than 3mg/dl - Normal AST/ALT, Alk Phos - Fasting for 24 hours causes elevations in unconjugated bilirubin - Liver biopsy is unnecessary, usually normal	Jaundice improves with rest and healthy diet
Crigler-Najjar syndrome type I and II	- Rare, autosomal recessive disorder - Type I: severe jaundice and neurologic impairment from kernicterus - Type II: patients have less severe bilirubin elevations - Reduced hepatic glucuronosyl transferase activity - Unconjugated bilirubin may rise to <20 mg/dL during fasting or illness	None required, or phenobarbital for patients with type II
Dubin-Johnson syndrome	- Rare except in Sephardic Jews (1:3000) - Mild chronic conjugated hyperbilirubinemia - Defect in organic anion transport in hepatocytes - Icterus only noted during pregnancy, illness, or with oral contraceptive pills - Diagnosed by finding increased conjugated bilirubin with otherwise normal liver function tests	None required
Rotor syndrome	- Rare defect in hepatic storage of conjugated bilirubin, which leaks into the plasma - Similar to Dubin-Johnson, but can be differentiated by urinary coproporphyrin analysis	None required

4.4.3 Common and commonly confused causes of jaundice

Clinical findings	Mechanism of disease	Workup & treatment
Glucose-6-Phosphate Dehydrogenase Deficiency		
- The most common enzymatic disorder of red blood cells in humans, affecting 200 to 400 million people. - X-linked - Characterized by episodic anemia due to hemolysis of older RBCs after exposure to oxidative drugs (including sulfa drugs and the antimalarial drug primaquine), infections, or certain foods (favism).	- Deficient G6PD causes low levels of glutathione in reduced form leading to ↑ RBC oxidative damage (Heinz body deposition). RBCs become rigid and nondeformable, making them susceptible to stagnation and destruction by reticuloendothelial macrophages in the marrow, spleen and liver.	**Workup:** ↓Hct, ↑LDH, ↑ unconjugated bilirubin **Treatment:** Symptoms are usually mild or self-limited. Avoidance of inciting oxidative drugs or foods usually suffices.
Gilbert's Syndrome		
- The most common inherited disorder of bilirubin glucuronidation - Presents in young adults as mild, predominantly unconjugated hyperbilirubinemia with otherwise normal lab tests	- ↓ bilirubin conjugation secondary to underactive hepatic bilirubin UGT enzyme leads to high levels of unconjugated bilirubin.	**Work-up:** Hct and LDH in normal range, ↑ unconjugated bilirubin **Treatment:** No treatment is necessary. Recommend reduced stress and adequate fluid intake.

4.5 Ascites

4.5.1 Paracentesis tubes

Hematology purple top	Cell count, differential
Chemistry red or yellow top	Total protein, albumin, glucose, LDH, amylase, triglyceride, bilirubin
Microbiology 10ml/culture bottle	Gram stain, culture (culture bottles), TB culture and smear (fungal collection tubes)
Pathology	Cytology
Useless	pH, lactate, fibronectin, cholesterol

4.5.2 Analysis of ascites fluid

	SBP	Exudate	Exudate	Transudate
Common Causes	-	Cirrhosis 81%	Heart Fail. 3% Pericarditis Budd-Chiari	Cancer 10% TB 2% Nephrotic 1% Pancreatic 1% Other 2%
Fluid appearance	Turbid or purulent	Straw-colored	Straw-colored	Variable
Cell count	PMN >250/µl, 50-70% of WBC	WBC < 250	WBC < 1000/µl	TB: Lymphocyte 250-4000 Peritoneal carcinomatosis WBC > 1000/µl
SAAG (g/dL)	usually ≥ 1.1	≥ 1.1	≥ 1.1	< 1.1
Total ascitic protein (g/dL)	< 1	< 2.5	≥ 2.5	> 2.5
LDH fluid: serum	> 0.6	< 0.6	< 0.6	> 0.6

- **SAAG (Serum-Ascites Albumin Gradient):** >1.1 g/dL indicates portal hypertension with 97% accuracy[1]
- **SBP (Spontaneous Bacterial peritonitis):** Initial treatment for SBP is **Cefotaxime** 2grams IV q 8hrs. Give IV albumin 1.5 g/kg at diagnosis followed by 1g/kg on day 3.
- **Fluid appearance:** If the ascites fluid is as brown as molasses and the [bilirubin] is greater than serum bilirubin, the patient probably has a ruptured gallbladder or perforated duodenal ulcer.
- **Perforation:** Evaluate for perforation if PMN >250 cells/mm^3 + total protein >1 g/dL, glucose <50, LDH > upper limit of normal for serum; key feature is a polymicrobial gram stain.
- **Bloody tap:** Subtract 1 WBC for every 750 RBC, subtract 1 PMN for every 250 RBC.

[1] Runyon BA, Montano AA, Akriviadis EA et al. The serum-ascites albumin gradient is superior to the exudate-transudate concept in the differential diagnosis of ascites. Annals of Internal Medicine 1992 Aug 1; 117(3):215-20.

4.6 Pancreatitis

4.6.1 Prognostic signs in pancreatitis - Ranson's criteria

On admission	During 48 hours	# of criteria : % mortality
1. Age > 55 years 2. WBC > 16,000 3. Glucose > 200 mg/dL 4. AST > 250 IU/L 5. LDH >350 IU/L	1. PaO_2 < 60 mm Hg 2. Drop in Hct > 10 % 3. BUN increases > 5 mg/dL despite fluids 4. Calcium < 8 mg/dL 5. Fluid sequestration > 6L 6. Base deficit > 4 MEq/L	3: 1% 3-4: 15% 5-6: 40% >7: 90-100%

4.6.2 Atlanta criteria for severe acute pancreatitis

1. >3 Ranson's criteria
2. >8 Apache II points
3. Organ failure
- Shock (systolic BP <90 mmHg) - Pulmonary insufficiency (PaO_2 < 60 mmHg) - Renal failure (Cr > 177 µmol/L after rehydration) - GI bleeding (> 500 mg/24hr) - DIC (platelets <100,000/mm^3, fibrinogen <1.0 g/L, fibrin split products)
4. Serum calcium <1.87 mmol/L
5. Local complications:
- Necrosis, abscess, pseudocyst
Patient has severe acute pancreatitis if any ONE of the above is present. Source: Gan, May, Raboud et al. American Journal of Gastroenterology 1998 (6):1278-83. Whitcomb DC. N Engl J Med 2006;354:2142-50.

4.6.3 CT scan classification

Class	Findings
A	Normal pancreas
B	Focal or diffuse enlargement
C	Gland abnormalities, mild peripancreatic abnormalities, scan haziness
D	Fluid collection in a single location, phlegmon
E	≥ 2 fluid collections or presence of gas in or around pancreas
Source: Balthazar EJ et al. Acute Pancreatitis: Value of CT in establishing diagnosis. Radiology 1990; 174:331	

4.6.4 Clinical presentation

History	RUQ pain radiating to back, NV, fever, h/o alcohol use, surgery, biliary colic, high triglycerides
Physical	Abdominal tenderness, guarding rigidity, ↑ HR, ↑ RR, ↓ BP, mild jaundice, diminished bowel sounds, poss. basilar rales esp. in left lung (inflammation), muscle spasms (↓ Ca), internal hemorrhage in severe cases (Grey-Turner's sign-flank discoloration, Cullen's sign: periumbilical discoloration)
Causes	Major: EtOH, biliary stone disease Minor: Drugs (azathioprine, corticosteroids, sulfonamides, thiazides, furosemides, NSAIDs, mercaptopurine, methyldopa, and tetracyclines); Viruses (mumps, coxsackie virus, CMV, hepatitis virus, EBV, and rubella); mycoplasma; hypertriglyceridemia (>1000mg/U); procedures (surgery, ERCP); PUD; cancer; scorpion and snake bites

4.6.5 Keys to therapy in pancreatitis

Fluids	Aggressive IVF hydration with crystalloids. Patients often require >5 L of fluids.
Nutrition	Bowel rest in initial phase, but, if tolerated, begin PO feeding early. Parenteral nutrition may be necessary if PO intake is not tolerated for prolonged duration.
Medication	• **Pain:** Pain control is essential. Use opioids as necessary. • **Antibiotics:** Use in severe cases with high suspicion of infection, or phlegmon visible on CT. Treat with **imipenem** for 7-10 days.
Procedures	CT-guided aspiration of necrotic tissue and/or ERCP for stone removal may be needed. Consult necessary.
Specialist consults	• GI Consult: if pts not tolerating PO after 3-4 days, or if biliary obstruction is suspected • ICU Consult: severe pancreatitis as defined by Atlanta Criteria. • Surgery/interventional radiology consult: If suspected infection with necrotic pancreatic tissue.
Over 80% of pancreatitis cases respond well to conservative treatment with fluids and pain medication.	

4.7 Biliary Dysfunction

	Primary biliary cirrhosis	Primary sclerosing cholangitis
General	Autoimmune destruction of the small biliary ducts within the liver, often progressing to cirrhosis	Fibrosis and structuring of medium and large intrahepatic and extrahepatic biliary ducts that can lead to end-stage liver disease
Sex	95% female	70% male
Age at onset	30 - 65	40
Symptoms	Fatigue, pruritus, hyperpigmentation, xanthomas	Asymptomatic, fever, fatigue, and pruritus
Lab test	Marked elevation of alk phos, **antimitochondrial antibodies** are the hallmark, hyperlipidemia, ANA	Elevated alk phos, bilirubin, **P-ANCA** (~60%)
Liver biopsy	Confirms the diagnosis. Helps stage the disease.	Rarely diagnostic
Imaging	Not needed	Characteristic **multifocal structuring on cholangiography** ERCP
Prognosis	Normal life expectancy with treatment	Median survival of 12 years from time of diagnosis without liver transplant
Associated diseases	Rheumatoid arthritis, CREST, thyroid dysfunction, Celiac disease	Strong association (80%) with **ulcerative colitis,** increased risk of cholangiocarcinoma (10-15% lifetime), and colon cancer
Treatment	Ursodeoxycholic acid 13-15 mg/kg/day	Ursodeoxycholic acid is not recommended, but controversial.* Consider enrollment in trial. For advanced liver disease consider liver transplantation.

*Source: 2010 American Association for the Study of Liver Diseases (AASLD) Primary Sclerosing Cholangitis. Chapman R, Fevery J, Kalloo A, et al. Hepatology 2010 51(2): 660-678

4.8 Inflammatory Bowel Disease

	Ulcerative colitis	Crohn's disease
Type of involvement	Diffuse, no skip areas	Skip areas
Depth of involvement	Mucosa & submucosa	Transmural
Rectal involvement	95%	50%
Perianal disease	-	+
Fistulas	-	+
Ileal involvement	-	+
Aphthous & linear ulcers	-	+
Cobblestone appearance	-	+
Ulceration	Fine, superficial	Deep with submucosal extension
P-ANCA	70%	Occasional
Anti-saccharomyces Ab	Occasional	> 50%
Risk of colon CA	++	+
Granulomas	-	Non-caseating
Extraintestinal manifestations	Arthritis, iritis, erythema nodosum, pyoderma gangrenosum	
Medical options	**Ulcerative proctitis:** 5-ASA suppositories Consider adding: rectal steroid enemas, steroid foam, 5-ASA enemas **Ulcerative colitis:** Oral 5-ASA and/or rectal 5-ASA enemas or steroid foam For severe disease consider adding enema or IV steroids, or TNF-α inhibitors	**Mild to moderate disease:** Oral 5-ASA or sulfasalazine Consider adding: antibiotics Flagyl +/- Cipro **Severe:** IV steroids, immunosuppressive drugs, TNF-α inhibitors **Fistulas:** TNF-α inhibitors

4.9 Celiac Disease (Gluten-Sensitive Enteropathy)

Prevalence	1% of whites of northern European ancestry, 1:300 in USA.
Definition	Villous atrophy, symptoms of malabsorption such as steatorrhea, weight loss or other nutrient deficiency and resolution of symptoms upon withdrawal of gluten-containing foods.
Age at presentation	Infancy to age 60.
Associated conditions	Dermatitis herpetiformis, diabetes mellitus type I, selective IgA deficiency, Down syndrome, elevated AST/ALT.
Clinical manifestations	Diarrhea with bulky, foul-smelling, floating stools. Malabsorption with weight loss and growth failure in children.
Non-GI complications	Iron deficiency anemia, arthritis, neuropsychiatric disease from deficiency of B vitamins, osteoporosis from calcium and vitamin D deficiency, hyposplenism, kidney disease.
Diagnosis	Endoscopy with biopsy is the gold standard; also consider capsule endoscopy, serology (tissue transglutaminase and IgA levels), and HLA type (can help rule out celiac disease).
Treatment	• Dietary counseling: wheat, rye, and barley should be avoided. • Soy beans, tapioca, rice, corn, buckwheat and potatoes are safe • Vitamin supplementation • Steroids or immunosuppressives may be necessary for refractory disease

4.10 Upper GI dysfunction

4.10.1 Peptic ulcer disease (PUD)

	Chronic gastritis	Gastric ulcers	Duodenal ulcers
Etiology	Type A (fundal): autoimmune Type B (antral): H. pylori, NSAIDS	H. pylori (70%), Malignancy (10%)	H. pylori (90%) Increased acid production
Symptoms	Asymptomatic, pain, nausea/vomiting, anorexia, upper GI bleed	Abdominal pain worse with food intake	Abdominal pain 1-3 hrs postprandial, relieved by food/ antacids
Diagnosis	Upper endoscopy	Endoscopy with biopsy for H. pylori	Endoscopy with biopsy for H. pylori
Acid level	+/-	Low to normal	Increased (in 80%)
Treatment	Treat cause: H. pylori, stop NSAIDS, B12 for pernicious anemia	Treat H. pylori if identified on endoscopy	Treat H. pylori if identified on endoscopy, stop smoking
Treatment for H. pylori: Amoxicillin 1g BID, **clarithromycin** 500mg BID, **proton pump inhibitor** BID x 7-14 days. In pts with PCN allergy substitute **metronidazole** 500mg BID for amoxicillin.			

4.10.2 Barrett's esophagus

Diagnosis	Finding columnar epithelium in the distal esophagus Histology reveals specialized intestinal metaplasia
Screening endoscopy	White males are at highest risk Patients with GERD that fail empiric therapy and present with "red flag" symptoms suggesting complicated disease: Anorexia, weight loss, dysphagia, odynophagia, bleeding, iron deficiency
Risks	0.5% annual risk of developing adenocarcinoma of the esophagus or gastroesophageal junction
Intervention	Perform biopsy to evaluate for dysplasia, then proceed as follows: - No dysplasia: Repeat endoscopy in 1-2 years - Low-grade dysplasia: Intensive therapy followed by endoscopy in 6 mo - High-grade dysplasia: Surgery or endoscopic therapies
Definitive treatment	High-grade dysplasia: Esophagectomy Low-grade lesions should be followed closely with endoscopic surveillance

4.11 5 Board-Style Questions

1) A 40-year-old male patient has a history of celiac sprue for 10 years, controlled on a gluten-free diet, now presents with abdominal pain, fever, and weight loss. What is the likely cause?
2) A 35-year-old woman has a history of GERD for 2 years. Manometry shows absence of peristalsis in the body of the esophagus and decreased lower esophageal sphincter tone. What diagnosis should be considered in this patient?
3) A 20-year-old male college student presents with cough, and fever around the time of finals. On routine labs he is found to have an elevated bilirubin of 4 mg/dL with a direct bilirubin of 0.2. AST is 32. Alt is 27, and alkaline phosphatase is 100. What disease does this patient have?
4) A 65-year-old man with HTN and diabetes mellitus type II presents with new onset foot drop on the left and wrist drop on the right. The only findings on his labs are an elevated creatinine at 1.4 and HBsAG+. What is the cause of this patient's symptoms?
5) 38-year-old female presents to the emergency department complaining of severe watery diarrhea. The potassium is found to be 2.3. There is a low osmolal gap, as well as hypochlorhydria. What diagnosis should be considered in this patient?

5 Geriatrics

5.1 Dementia in the Elderly

DSM IV criteria for dementia	
1	Memory impairment
2	At least one of the following: Aphasia, apraxia, agnosia, disturbance in executive functioning
3	The disturbance in 1 and 2 significantly interferes with work, social activities, or relationships
4	Disturbance does not occur exclusively during delirium

From American Psychiatric Association Diagnostic and Statistical Manual, 4th ed, APA Press, Washington DC, 1994.

Initial testing in dementia	
Imaging	CT or MR scans in the routine initial evaluation are appropriate
Depression	Screening for depression is appropriate
Labs	B12, TSH, RPR
Other	There are no CSF or other biomarkers for routine use in determining the diagnosis of Alzheimer's disease at this time

Knopman DS, DeKosky ST, Cummings JL, et al. Practice parameter: Diagnosis of dementia (an evidence-based review). Report of the Quality Standards Subcommittee of the American Academy of Neurology. Neurology 2001; 56:1143.

FDA approved drugs

Drug name	Brand name	Approved For	FDA Approved
1. donepezil	Aricept	All stages	1996
2. galantamine	Razadyne	Mild to moderate	2001
3. memantine	Namenda	Moderate to severe	2003
4. rivastigmine	Exelon	Mild to moderate	2000
5. tacrine	Cognex	Mild to moderate	1993

Source: http://www.americangeriatrics.org/health_care_professionals/clinical_practice/clinical_guidelines_recommendations/ then click on Guideline for Alzheimer's Disease Management (California Workgroup on Guidelines for Alzheimer's Disease Management, 2008) - AGS Participated

Pharmacologic treatment of Alzheimer Disease (AD)*	
Cholinesterase inhibitors	Should be considered in patients with mild to moderate AD, although studies suggest a small average degree of benefit.
Vitamin E	May slow the progression of AD. Rec. dose: 1000 IU PO bid
Selegeline	Its use is supported by one study, but has a less favorable risk-benefit ratio. Recommended dose: 5mg PO bid
Estrogen	Not recommended in the treatment of AD

*There are no adequately controlled trials demonstrating pharmacologic efficacy for any agent in ischemic vascular (multi-infarct) dementia

Source: Doody RS, Stevens JC, Beck C, et al. Practice Parameter: Management of dementia (an evidence-based review): Report of the Quality Standards Subcommittee of the American Academy of Neurology. Neurology 2001; 56:1145-1166.

Differential diagnosis

Dementia syndrome	Pathogenesis	Clinical features	Diagnosis	Treatment
Alzheimer disease	Extracellular deposition of amyloid beta-protein. Intracellular neurofibrillary tangles, and loss of neurons	Progressive loss of memory, personality changes, global cognitive dysfunction and functional impairment	Based on clinical grounds	Cholinesterase inhibitors with Memantine
Vascular dementia	Large artery infarctions, small artery infarctions (lacunar infarct), or chronic subcortical ischemia	Abrupt onset with stepwise deterioration	Prominent executive dysfunction, history of stroke, and vascular risk factors should suggest the diagnosis and prompt a neuro-imaging study.	Secondary stroke prevention with Aspirin, and blood pressure control. Empiric cholinesterase inhibitors with Memantine

Pick's disease (and other fronto-temporal dementias)	Focal atrophy of the frontal and temporal lobes in the absence of Alzheimer pathol. Pick bodies are silver-staining intracytoplasmic inclusions	Gradual and progressive behavior change and language dysfunction	Prominent behavioral and language changes	Treatment of symptoms
Dementia with Lewy bodies	Lewy bodies are round, eosinophilic, intracytoplasmic inclusions in the nuclei of cortical neurons	Progressive dementia with visual hallucinations, and motor features of parkinsonism	Based on clinical grounds	Behavior therapies are preferred, then cholinesterase inhibitors. Low-dose atypical neuroleptics for psychotic symptoms

Differentiating delirium from dementia		
Features	**Delirium**	**Dementia**
Onset	acute, abrupt	gradual
Course, duration	acute illness, lasting days to weeks	chronic illness, progressing over years
Attention	strikingly short	not reduced (except for severe dementia)
Disorientation	early	later in the illness, after months or years
Consciousness	clouded, altered, changing level	clear until terminal stage
Psychomotor changes	marked (hyperactive or hypoactive)	occurring late
Physiologic changes	prominent	less prominent
Sleep-wake cycle	disturbed, hour-to-hour variation	disturbed, day-night reversal
Variability	variable from moment to moment	stable from day to day
Reversibility	usually reversible, often completely	generally irreversible

5.2 Urinary Incontinence

	Symptoms	Mechanism	Treatment
Urge	Incontinence preceded by an intense urge to urinate	Uninhibited bladder contractions due to detrusor overactivity	Bladder retraining. Anticholinergic drugs (**tolterodine, oxybutynin**)
Stress	Leakage when intraabdominal pressure is increased, or with exertion, laughing, coughing, bending, or sneezing	Reduced sphincteric resistance due to impaired urethral support from the pelvic endofascia and muscles	Kegel pelvic muscle exercises. Estrogen cream or ring applied locally to strengthen urethral tissue. Surgery for cystocele. **Duloxetine**
Mixed	Leakage and urgency associated with exertion, laughing, coughing, bending, or sneezing	Detrusor overactivity and impaired urethral sphincter function	As above
Overflow (urethral obstruction)	Dribbling and/or continuous leakage associated with incomplete bladder emptying	Outlet obstruction often by benign prostatic hypertrophy. Post-void residual is increased	**tamsulosin finasteride** for BPH
Overflow (detrusor instability)	Dribbling and/or continuous leakage associated with incomplete bladder emptying	Impaired detrusor contractility- idiopathic or neurologic. Post-void residual is increased	Supportive Voiding maneuvers Catheterization

5.3 Falls in the Elderly

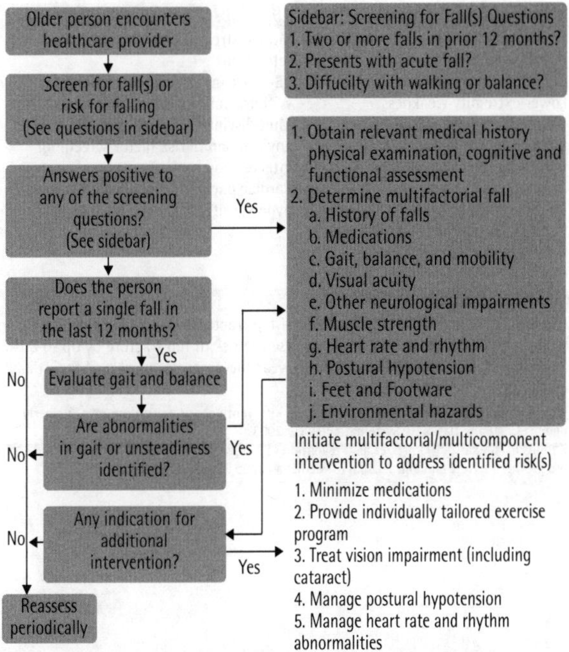

Source: Summary of the Updated American Geriatrics Society/British Geriatrics Society clinical practice guideline for prevention of falls in older persons. J Am Geriatr Soc. 2011 Jan;59(1):148-57. Complete AGS/BGS guidelines available online at: http://www.americangeriatrics.org/health_care_professionals/clinical_practice/clinical_guidelines_recommendations/2010/

5.4 Falls - Risk Factors and Prevention

Risk factors for falls	Fall prevention steps[1]
- Female gender - Past history of a fall - Cognitive impairment - Lower extremity weakness - Balance problems - Medications (commonly benzodiazepines or opioids) - Arthritis - History of stroke - Orthostatic hypotension - Dizziness - Anemia	- Muscle strengthening and balance retraining - 15-week Tai Chi exercise program - Withdrawal of psychotropic medications - Multidisciplinary, multifactorial, health/ environmental risk factor screening/ intervention programs - Cardiac pacing for fallers with carotid sinus hypersensitivity
Hip fracture prevention[2]	
- Hip protectors reduce the general risk of hip fractures by 60%. If they are being worn at the time of the fall they decrease the risk of hip fracture by up to 80%. - 31% of people in this study refused to wear the protector as part of their daily clothing	

1. Gillespie LD, Gillespie WJ, Robertson MC, et al. Interventions for preventing falls in elderly people. Cochrane Database Systematic Review 2003.
2. Kannus P, Parkkari J, Neimi S, et al. Prevention of hip fractures in elderly people with use of a hip protector. New England Journal of Medicine, 2000;343:1506-13.

5.5 Insomnia in the Elderly

Medical DO	Neurological DO	Psychiatric DO	Primary sleep DO	Other
- Congestive heart failure - Ischemic heart disease - Nocturnal angina - COPD - Asthma - Peptic ulcer disease - Reflux esophagitis	- Stroke - Alzheimer's disease - Parkinson - Brain tumors - Traumatic brain injury - Peripheral neuropathy - Headache syndromes (migraine, cluster)	- Depression - Anxiety - Schizophrenia	- Idiopathic - Circadian rhythm DO - Restless leg syndrome - Periodic limb movements - Inadequate sleep hygiene - Altitude insomnia - Insufficient sleep - Central sleep apnea	- Alcohol - Drug-related
To be considered chronic, symptoms of insomnia have to persist for > 3 months.				

Sleep hygiene education for insomnia
- Improve the sleep environment: noisy pets, snoring bed partner - Comfortable bed and room temperature - Turn the clock away; reduce fixation on bedside clocks - Avoid alcohol, nicotine or caffeine - Encourage exercise, but not too close to bedtime

Insomnia medications				
Medication	**Dur. of action**	**Half-life**	**Indications**	**Dose**
Benzodiazapines				
temazepam (Restoril)	Intermediate	8–15 h	Mainly for sleep maintenance	7.5–30 mg
estazolam (Prosom)	Intermediate	10–24 h	Mainly for sleep maintenance	0.5–2 mg
triazolam (Halcion)	Short	2–5 h	Mainly for sleep-onset insomnia	0.125–0.25
Non-Benzodiazepines				

eszopiclone (Lunesta)	Intermediate	5–7 h	Mainly for sleep maintenance	1–3 mg
zolpidem (Ambien)	Short	3 h	Mainly for sleep-onset insomnia	5–10 mg
zaleplon (Sonata)	Ultrashort	1 h	Sleep-onset or sleep mainten.	5–20 mg
Melatonin receptor agonists				
ramelteon (Rozerem)	Short	2–5 h	Mainly for sleep-onset insomnia	8 mg
Source: Silber MH, Chronic Insomnia, New England Journal of Medicine 2005; 353:803-10.				

5.6 Visual Impairment

Global causes of blindness in 2002	Percent
Cataract	47.8%
Glaucoma	12.3%
Age-related macular degeneration	8.7%
Corneal opacities	5.1%
Diabetic retinopathy	4.8%
Childhood blindness	3.9%
Trachoma	3.6%
Resnikoff S, Pascolini D, Etya'ale D, et al. Global data on visual impairment in the year 2002, Bulletin of the WHO 2004;82:844-851.	

Common causes of visual impairment in the elderly		
Condition	**Mechanism**	**Treatment**
Presbyopia	Hardening of the lens with age	Corrective lenses, surgery
Cataracts	Opacity of the lens	Surgery
Age related macular degeneration	Dry: Atrophic Wet: Neovascularization or exudative	Dry: Antioxidants Wet: Laser therapy, photodynamic therapy, VEGF inhibitors
Glaucoma	Optic neuropathy characterized by elevated intraocular pressure	Acute angle closure glaucoma is an emergency that must be treated within 24 hrs to prevent permanent blindness
Diabetic retinopathy	Chronic hyperglycemia with accumulation of advanced glycosylation end products in the extracellular fluid	Glycemic control, antihypertensive therapy, ACE inhibitors, antiplatelet agents, steroids, laser, surgery

5.7 Auditory Impairment

Presbycusis	Treatment
Sensorineural hearing loss associated with aging Affected by lifetime noise exposure, genetics, medications, and infections Usually more pronounced after age 50 Usually bilateral	Hearing aids Cochlear implants

5.8 Pressure Ulcers

Stage	Characteristics	Treatment
1	Area of persistent redness on intact skin with any of the following changes: - Skin temperature (warmth or coolness) - Tissue consistency (firm or boggy) - Sensation (pain, itching)	Preventive measures, relieve pressure with frequent turning and cushions
2	Partial-thickness skin loss involving the epidermis and/or dermis. Appears as an abrasion, blister or shallow ulcer	Occlusive or semipermeable dressings that will maintain a moist wound environment. Avoid wet-to-dry dressings
3	Full-thickness skin loss which may extend down to, but not through the underlying fascia. Appears as a deep crater with or without undermining of the adjacent tissue	Correcting nutritional deficiencies, managing tissue pressure, removing necrotic tissue, managing wound infections, and maintaining a moist wound environment
4	Full-thickness skin loss with extensive destruction, tissue necrosis, or damage to the muscle, bone or supporting structures	Same as stage 3. May include surgical debridement

Based on National Pressure Ulcer Advisory Panel definitions

5.9 5 Board-Style Questions

1) A 55-year-old woman reports feeling tired while at work. Her husband states that her legs have "jerking movements" while she is sleeping. These symptoms occur about 10 nights per month. What medication would you offer this patient?
2) An 84-year-old man has recurrent syncope. Symptoms occur when he wears a tight collar shirt or when he turns his head far to the right. How should this patient be treated?
3) An 85-year-old patient admitted after an intertrochanteric hip fracture undergoes surgical repair and now requests Benadryl to help sleep at night. What are the four reasons not to give this patient Benadryl as a sleep aid?
4) The same elderly patient who recently had hip surgery has been receiving Demerol for pain. He now develops new onset seizures. What is the cause?
5) What immunizations are recommended for a 72-year-old patient in good health?

6 Hematology

6.1 Anemia

Initial Assessment	
Step 1: Lab tests	Hemoglobin (Hb) concentration, MCV & RDW, reticulocyte count, peripheral blood smear
Step 2: Use MCV to classify the anemia	Microcytic (MCV < 80), normocytic (MCV 80-100), macrocytic (MCV >100)
Step 3: Identify cause	Additional tests to identify the precise cause of anemia
Step 4: Treatment	Apply appropriate treatment and evaluate response to therapy

Determining Anemia Type

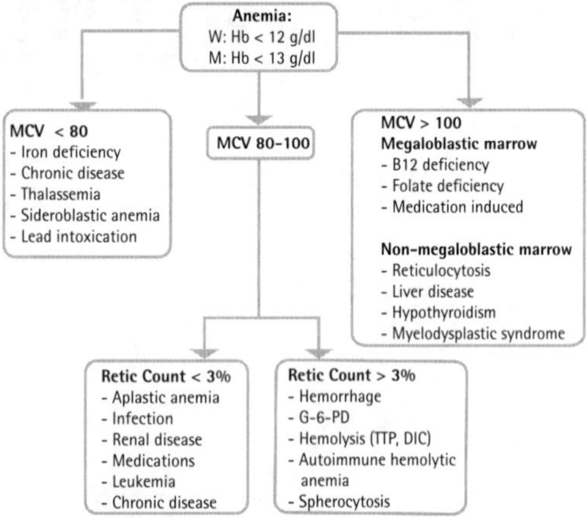

Identifying Possible Anemia Causes	
↓ RBC production	
Stem cell failure	- Aplastic anemia - Myelodysplastic syndromes or leukemia
Progenitor cell failure	- Pure red cell aplasia - Anemia of renal failure - Anemia of chronic disease - Endocrine cause (hypothyroidism)
Precursor cell failure	- Megaloblastic anemia - Dietary deficiency (iron deficiency) - Hemoglobinopathy (thalassemia) - Enzyme deficiency (G-6-PD) - Medication/drug (EtOH)
↑ RBC destruction	
Hereditary	- Membrane defects (hereditary spherocytosis) - Globin defects (sickle cell disease) - Enzyme defects (pyruvate kinase deficiency)
Acquired	- Traumatic - Microangiopathic (TTP) - Antibody-mediated - Hypersplenism - Acute blood loss - Paroxysmal nocturnal hemoglobinuria

6.1.1 Microcytic anemia

Iron Studies				
Disorder	**Serum Iron**	**TIBC**	**Ferritin**	**Marrow Iron**
Iron deficiency	↓	↑	↓	↑↓
Chronic disease	↓	↓	↑	↔

Differential Diagnoses			
Disorder	**Common causes**	**Diagnosis**	**Treatment**
Iron deficiency	Blood loss, malabsorption	Low serum ferritin	Ferrous sulfate 325 mg PO TID + Vit C
Chronic disease	Infection, inflammation, malignancy	Low serum iron and TIBC	Treat underlying disease. Give EPO if low erythropoietin
Thalassemia	Reduced or absent production of a globin chain	Family history, disproportionately high RBC count	Varies by type
Sideroblastic	Drug-induced, myelodysplastic syndrome	Ringed sideroblasts in the bone marrow	Stop offending drug or EtOH. Approach like MDS
Lead poisoning	Paint, batteries, work exposure	Blood lead level	Stop exposure. Chelation if Pb > 80 µg/dl

6.1.2 Thalassemia

Introduction	
General info	Each hemoglobin molecule (Hb) is a tetramer composed of two separate pairs of identical globin chains. Globin types include β, α, and δ. Adult hemoglobin is approx. 96% HbA ($\alpha_2\beta_2$) and 2.5% HbA_2 ($\alpha_2\delta_2$).
Pathophysiology	Thalassemia results from an inherited defect in the synthesis of one or more globin chains.
Clinical	The result is ineffective erythropoiesis, defective hemoglobin production, hemolysis and anemia. Previously undiagnosed adults may present with mild anemia and a disproportionately low MCV.

Types			
Type	**Genetic variant**	**Clinical findings**	**Population at risk**
Alpha-thalassemia			
Normal	$\alpha\alpha$ / $\alpha\alpha$	Normal	Alpha–thalassemias are widespread in Africa, the Mediterranean, the Middle East, and Southeast Asia.
Silent carrier	α- / $\alpha\alpha$	Normal	
Alpha-thalassemia trait	α–/α– or —/$\alpha\alpha$	↓ MCV, ↓ MCH	
HbH disease	--/α-	Hypochromic, marked hemolytic anemia & splenomegaly	
Hb Barts (hydrops fetalis)	-- / --	Incompatible with life, infant dies within hrs	
Beta-thalassemia			
Beta-thalassemia minor	Heterozygous carrier	↓Hb 9-11 g/dl, ↓MCV 50-70 fl, ↓MCH 20-22 pg	Beta-thalassemia occurs sporadically in all races, most commonly in populations from the Mediterranean, Middle East, India, Pakistan, Southeast Asia, southern Russia, and China.
Beta-thalassemia intermedia	Heterozygous	Ranges from severe transfusion-dependent anemia to mild anemia (Hb 10-12 with ↓ MCV)	
Beta-thalassemia major	Homozygous or compound heterozygous state	Total absence of beta chain production, Hb F is the only Hb produced; transfusions are required in the first months of life. Hb ranges 2-3 g/dl	

6.1.3 Other microcytic anemias

Disease	Definition	Pathogenesis	Findings	Treatment
Anemia of chronic renal failure	Anemia in pts with uremia	Reduced production of erythropoietin (EPO)	Normocytic, normochromic anemia. Iron and Folic acid may be low due to dialysis.	EPO replacement
Anemia of chronic disease	Anemia lasting > 2 mo, associated with chronic infection, inflam. disease, or neoplasm.	↓ RBC lifespan Less iron available for Hemoglobin production ↓ production of EPO	Low serum Iron Normal TIBC Normal ferritin Increased storage of iron in marrow	No tx required Iron is contra-indicated Replace EPO if low

6.1.4 Megaloblastic anemia - categories

General Categories	
Category	**Causes**
Abnormalities of DNA metabolism	Vitamin B12 (cobalamin)/ folate deficiency Drugs: - Hydroxyurea - Zidovudine (AZT) - Chemotherapy medications
Shift to immature or stressed RBCs	Reticulocytosis ↑ erythropoietin Aplastic anemia / Fanconi´s anemia Pure red cell aplasia
Primary bone marrow disorders	Myelodysplastic syndromes Congenital dyserythropoietic anemias Large granular lymphocyte leukemia
Lipid abnormalities	Liver disease Hypothyroidism Hyperlipidemia
Unknown mechanisms	Alcohol Multiple myeloma and other plasma cell disorders

6.1.5 Megaloblastic anemia - causes

Cause	Clin. features	Causes	Lab tests	Treatment
Vitamin B12 deficiency	Neurologic deficits: - Dementia - Psychosis	Impaired absorption most commonly from pernicious anemia	↓ cobalamin ↑ methyl-malonic acid ↑ homo-cysteine	1000 µg of vitamin B12 IM daily x 2 weeks, then weekly until Hct is normal, and then monthly for life
Folate deficiency	No neurologic findings	Inadequate diet, reserves are small, so deficiency develops rapidly	↓ serum folate (<2 ng/mL) confirms the diagnosis	Folic acid 1-5 mg daily. Must rule out concurrent B12 deficiency, if present, is treated to prevent irreversible neurologic deficits
Drug-induced	No neurologic findings	Common drugs: Methotrexate, trimethoprim, hydroxyurea and phenytoin	↓ serum folate (<2 ng/mL) confirms the diagnosis	Withdrawal of medication or treatment with folinic acid or folic acid (depends on the medication)

6.1.6 Sickle cell anemia

Crises	
Crisis	**Clinical features and management**
Acute painful episode	Lasts 2-7 days Most common type of crisis Management: - Aggressive pain relief - Hydration - Supplemental oxygen - Rule out infection/thrombosis
Acute severe anemia	**Aplastic crisis:** - Transient arrest of erythropoiesis with <1% reticulocytes - Often follows infections, including parvovirus B19, streptococcal, and EBV **Splenic sequestration crisis:** - Sudden massive pooling of RBCs in the spleen - Mortality is 10-15%
Chest syndrome	Chest pain + new infiltrate on CXR + fever Most frequent cause of death in adults Targets of treatment include pneumonia, thrombosis, and embolism.
Other	**Infection:** a major cause of morbidity and mortality, especially in children. Encapsulated organisms including *S. pneumoniae, H. influenza, and N. meningititis* should be suspected **Priapism:** emergent urology consult **Myocardial infarction** **Hepatic dysfunction** **Renal dysfunction** **Retinopathy**

6.2 Cytopenias

	Definition	Common causes	Tests	Must not miss
Neutropenia	ANC <1500/µl **Severe:** ANC <500/µl	- Medication - Infection - Chemotherapy	- CBC with differential - Viral testing (HIV, - Hepatitis, Monospot) - May consider - Bone marrow biopsy	Acute onset of severe neutropenia with fever requires prompt cultures, IV fluids and antibiotics (neutropenic fever)
Thrombocytopenia	Platelet count <150,000/µl **Surgery bleed risk:** < 50,000/µl **Spontaneous bleeding:** < 10,000/µl	TTP/HUS HIT DIC ITP Medications Infection/Sepsis Alcohol HIV Hypersplenism Liver Disease Multifactorial	CBC Peripheral smear Viral testing (HIV) Blood cultures May consider bone marrow biopsy Liver spleen scan to evaluate for hypersplenism	TTP requires emergent plasma exchange otherwise the have mortality rate approaches 90%. HIT is associated with both venous and arterial thrombosis. DIC is associated with life-threatening hemorrhage and is associated with a mortality rate of 30-80%

6.3 Cythemia

	Definition	common causes	tests	Must not miss
Neutrophilia	ANC > 7500/µl	- Infection - Stress - Smoking - Pregnancy - Following exercise - Glucocorticoids - Chronic myelogenous leukemia (CML)	- CBC with differential - Blood cultures - BUN and creatinine - Hemolysis (bilirubin) - Troponin I - BCR/ABL testing for CML	Myocardial infarction as well as hemorrhage can cause neutrophilia and are often overlooked
Eosinophilia	> 600cells/µL **Severe:** > 5,000/µL	- #1 worldwide: Infection with helminths (hookworm) - Asthma - Allergic rhinitis - Medication-induced - Neoplasms	- Stool for O & P - Pulmonary function tests - HIV - Lymph node biopsy for Hodgkins disease	Eosinophilia may be a marker for adrenal insufficiency, especially in the critically ill. It is also associated with atheroembolic disease
Thrombocythemia	>500,000/µl **Extreme:** >1,000,000/µl	- Infection - Post surgical - Malignancy - Acute blood loss - Iron deficiency - Essential thrombocythemia (ET)	- Peripheral smear - CBC - Serum ferritin - ESR/C-reactive protein - Hemolysis studies - JAK2 gene mutation present in 50-75% of patients with ET	Prompt reduction of platelet counts is required for patients with ET with and evidence of cerebrovascular or microvascular ischemia

Polycythemia	↑ RBC mass Hb >16.5 in women and >18.5 g/dL in men	- COPD - Sleep apnea - Morbid obesity - Smoking - Polycythemia vera (PV)	- Repeat CBC - CXR (pulmonary disease) - Liver function tests (hepatoma) - U/A (renal cell carcinoma) - Erythropoietin level - JAK2 gene mutation in 97% of patients with PV	Thrombotic events in polycythemia vera may be threatening

6.4 Leukemia

Key characteristics	Expected prognosis	General treatments
Acute Myelogenous Leukemia (AML)		
Most common leukemia in adults **Auer rods** may be present Average age at presentation is 65 **M7** associated with Down syndrome 12,000 new cases/year in USA	Varies with age and AML subtype Better survival in younger patients Overall ~30% cure rate	Anthracycline-based chemotherapy (**daunorubicin, idarubicin**) - along with **cytarabine** (Ara-C) Bone marrow transplant **M3-APL** subtype of AML is treated with **all-trans retinoic acid** with cure rates from 80-85%

Chronic myelogenous leukemia (CML)		
Average age at presentation is 50 **Philadelphia chromosome** is pathognomonic: translocation of abl gene from chromosome 9 to 22 (BCR/ABL) tested from peripheral blood 4,500 new cases/year in USA	Without treatment, universally progresses to blast crisis blast crisis and acute leukemia. With treatment, and close followup, prognosis is generally excellent	**Imatinib** (Gleevac) inhibits activity of the mutant tyrosine kinase product of the bcr-abl gene. This **targeted therapy** has a ≥ 90% response rate **Dasatinib** (Sprycel) and Nilotinib (Tasigna) are also approved, and more potent inhibitors of BCR/ABL tyrosine kinase.
Acute lymphocytic leukemia (ALL)		
Most common leukemia in children Peak age at diagnosis 3-4 years 4,000 new cases/year in USA	80% cure rate in children, much lower in adults. Most adults will eventually relapse	For adults: intensive chemotherapy to first induce remission, then consolidation to eliminate residual disease, and finally, maintenance. This usually requires ~2.5 years. Consider bone marrow transplantation.
Chronic lymphocytic leukemia (CLL)		
Presents in patients older than 50 years **Mature lymphocytes** on peripheral smear with smudge cells Expresses **CD-5** 10,000 new cases/year in USA	When only lymphocytosis is present median survival is 150 months. When anemia and thrombocytopenia are also present, the median survival decreases to 9 months	Low-risk disease can be monitored. High-risk disease can be treated with alkylating agents or nucleoside analogs

6.5 Anticoagulation and antithrombosis

6.5.1 Venous thromboembolism prophylaxis

Recommendations for Prophylaxis of Venous Thromboembolism per ACCP, 2008			
VTE Risk Level	**Examples**	**Suggested Prophylaxis**	**DVT Risk[1]**
Low risk	Minor surgery in mobile patients Fully mobile medical patients	No specific prophylaxis: early and aggressive ambulation	< 10%
Moderate risk	Most general, open gynecologic or urologic surgical patients Medical patients on bed rest or who are sick	LMWH (at recommended doses) or Low-dose UFH (bid or tid) or Fondaparinux	10%-40%
High risk	Hip or knee arthroplasty, hip fracture surgery Major trauma, spinal cord injury	LMWH (at recommended doses) or Fondaparinux or Vitamin K antagonists (INR 2-3)	40%-80%
Moderate to high risk plus high bleeding risk	As above for moderate and high risks	Mechanical prophylaxis[2]	10%-80%

LMWH = low-molecular-weight heparin; UFH = unfractionated heparin; INR = international normalized ratio
[1]Represents DVT risk without thromboprophylaxis
[2]Mechanical prophylaxis includes the use of intermittent pneumatic compression devices, a venous foot pump, or graduated compression stockings; careful attention should be given to the proper use of (eg, correct sizing), and optimal adherence with, these methods; consider switching to anticoagulant prophylaxis when bleeding risk decreases.

6.5.2 Hypercoagulable states

When to suspect	What test to order	Treatment
- Age <50 with family history - Cerebral venous thrombosis - 2nd or 3rd trimester pregnancy loss May consider testing: VTE in association with OCP/HRT or pregnancy - Patients >50 with first spontaneous VTE	- Antithrombin III - Protein C and protein S - Prothrombin G20210A - Factor V Leiden - Antiphospolipid antibodies (anticardiolipin IgG and IgM, lupus anticoagulant) - +/- Factor VIII coagulant activity	- Goal INR: 2-3 - Superficial vein thrombosis → treat for at least 4 weeks - 1st episode provoked (obvious cause) → treat for at least 3 months - 1st episode unprovoked → treat for at least 3-6 months - 2nd episode, life-threatening, active cancer, or persistent risk factors → lifelong - PE treat for at least 6-12 months
Source: Bates et al. NEJM 2004:351:268-277, NCCN practice guidelines v 1.2010		

6.5.3 Managing elevated INR

Recommendations for Managing Elevated INR or Bleeding in Patients Receiving Warfarin	
Condition	**Description**
INR above therapeutic range but <5.0; no significant bleeding	Lower dose or omit dose, monitor more frequently, and resume at lower dose when INR therapeutic; if only minimally above therapeutic range, no dose reduction may be required.
INR >5 but <9.0; no significant bleeding	Omit next 1-2 doses and give vitamin K (1-4 mg PO), particularly if at increased risk of bleeding. If more rapid reversal is required because the patient requires urgent surgery, vitamin K (2-4 mg orally) can be given with the expectation that a reduction of the INR will occur in 24 h. If the INR is still high, additional vitamin K (1-2 mg orally) can be given.
Modified from: Ansell J, Hirsh J, Bussey H, et al. Chest 2004;126(s)204-233.	

INR >9 but no significant bleeding	Hold dose when INR therapeutic warfarin therapy and give higher dose of vitamin K (5-10 mg PO) with the expectation that the INR will be reduced substantially in 24-48 h. Monitor more frequently and use additional vitamin K if necessary. Resume therapy at lower dose.
Serious or life-threatening bleeding at any elevation of INR	Hold warfarin therapy and give vitamin K (10mg by slow IV infusion), supplemented with FFP or prothrombin complex concentrate. Recombinant factor VIIa is alternative. Vitamin K can be repeated every 12 h.
Modified from: Ansell J, Hirsh J, Bussey H, et al. Chest 2004;126(s)204-233.	

6.5.4 Coagulation cascade and anticoagulants

Coagulation Cascade and Anticoagulant Mechanisms of Action

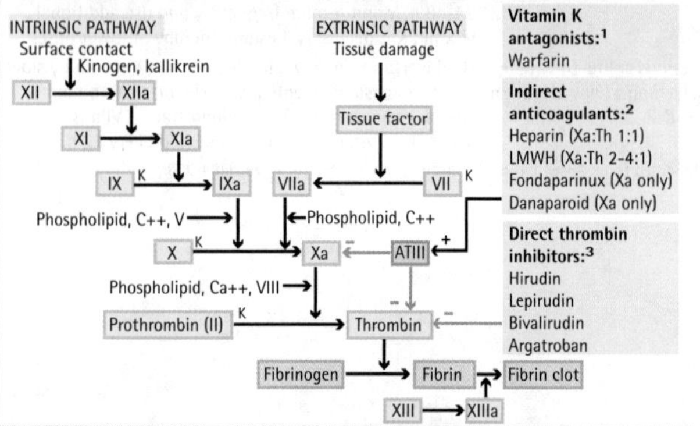

1. Vitamin K antagonists interfere with the cyclic interconversion of vitamin K and its 2,3 epoxide leading to defective vitamin K-dependent factor formation (prothrombin, VII, IX, X).
2. Indirect anticoagulants activate antithrombin III (ATII), selectively accelerating its inactivation of factors Xa and thrombin. Heparin inactivates factor Xa and thrombin in an appx. 1:1 ratio, LMWH in a 2-4:1 ratio (depending on molecular size), and fondaparinux and danaparoid inactivate only factor Xa.
3. Direct thrombin inhibitors directly inhibit the enzymatic activity of thrombin.

6.5.5 Platelet activation and antiplatelet agents

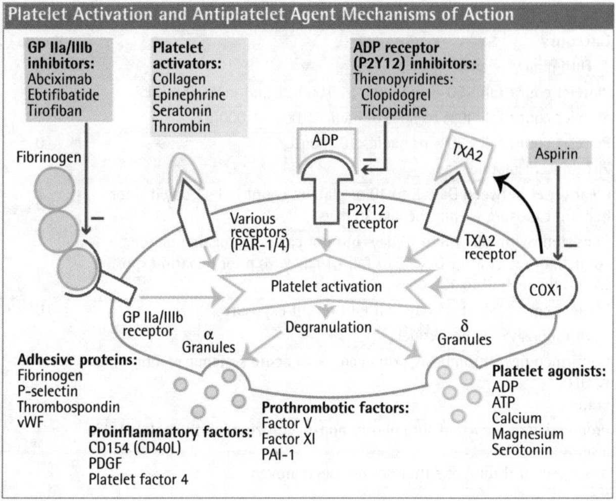

6.6 Heparin-Induced Thrombocytopenia (HIT)

Pretest Scoring System Probability of HIT – The 4 Ts	
Category	**Points**
1. Thrombocytopenia	
Platelet count fall >50% and nadir ≥20,000/μL and < 100,000/μL	2
Platelet count fall 30% to 50% or nadir 10,000-19,000/μL	1
Platelet count fall <30% or nadir <10,000/μL	0
2. Timing of platelet fall	
Clear onset between Days 5 to 10 or platelet count fall ≤1 day if prior heparin exposure within the last 30 days	2
Consistent with fall at 5 to 10 days but not clear (eg, missing platelet counts), or onset after Day 10 or fall ≤1 day with prior heparin exposure within the last 30 to 100 days	1
Platelet count fall at <4 days without recent exposure	0
3. Thrombosis or other sequelae	
Confirmed new thrombosis, skin necrosis, or acute systemic reaction post-IV UFH bolus	2
Progressive or recurrent thrombosis, non-necrotizing (erythematous) skin lesions, or suspected thrombosis that has not been proven	1
None	0
4. oTher causes for thrombocytopenia	
None apparent	2
Possible	1
Definite	0

Scoring: Add points (0 to 2) for each of the 4 categories to determine the total score.
Interpretation: 0–3: low pretest HIT prob; 4–5: intermediate pretest HIT prob; 6–8: high pretest HIT prob; Note: Scores do not supersede clinical judgment.
Adapted from Lo GK, et al. Evaluation of pretest clinical score (4 Ts) for the diagnosis of heparin-induced thrombocytopenia in two clinical settings. *J Thromb Haemost.* 2006;4:759–765.

6.7 Transfusion Basics

Clinical findings	Findings	Action
Immediate Reactions		
Acute hemolytic reaction	Usually due to ABO incompatibility Patients develop fever, low back pain, chest tightness, hypotension, nausea or vomiting Intravascular hemolysis may lead to DIC or ischemic necrosis	Terminate transfusion immediately Send sample back to blood bank for analysis Monitor closely for acute renal failure Begin IV hydration to **maintain urinary output >100 ml/hr**
Febrile reaction	1/3 of all transfusion reactions May be secondary to hemolytic reaction, sensitivity to leukocytes or platelets, bacterial pyrogens. May be prevented by using **leukocyte filter** and **premedication** with Benadryl 25mg PO and Tylenol 650mg PO	The transfusion is usually terminated and the patient premedicated before the next transfusion, where a leukocyte filter is used or leukocyte-reduced cells are transfused.
Pulmonary hypersensitivity reaction	Within 4 hours of transfusion a patient develops fever, chills, respiratory distress, tachycardia, pulmonary edema and bilateral pulmonary infiltrates on CXR Results from leukocyte incompatibility Symptoms resolve in 24 hrs	Supportive care
Allergic reactions	Development of pruritus, urticaria, and possibly angioedema and bronchospasm Caused by hypersensitivity to plasma proteins	Terminate transfusion **Benadryl** for urticaria and pruritus **Epinephrine** 0.4mg SC 1:1000 or anaphylaxis

Clinical Findings	Findings	Action
Immediate Reactions		
Anti-IgA in IgA deficient recipient	- Severe anaphylaxis may occur in patients with IgA deficiency who have IgA antibodies. - Reaction can occur with as little as 10 mL of plasma - Can be prevented by using washed RBCs	Terminate transfusion Epinephrine if necessary
Bacterial contamination	Symptoms of infection beginning immediately or within 30 minutes of beginning transfusion	Terminate transfusion Gram stain should be examined from transfused blood Initiate broad spectrum antibiotics until organism is identified
Delayed Reactions		
Delayed hemolytic reaction	4-14 days after transfusion patient develops jaundice, fall in hemoglobin, and positive direct Coombs test Caused by antibodies not detected on the screen or cross-match	Usually mild and do not require treatment
Post-transfusion purpura	Thrombocytopenia caused by antibodies to a platelet-specific antigen	Close monitoring
Transmission of disease	Risk of hepatitis B: 1: 58,000 to 1: 269,000 Risk of hepatitis C: 1: 1,900,000 Risk of HTLV: 1: 2,000,000 Risk of HIV: 1: 2,100,000	Inform patients

6.8 4 Board-Style Questions

1) A 40-year-old man reports episodes of dark urine in the morning. Urine dipstick is positive for blood, but there are no RBCs seen on microscopic evaluation. He is anemic with an elevated total bilirubin, but a direct Coombs test is negative, and there are no schistocytes on a peripheral smear. Reticulocyte count is elevated at 8%. Red cell testing reveals the absence of CD-55 and CD-59 antigens. What diagnosis has been confirmed?
2) A patient with sickle cell disease presents with the sudden onset of left hip pain. There was no trauma to the hip, and an x-ray is normal. What test should be performed next?
3) A patient with a long history of anemia due to chronic renal failure presents with a new-onset seizure. What medication is the most likely to cause the seizure in this patient?
   a) Atenolol
   b) Erythropoietin
   c) Renagel
   d) Lipitor
4) A 73 year old man with ITP (idiopathic thrombocytopenic purpura) is no longer responding to steroids. His blood type is Rh+. Based on this finding, what medication may be considered?

7 HIV

7.1 General Information

Acute HIV infection

- May present with non-specific symptoms that resolve spontaneously
- Patients are highly infectious due to high viral load in blood and genital secretions
- There is **no detectable antibody**
- Diagnosis confirmed by demonstrating an **elevated viral load** (usually >100,000 copies/ml) or **positive p24 antigen**
- Antibodies will become positive ~12 days after onset of symptoms

HIV Screening and Testing Guidelines*

Adolescent and adult patients in all health-care settings:

- HIV screening is recommended for patients ages 13-64 years in all health-care settings after the patient is notified that testing will be performed unless the patient declines (opt-out screening).
- Persons at high risk for HIV infection should be screened for HIV at least annually. High-risk groups include:
  - IV drug users
  - Persons who exchange sex for money or drugs
  - Man who have sex with men or heterosexual persons who themselves or whose sex partners have had more than one sex partner since their most recent HIV test
  - Partners of persons in above groups or of known HIV patients
- All patients with signs or symptoms consistent with HIV infection or an opportunistic illness characteristic of AIDS should be tested for HIV (especially if recent high-risk behavior). When acute retroviral syndrome is a possibility, a plasma RNA test should be used in conjunction with an HIV antibody test to diagnose acute HIV infection.
- Separate written consent for HIV testing should not be required; general consent for medical care should be considered sufficient to encompass consent for HIV testing.
- Prevention counseling should not be required with HIV diagnostic testing or as part of HIV screening programs in health-care settings.
- HIV testing must be voluntary and free from coercion. Patients must not be tested without their knowledge.
- HIV testing is recommended and should be routine for persons attending STD clinics and those seeking treatment for STDs in other clinical settings.
- Access to clinical care, prevention counseling, and support services is essential for persons with positive HIV test results.

Pregnant women and newborns:

- All pregnant women in the United States should be screened for HIV infection as early as possible during the pregnancy. HIV screening should be included in the routine panel of prenatal screening tests for all pregnant women.
- HIV screening is recommended after the patient is notified that testing will be performed unless the patient declines (opt-out screening).
- Pregnant women should receive oral or written information that includes an explanation of HIV infection, a description of interventions that can reduce HIV transmission from mother to infant, and the meanings of positive and negative test results and should be offered an opportunity to ask questions and to decline testing.
- Any woman with undocumented HIV status at the time of labor should be screened with a rapid HIV test unless she declines (opt-out screening).
- When a woman's HIV status is still unknown at the time of delivery, she should be screened immediately postpartum with a rapid HIV test unless she declines (opt-out screening).
- When the mother's HIV status is unknown postpartum, rapid testing of the newborn as soon as possible after birth is recommended so antiretroviral prophylaxis can be offered to HIV-exposed infants. Women should be informed that identifying HIV antibodies in the newborn indicates that the mother is infected.
- Repeat screening in the third trimester (<36 weeks) is recommended in certain jurisdictions with elevated rates of HIV infection among pregnant women.
- Separate written consent for HIV testing should not be required; general consent for medical care should be considered sufficient to encompass consent for HIV testing.

*Adapted from Branson BM, et al. Revised Recommendations for HIV Testing of Adults, Adolescents, and Pregnant Women in Health-Care Settings. CDC MMWR Recommendations and Reports. September 22, 2006;55(RR14):1-17.

7.2 HIV Testing (HIV-1)

Test	Description	Accuracy
Enzyme immunoassay (EIA)	- Initial screening test - Positive test should be confirmed with a Western blot	- Sensitivity >99.3%-99.7%
Western blot	- Requires detection of at least 2 of the following: p24, gp41, and gp120/160 - Can detect HIV-2	- Sensitivity 99.3% - Specificity 99.7%
Quantitative HIV RNA	- Uses reverse transcription and then amplification by PCR.	- Sensitivity and specificity depend on CD4 counts - If CD4 < $200/mm^3$: Sensitivity 98%-100%
Rapid HIV	- Results available in minutes - Test for HIV antibodies - Requires confirmatory testing	- Sensitivity >99.3% - Specificity >98.6%
Primary Care Guidelines for the Management of Persons Infected with Human Immunodeficiency Virus: 2009 Update by the HIV Medicine Association of the Infectious Diseases Society of America		

7.3 Initiating Antiretroviral Therapy (ART) in Treatment-Naïve Patients

CD4 Count-Based Recommendations for ART Initiation		
CD4 (cells/mm^3)	Comments	Level of evidence
<350	ART should be initiated in all patients with AIDS-defining illness or CD4 <350 cells/mm^3	A-I
350-500	Advisory panel was divided: 55% voted for strong recommendations of starting ART (A); 45% voted for moderate recommendation (B)	A/B-II
>500	Advisory panel was divided: 50% favor starting ART at this stage of HIV disease (B); 50% view initiating therapy at this stage as optional (C)	B/C-III
Initiate ART Regardless of CD4 Count in The Following Groups:		
Conditions		Level of evidence
HIV-associated nephropathy (HIVAN)		A-II
Hepatitis B virus (HBV) coinfection when treatment of HBV is indicated		A-III
Pregnant women who do not meet criteria for treatment with the goal to prevent perinatal transmission		A-I
Other Recommendations		
Patients initiating ART should be willing and able to commit to lifelong treatment and should understand the benefits and risks of therapy and the importance of adherence		(A-III)
Patients may choose to postpone therapy, and providers, on a case-by-case basis, may elect to defer therapy based on clinical and/or psychosocial factors		-

Rating of Recommendations: A = Strong; B = Moderate; C = Optional
Rating of Evidence: I = data from randomized controlled trials; II = data from well-designed nonrandomized trials or observational cohort studies with long-term clinical outcomes; III = expert opinion
Source: Guidelines for the Use of Antiretroviral Agents in HIV-1-Infected Adults and Adolescents January 10, 2011. (http://aidsinfo.nih.gov/contentfiles/AdultandAdolescentGL.pdf).

7.4 Sites of Action of Anti-Retroviral Drugs

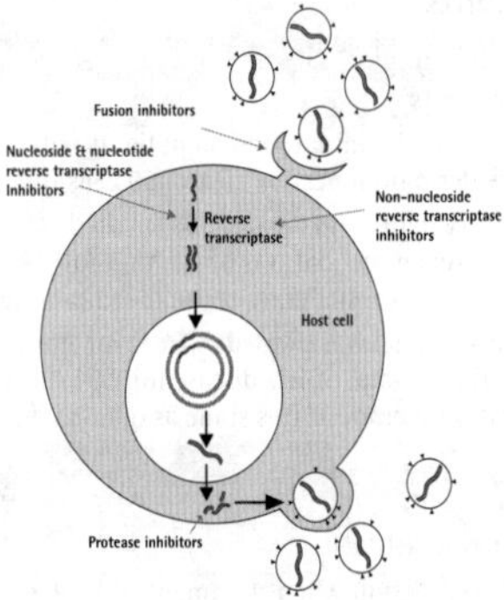

7.5 HIV Drugs

Drug (abbreviation)	Brand	Key Side-Effects
Nucleoside and nucleotide reverse transcriptase inhibitors (NRTIs)		
abacavir (ABC)	Ziagen	Hypersensitivity syndrome in 5-8% of patients: Rash can be fatal if patient is re-challenged with abacavir
didanosine (ddI)	Videx	Severe lactic acidosis, pancreatitis, and peripheral neuropathy
emtricitabine (FTC)	Emtriva	-
lamivudine (3TC)	Epivir	-
stavudine (d4T)	Zerit	Severe lactic acidosis, pancreatitis, and peripheral neuropathy
tenofovir (TDF)	Viread	Avoid in patients with renal failure
zalcitabine (ddC)	Hivid	-
zidovudine (ZDV, AZT)	Retrovir	Headache, anemia with ↑MCV, myopathy, thrombocytopenia

Non-nucleoside reverse transcriptase inhibitors (NNRTIs)		
delavirdine (DLV)	Rescriptor	-
efavirenz (EFV)	Sustiva	CNS toxicity including vivid dreams, rash
nevirapine (NVP)	Viramune	Hepatic necrosis usually in the first 6 weeks of treatment. May cause Stevens-Johnson syndrome and toxic epidermal necrolysis, rash.
Protease inhibitors (PIs)		
amprenavir (APV)	Agenerase	-
atazanavir (ATV)	Reyataz	Rash
darunavir (DRV)	Prezista	-
fosamprenavir (FPV)	Lexiva	Rash
indinavir (IDV)	Crixivan	Nephrolithiasis, interstitial nephritis
lopinavir/ritonavir (LPV/r)	Kaletra	-
nelfinavir (NFV)	Viracept	-
ritonavir (RTV)	Norvir	Gastrointestinal intolerance
saquinavir (SQV)	Fortovase Invirase	-
tipranavir (TPV)	Aptivus	-
Fusion inhibitors		
enfuvirtide (T-20)	Fuzeon	-
Fixed dose combinations		
zidovudine + lamivudine	Combivir	-
zidovudine + lamivudine + abacavir	Trizivir	-
lamivudine + abacavir	Epzicom	-
emtricitabine + tenofovir	Truvada	-

7.6 Initial HAART Regimen Approaches*

Option 1	**2 NRTIs + 1 NNRTI** - Start with zidovudine (ZDV, AZT) + lamivudine (3TC) + efavirenz (EFV) - Since Combivir = AZT + 3TC, the patient can start with Combivir + Sustiva - 1st trimester of pregnancy: AZT + 3TC + nevirapine
Option 2	**2 NRTIs + ritonavir-boosted PIs** - Start with zidovudine (ZDV, AZT) + lamivudine (3TC) and add ritonavir (RTV) + lopinavir (LPV) - As combination pills the patient may take Combivir + Kaletra or Combivir + Sustiva. The simplest regimen is Atripla (efavirenz/emtricitabine/tenofovir) one tablet per day.

*Triple drug therapy is currently the initial standard approach. Patients are started on 2 NRTIs + 1 NNRTI or 2 NRTIs + PI-boosted low-dose ritonavir
HAART = highly active antiretroviral therapy (defined as at least 3 ART agents)

7.7 HAART Drug-Drug Interactions

Medications	Interactions
Antifungals - voriconazole	Should not be combined with NNRTIs or PIs
Antibiotics for TB - rifampin - rifabutin - clarithromycin	Used with caution due to reduction in concentration of PIs
Erectile dysfunction - sildenafil - tadalafil - vardenafil	Doses will need to be reduced when used concomitantly with PIs
Herbal medications - St. John's wort - Supplemental garlic	Should not be combined with PI or NNRTI-based HAART

HMG-CoA reductase inhibitors - simvastatin - lovastatin	Should not be combined with PIs
Oral contraceptives	Used with caution in patients on HAART due to the variations in effects on estradiol levels
Psychotropic medications benzodiazepines - alprazolam - midazolam - triazolam	Should not be combined with PIs

7.8 Common CD4 Count-Related Disease

CD4 count	Disease
>500	Vulvovaginal candidiasis Non-HIV-related infections
200 - 500	Recurrent HSV, zoster, recurrent bacterial infections, TB, thrush, lymphoma, Kaposi sarcoma, oral hairy leukoplakia, seborrheic dermatitis
50 - 200	Pneumocystis jiroveci pneumonia (formerly Pneumocystis carinii pneumonia or PCP)
<50	MAC, CMV retinitis, cryptococcus, cryptosporidia, histoplasmosis, toxoplasmosis, PML, CNS lymphoma, AIDS dementia

7.9 HIV Prophylaxis

CD4 count	Action	Antibiotic
<200	Begin PCP prophylaxis	TMP-SMX (Bactrim) 1 double-strength tablet daily
<100	Begin toxoplasmosis prophylaxis	TMP-SMX (Bactrim) 1 double-strength tablet daily
< 50	Begin disseminated MAC proph.	azithromycin 1200 mg qweek

7.10 Opportunistic Infection Treatments

Opport. infect.	First-line treatment	Alternative treatment
PCP - Pneumocystis jiroveci pneumonia	**trimethoprim-sulfamethoxazole (TMP-SMX, Bactrim)** IV dosing: Total daily dose is based on TMP: 15-20 mg/kg/day. The dose is divided and given every six or eight hours x 21 days. PO dosing: 2 double-strength tablets every eight hours x 21 days + **prednisone,** if PaO2 < 70 mmHg on room air or A-a gradient > 35 mmHg: 40 mg PO bid for 5 days 40 mg PO qday for 5 days 20 mg PO qday for 11 days	**pentamidine** 4 mg/kg/day IV for 21 days
Toxoplasmosis	**pyrimethamine** 200mg loading dose followed by 75 mg/day PO + **sulfadiazine** 6-8 g/day PO in four divided doses + **leucovorin** 10-25mg/day PO Treat for **six weeks** or more	**pyrimethamine** 200mg loading dose followed by 75 mg/day PO + **clindamycin** 600-1200mg IV or 450mg PO 4 times/day + **leucovorin** 10-25mg/day PO
Crypto-sporidiosis	Antiretroviral therapy to reconstitute immunity	**nitazoxanide** 1000 mg twice daily for 2–8 weeks
Microsporidiosis	Antiretroviral therapy to reconstitute immunity	**albendazole** 400mg twice daily for 2–4 weeks

Opport. infect.	First-line treatment	Alternative treatment
Mycobacterium tuberculosis	First 8 weeks, directly observed therapy: **isoniazid** 5mg/kg (max 300mg) **+ rifabutin** 300mg PO qday **+ pyrizinamide** 20-25mg/kg PO qday **+ ethambutol** 15-20mg/kg PO qday Next 18 weeks: **isoniazid** 5mg/kg (max 300mg) **+ rifabutin** 300mg PO tiw	Resistant to INH: **rifamycin** + **pyrizinamide** + **ethambutol** for 6 months
Mycobacterium avium complex	**clarithromycin** 500 mg PO bid + **ethambutol** 15 mg/kg PO qday **+/- rifabutin** 300mg PO qday	**azithromycin** 500-600mg PO qday **+ ethambutol** **+/- rifabutin**
Bacterial pneumonia	**cefotaxime** 1-2g IV q8-12h **or ceftriaxone** 1-2 g IV qday **+/- azithromycin** 500mg PO qday x 1d, then 250mg PO days 2-5	Fluoroquinolone with extended activity against pneumococcus (**levofloxacin, or moxifloxacin**)
Bacterial enteritis	**ciprofloxacin** 500-750mg PO bid (or 400 mg IV bid) for 7-14 days	**azithromycin** 500mg PO qday
Bartonellosis	Non-CNS: **erythromycin** 500mg PO qid **or doxycycline** 100mg PO/IV q12h for 3 months	Non-CNS: **azithromycin** 500mg PO qday for 3 months
Syphilis	Of unknown duration without CNS involvement: **benzathine penicillin G** 2.4 million units weekly for 3 weeks	Of unknown duration without CNS involvement: **doxycycline** 100mg PO bid for 28 days
Oropharyngeal candidiasis	**fluconazole** 100mg PO daily **or itraconazole** oral solution 200mg PO daily for 7-14 days	**clotrimazole** troches 10mg PO 5 times/day for 7-14 days

Opport. infect.	First-line treatment	Alternative treatment
Esophageal candidiasis	**fluconazole** 100mg (up to 400mg) PO/IV qday x14-21 days	**voriconazole** 200mg PO/IV bid for 14-21 days
Cryptococcus meningitis	**amphotericin B** 0.7 mg/kg body weight IV qday **+/- flucytosine** 25 mg/kg PO qid for 2 weeks	**liposomal amphotericin B** 4mg/kg IV qday **and/or flucytosine** 25mg/kg PO qid for 2 weeks
Histoplasmosis	Severe disseminated disease: **amphotericin B** 0.7 mg/kg IV qday for 3-10 days followed by **itraconazole** 200mg PO bid for 12 weeks	**itraconazole** 400mg IV qday for 3-10 days followed by itraconazole oral solution 200mg po bid for 12 weeks
Coccidiomycosis	**amphotericin B** 0.5-1.0 mg/kg IV qday until there is clinical improvement (usually total dose 500-1,000mg)	**amphotericin B** 0.5-1.0 mg/kg IV qday **+ fluconazole** 400-800 mg po qday
Aspergillosis	**voriconazole** 400mg IV for 2 days, then 200mg PO bid until there is clinical response	**amphotericin B** 1.0 mg/kg IV qday
CMV retinitis	Immediate sight-threatening lesions: **ganciclovir** intraocular implant + **valganciclovir** 900 mg po qdaily	Sight not threatened: **ganciclovir** 5mg/kg IV bid for 14-21 days then 5 mg/kg qday
Herpes simplex	Orolabial lesions and initial or recurrent genital HSV: **famciclovir** 500mg PO bid **or valacyclovir** 1g PO bid **or acyclovir** 400mg PO tid for 7-14 days	**foscarnet** 120-200 mg/kg IV divided in 2-3 doses per day until there is clinical response
Varicella zoster	Local dermatomal involvement: **famciclovir** 500mg **or valacyclovir** 1g PO tid for 7-10 days	Extensive cutaneous lesions: **acyclovir** 10mg/kg IV q8h until lesions have resolved

Opport. infect.	First-line treatment	Alternative treatment
Human papillomavirus	Condyloma acuminata (genital warts) **podofilox** 0.5% solution or 0.5% gel to lesions bid x 3 days, repeat weekly for up to 4 weeks	**Liquid nitrogen** cryotherapy, repeat every 1-2 weeks for up to 3-4 times
Hepatitis C	**Peg interferon alfa-2b** (1.5 mcg/kg) subQ weekly **+ ribavirin** (wt <75kg) 400mg in am and 600mg in pm for 48 weeks in genotype 1	**Peginterferon alfa-2a** 180mcg subQ weekly **+ ribavirin**
Hepatitis B	**lamivudine** 150 mg PO bid as part of antiretroviral therapy	**adefovir** 10mg/day in addition to antiretroviral therapy

7.11 Virologic Failure

Definition	Causes	Action
- Inability to achieve a viral load <50 copies/mL by 24 weeks of treatment - Any sustained return of the viral load to >50 copies/mL	Drug resistance or failure of drugs to reach their target: - Adherence - Drug-drug interactions - Altered pharmacology	**Resistance:** Resistance testing and modifying patient's regimen **Adherence:** Pill counting, counseling, if possible reduce the dose frequency and number of pills, support groups

7.12 Diarrhea in AIDS patients

Category	Specific cause	Tests
Protozoal/fungal	Microsporidium, Cryptosporidium, Isospora, Giardia, Entamoeba, leishmaniasis, blastocystitis, Cyclospora, histoplasmosis, coccidiomycosis, candidiasis	Mulitiple stool cultures and examination for ova and parasites. >3 specimens increases the yield. Acid fast smear for Crypto, Isospora and Cyclospora. Trichrome staining for Microsporidium
Viral	CMV, HSV, adenovirus, rotavirus, Norwalk	CMV diagnosis may require endoscopy
Bacterial	Salmonella, Campylobacter, Mycobacterium avium complex (MAC), Mycobacterium tuberculosis (TB), Clostridium difficile (C. diff), Shigella, bowel bacterial overgrowth	Stool culture for bacteria C. difficile toxin assay Fungal blood cultures for MAC Endoscopy may be required if all cultures are negative
Malignancy	Lymphoma, Kaposi sarcoma	Endoscopy with biopsy may confirm the diagnosis
Pancreatic insufficiency	CMV, MAC, drug-induced (didanosine, pentamidine), tumor invasion (lymphoma, KS)	Check amylase and lipase. Try to modify patient's HAART regimen. ERCP may be required to confirm diagnosis
Idiopathic	AIDS enteropathy	Difficult to diagnose

7.13 Needle-Stick Post-Exposure Prophylaxis

Patient HIV status	Solid needle and superficial injury	Large-bore, hollow needle, deep puncture, visible blood on device
HIV + - Asymptomatic - Viral load <1500 RNA copies/ml	2-drug prophylaxis	3-drug prophylaxis
HIV + - Symptomatic - AIDS - Acute seroconversion - High viral load	3-drug prophylaxis	3-drug prophylaxis
Unknown HIV status	Generally, no post-exposure prophylaxis is advised, 2-drug prophylaxis is given if patient has HIV risk factors	Generally, no post-exposure prophylaxis is advised, 2-drug prophylaxis is given if patient has HIV risk factors
HIV-negative	No prophylaxis advised	No prophylaxis advised
Sample prophylactic regimens		
Two-drug regimens	[ZDV + 3TC] or [ZDV + FTC] or [TDF + 3TC] or [TDF + FTC]	
Three-drug regimens	[two-drug regimen + LPV/r Kaletra)] or [two-drug regimen + SQV/r or EFV]	
Duration	4 weeks	
Monitoring	Check HIV serology at baseline, 6 weeks, 12 weeks, and 6 months. Check for Hepatitis C coinfection	
Risk	Average risk of HIV seroconversion is 3/1000 with no prophylaxis. The risk is reduced 80% when post-exposure prophylaxis is given promptly	

7.14 5 Board-Style Questions

1) What vaccines are contraindicated in patients with advanced AIDS?
2) A 48-year-old man diagnosed with HIV 10 years ago, with a recent CD4 count of 320 and on HAART, has noticeable accumulation of visceral fat in the abdominal area and development of a buffalo hump. He has developed temporal wasting, insulin resistance, and worsening of his lipid profile. What is the name of this constellation of findings?
3) A 38-year-old woman with AIDS and a low CD4 count of 28 presents to the emergency department complaining of fever. She is found to have hepatosplenomegaly and transaminitis. Chest x-ray reveals enlarged hilar lymphadenopathy and multiple pulmonary nodules. This patient is a resident of Ohio. What diagnostic test will confirm the diagnosis?
4) An HIV+ man comes to your office because his partner was admitted to a local hospital with active tuberculosis. Your patient's PPD is negative. Does he require any treatment at this time?
5) A 27 year old man who works for a large multinational corporation has lived in South Africa for the past 8 years. His work requires that he travel between Europe, South Africa, and the United States. He presents to your office complaining of the abrupt onset of fever, lymphadenopathy, and a sore throat. He is otherwise in good health. He exercises regularly and eats a varied diet, low in saturated fat. On further questioning the patient reports high risk sexual behavior.
   Why is establishing the diagnosis of primary HIV infection important, and what testing should be performed at this time?

8 Infectious Diseases

8.1 Bone

Infection site/diagnosis	Usual organisms	Primary treatment
Osteomyelitis/ Adult	- *P. aeruginosa* - *Staphylococcus* - *Salmonella* - *Serratia* - *Enterococcus*	Treat based on bone and blood cultures. Generally treat with parenteral antibiotics for 4-6 weeks
Osteomyelitis/ With sickle cell anemia or thalassemia	- *Salmonella* and other G- bacilli	ciprofloxacin 400 mg IV q12h
Osteomyelitis/ Contiguous with vascular insufficiency from diabetic foot ulcer	- Polymicrobial (G+ cocci, G- bacilli and anaerobes), - Group B *Streptococcus*	Debride and obtain bone culture; revascularize if possible; give specific Abx based on cultures for 6 weeks
Osteomyelitis/Nail puncturing a tennis shoe	- *P. aeruginosa*	ciprofloxacin 400 mg IV q12h OR levofloxacin 750 mg PO qday
Osteomyelitis/ Animal bite	- *Pasteurella*	ampicillin-sulbactam 3 g IV q6h
Osteomyelitis/ Human bite	- *Eikenella*	ampicillin-sulbactam 3 g IV q6h
Osteomyelitis/Chronic > 2 weeks with presence of necrotic bone	- *S. aureus* - *Enterobacteriaceae* - *P. aeruginosa*	Empiric therapy is not indicated. Treatment based on biopsy and culture results

8.2 Breast

Infection site/diagnosis	Usual organisms	Primary treatment
Mastitis without abscess	- Non-infectious - *S. aureus* - less frequently *S. Pyogenes*, *E. coli*, *Bacteroides*, *Peptostreptococcus*	- Hot compresses - analgesics (NOT NSAIDS!) dicloxacillin 500 mg PO qid - **OR** cefalexin 500 mg PO qid x 14d

8.3 CNS

Infection site/diagnosis	Usual organisms	Primary treatment
Encephalitis/ encephalopathy	- HSV - entero/arboviruses - West Nile virus - *Listeria* - cat-scratch disease (*Bartonella*) - rabies - HIV - *Toxoplasma gondii*	**HSV or VZV**: (empiric while awaiting results of CSF PCR for HSV) acyclovir 10 mg/kg IV q8h x 14-21d **CMV, HHV6:** ganciclovir 5mg/kg IV q12h x10-14d then 5mg/kg IV qd maintenance **Listeria**: ampicillin 2 mg IV q4h + gentamicin 5mg/kg/d IV divided q8h x 3-6 weeks; or TMP-SMX 15 mg/kg/d IV divided q6h x 6 weeks
Meningitis/aseptic (pleocytosis with hundreds of cells, CSF glucose normal, gram stain negative, cultures negative)	- Viral: Enteroviruses, HSV-2, LCM, HIV, arboviruses, mumps, influenza, parainfluenza, measles, EBV, CMV, HHV-6, West Nile virus - Bacterial: Leptospirosis, Lyme, rickettsial dx, endocarditis, TB, *Brucella* - Parasites: *Toxoplasma gondii* - Other: malignancy, CNS vasculitis, CNS sarcoidosis, drug-induced, Behcet's syndrome	Supportive care for most viral causes. Exceptions: Agammaglobulinemic patients with chronic enteroviral meningitis (IVIG) **HSV-2:** acyclovir 10 mg/kg IV q8h x 10-14d **VZV meningitis** in compromised host with severe infection: acyclovir 400 mg PO bid. **Acute HIV infection:** HAART **Leptospirosis:** doxycycline 100 mg IV q12h

Infection site/diagnosis	Usual organisms	Primary treatment
Acute bacterial meningitis Gram- Age: Preterm - 1 mo	- Group B *Strep* 49% - *E. coli* 18% - *Listeria* 7% - misc Gram- 10%	ampicillin + cefotaxime
Acute bacterial meningitis Gram- Age: 1 mo - 50 yrs	- *S. pneumoniae* - *H. influenzae*	Adult dosing: cefotaxime 2 g IV q4-6h **OR** cefriaxone 2 g IV q12h + dexamethasone 0.15 mg/kg IV q6h x 2-4d + vancomycin 500-750 mg IV q6h
Acute bacterial meningitis gram- Age: > 50 yrs or EtOH abuse or impaired cellular immunity	- *S. pneumoniae* - *Listeria* - Gram- bacilli	ampicillin 2 g IV q4h + ceftriaxone 2 g IV q12h + dexamethasone 0.15 mg/kg IV q6h x 2-4d + vancomycin 500-750 mg IV q6h
Acute bacterial meningitis with gram- bacilli	- *H. influenzae* - *Coliforms* - *P. aeruginosa*	cefepime 2 g IV q8h + gentamicin 2 mg/kg loading dose then 1.7 mg/kg q8h x 10d minimum treatment
PRO for *H. influenzae* type B for household and daycare contacts	- *H. influenzae* type B	rifampin 20 mg/kg PO (not to exceed 600mg) qd x 4 doses
Prophylaxis for close contacts with *N. meningitidis*	- *N. meningitidis*	rifampin 600 mg PO q12h x 4 doses (age >1month)
Acute bacterial meningitis with gram+ diplococci	- *S. pneumoniae*	ceftriaxone 2 g IV q12h + dexamethasone 0.15 mg/kg IV q6h x 2-4d + vancomycin 500-750 mg IV q6h
Acute bacterial meningitis with gram- diplococci	- *N. meningitidis*	ceftriaxone 2 gm IV q12h + dexamethasone 0.15 mg/kg IV q6h x 7d minimum treatment
Acute bacterial meningitis with gram+ bacilli or coccobacilli	- *Listeria monocytogenes*	ampicillin 2 gm IV q4h +/- gentamicin 2 mg/kg loading dose, then 1.7 mg/kg q8h x 14-21d

8.4 Ear

Infection site/diagnosis	Usual organisms	Primary treatment
Otitis externa with intact tympanic membrane	- *Pseudomonas* - *Enterobacteriaceae* - *Proteus* - *Staphylococcus* species - *Corynebacterium* - *Candida*	Eardrops: ofloxacin 0.3% solution 10 drops bid x 7-10 days or Cortisporin Otic® (hydrocortisone +polymyxin B +neomycin) 5 gtt tid-qid x 7-10d (prescribe suspension - the solution burns)
Otitis media, with certain diagnosis based on the presence of all the following: rapid onset, signs and symptoms of middle ear inflammation, middle ear effusion.	- viral 5-48% - bacteria 55% *S. pneumoniae* *H. influenzae* *M. catarrhalis* - no pathogen 25%, - bacteria + virus 15%	amoxicillin 90 mg/kg/day divided q8h or q12h x 10d (500mg PO tid) In child <3 months decrease dose to 20-30mg/kg/day divided q12h x 10d
Otitis media, age > 6mo with non-severe illness and diagnosis not certain	- viral 5-48% - bacteria 55% *S. pneumoniae* *H. influenzae* *M. catarrhalis* - no pathogen 25% - bacteria + virus 15%	Observation alone for 3 days. If symptoms worsen, begin: amoxicillin 90 mg/kg/d divided q8h or q12h x 10d

8.5 Eye

Infection site/diagnosis	Usual organisms	Primary treatment
Viral conjunctivitis	- Adenovirus (types 3 & 7 in children, 8, 11,& 19 in adults)	No treatment. If symptomatic, cold artificial tears may help. Highly contagious. Encourage hand washing. Low threshold for referral to ophthalmologist

Infection site/diagnosis	Usual organisms	Primary treatment
Bacterial conjunctivitis- With thick, globular, purulent white/yellow/ green discharge. Eyes stuck shut in the AM.	- *H. influenza* - *N. gonorrhoeae* - *C. trachomatis* - If tender pre-auricular LN think GC/*Chlamydia*	For GC/Chlamydia treat sexual partner, evaluate for other STD; ceftriaxone 1g IM x 1 dose + azithromycin 1 g PO x 1 dose. Can add trimethoprim-polymyxin B (Polytrim) sol'n 1 gtt q3h x 7-10d
Hordeolum (Stye)	- Sterile - If bacterial, S. aureus is the most common	Warm compresses x 15 minutes qid. If it does not resolve consult ophthalmologist
Chalazion	- Inflammatory disorders	Antibiotics are not indicated

8.6 Foot

Infection site/diagnosis	Usual organisms	Primary treatment
Diabetic foot ulcers/ mild, small, pulses present	- Polymicrobic: *S. aureus, Strep* species, coliforms, anaerobes	Glucose control + TMP-SMX DS 1 tablet PO bid x 1-2 weeks
Diabetic foot ulcers/ severe, limb-threatening, fever	- Polymicrobic: *S. aureus, Strep* species, coliforms, anaerobes	Glucose control + debridement + cultures and then: piperacillin-tazobactam 3.375 g IV q6h + vancomycin 1 g IV q12h
Onychomycosis	- *Trichophyton rubrum, Trichophyton mentagrophytes*	**Topical (not curative):** ciclopirox 8% (Penlac) topically bid x 48 weeks. (5-20% response rate) **Systemic:** terbinafine (Lamisil) 250 mg PO qd x 6 weeks (fingers) or 12 weeks (toes) OR itraconazole (Sporonox) 200 mg PO qd x 8 weeks (fingernails) or 12 weeks (toenails)

8.7 Gastrointestinal

Infection site/diagnosis	Usual organisms	Primary treatment
Cholecystitis	Often inflammatory and noninfectious, if infectious often polymicrobial: - *Enterobacteriaceae* 68% - *Enterococci* 14% - *Bacteroides* 10% - *Clostridium* species 7%	Treat with surgery + antibiotics With surgery only, treat for 24-48 hours. If surgery is delayed treat for 3-5 days piperacillin-tazobactam 3.375 g IV q6h or ampicillin-sulbactam 3.0 g IV q8h or ticarcillin-clavulanate 3.1g IV q12h
Gastroenteritis/ severe diarrhea, > 6 unformed stools/day +/- temp >101F, blood or fecal leukocytes	- *Shigella* - *Salmonella* - *C. jejuni* - *E. coli 0157:H7* - *C. difficile* - *E. histolytica* - *Cryptosporidia* - *Giardia lamblia*	Empiric: ciprofloxacin 500 mg PO q12h x3-5d or levofloxacin 500 mg PO qd x 3-5d
Gastroenteritis/ traveler's diarrhea	- Enterotoxigenic *E. coli* - *Shigella* - *Salmonella* - *Campylobacter* - *C. difficile* - *Amebiasis*	azithromycin 1 g PO x 1dose

Infection site/diagnosis	Usual organisms	Primary treatment
Gastroenteritis/ Specific pathogens	- *Shigella* - *Salmonella*: only treat if severe + age>50, valve disorder, severe atherosclerosis, cancer	ciprofloxacin 500 mg PO bid x 1-3d
	- AIDS, or Uremia	ciprofloxacin 500 mg PO bid x 5-7d
	- *C. jejuni*	erythromycin 500 mg po bid x 5d
	- *Giardia lamblia*	metronidazole 250-750mg PO tid x 7-10d
	- *E. coli* (EHEC)	No antibiotic
	- *C. difficile*	Stop implicated antibiotic, give metronidazole 500 mg PO tid x 10-14d
	- *Cyclospora*	TMP-SMX DS 1 PO bid x 7-10d
	- *E. histolytica*	metronidazole 750mg PO tid x 5-10d + paromomycin 500mg PO tid x 7d
	- *Isospora*	TMP-SMX DS 1 PO bid x 7-10d
	- *Aeromonas* & *Plesiomonas* (severe or prolonged)	ciprofloxacin 500 mg PO bid x 3d

Gastroenteritis/ parasitic, > 10 days in AIDS patient	- *Cyclospora*	TMP-SMX DS tab PO qid x 10d **OR** ciprofloxacin 500 mg PO bid x 10d
	- *Isospora*	TMP-SMX DS tab PO tid x 2-4 weeks
	- *Microsporidia*	albendazole 400 mg PO bid x 2-4 weeks
	- *Giardia lamblia*	metronidazole 250mg PO tid x 5d
	- *Cryptosporidium parvum*	azithromycin 600 mg PO qd x 28d or nitazoxanide 500-1000 mg PO bid x 3d
Gastroenteritis/ anoreceptive intercourse- colitis	- *Shigella* - *Salmonella* - *Campylobacter* - *E. histolytica*	ciprofloxacin 500 mg PO bid x 3d
Diverticulitis/perirectal abscess/peritonitis	- *Enterobacteriaceae* - *P. aeruginosa* - *Bacteroides* - *Enterococci*	**Outpatient - mild:** ciprofloxacin 750 mg PO bid + metronidazole 500mg PO q6h x 7-10d **Inpatient - moderate:** piperacillin/tazobactam 3.375 g IV q6h **OR** ampicillin/sulbactam 3.0 g IV q6h **Critical - ICU:** imipenem 500 mg IV q6h
Duodenal/gastric ulcer H. pylori-related	- *H. pylori*	Three-drug regimen: Prevpac 1 dose PO bid x 14d ; Prevpac = Lansoprazole (PPI) + clarithromycin 500mg PO bid + amoxicillin 1 g PO bid (eradication 85-90%)
Thrush/Oral candidiasis	- *Candida* species	**Topical:** clotrimazole 10 mg troches 5x day x 14d **Systemic:** fluconazole 200 mg PO x 1 day followed by 100 mg PO qd x 14d

Pseudomembranous colitis	- *Clostridium difficile*	Discontinue implicated antibiotic(s) + begin metronidazole 500mg PO tid x 10d **Alternative:** vancomycin 125 mg PO qid x 10d
Whipple's disease	- *Tropheryma whipple*	**Initial 14 days:** penicillin G 1.2M U IM qd **or** streptomycin 1g IM, then **For 1-2 yrs:** TMP-SMX DS tab PO bid

8.8 Genital Tract

Infection site/diagnosis	Usual organisms	Primary treatment
Chancroid	- *Haemophilus ducreyi*	azithromycin 1 g PO x 1 dose **OR** ceftriaxone 250 mg IM x 1d dose **OR** ciprofloxacin 500 mg PO bid x 3d
Urethritis/cervicitis/ proctitis (uncomplicated)	- *N. gonorrhoeae* - *C. trachomatis* - *Mycoplasma hominis* - *Ureaplasma* - *HSV* - *Trichomonas vaginalis*	Coverage for GC and chlamydia: ceftriaxone 250 mg IM x 1 dose + azithromycin 1 g PO x 1 dose **OR** ceftriaxone 250 mg IM x 1 dose + doxycycline 100 mg PO bid x 7d
Chlamydia (non-gonococcal urethritis)	- *C. trachomatis*	azithromycin 1 g PO x 1 dose **OR** doxycycline 100 mg PO bid x 7d
Disseminated gonococcal infection	- *N. gonorrhoeae*	ceftriaxone 1 g IV/IM qd x 7d or cefotaxime 1 g IV q8 x 7d
Granuloma inguinale	- *Klebsiella granulomatis*	TMP-SMX 1 DS tab PO bid for at least 3 weeks **OR** doxycycline 100 mg PO bid for at least 3 weeks **OR** ciprofloxacin 750 mg PO bid x 3weeks
Lymphogranuloma venereum	- *C. trachomatis*	Doxycycline 100mg PO Bid x 21 days

Infection site/diagnosis	Usual organisms	Primary treatment
Pelvic inflammatory disease	- *N. gonorrhoeae* - *Chlamydia* - *Bacteroides* - *Enterobacter* - *Streptococci*	**Outpatient:** Ceftriaxone 250mg IM x1 + Doxycyline 100mg PO Bid x 14 days with or without metronidazole 500 mg PO bid x 14d **Inpatient:** clindamycin 900 mg IV q8h + gentamicin loading dose 2mg/kg IV, then 5mg/kg qd for at least 24 h; after clinical improvement change to doxycycline 100mg PO bid to complete 14 days **Alternative:** cefoxitin 2 g IV q6h + doxycycline 100 mg PO q12h After clinical improvement changed to doxycycline 100 mg PO bid to complete 14 days
Pubic lice (crabs) & scabies	- *Pthirus pubis*	permethrin 1% or 5% lotion/ shampoo. Leave in for 10min, repeat q7d PRN **OR** lindane 1% lotion or shampoo. Leave lotion in for 12h (shampoo for 4 min), repeat q7d PRN (caution: neurotoxic!) Remove nits using special comb, disinfect all clothing and linen
Prostatitis	- *E. Coli* - *Klebsiella* - *Proteus* - *Enterococci* - *Pseudomonas* - *S. aureus* - *Strep. faecalis*	TMP-SMX 1 DS tab PO bid x 3-4wks **OR** doxycycline 100 mg PO bid x 3-4wks **OR** ciprofloxacin 500 mg PO bid x 3-4wks **OR** ofloxacin 400 mg PO bid x 3-4wks + optional alpha blocker to relieve symptoms: terazosin 0.4 mg PO qd

Infection site/Diagnosis	Usual Organisms	Primary Treatment
Syphilis/early primary, secondary, or latent < 1 year	- *Treponema pallidum*	Benzathine penicillin 2.4M U IM x 1 dose **OR** tetracycline 500 mg PO qid x 14d
Syphilis/> 1 year's duration	- *Treponema pallidum*	Benzathine penicillin 2.4M U IM qweek x 3 weeks **OR** tetracycline 500 mg PO qid x 28d
Neurosyphilis	- *Treponema pallidum*	**Asymptomatic:** Aqueous benzyl / procaine penicillin G 600,000 U IV qd x 15d **Symptomatic:** Crystalline penicillin G 2-4M U IV q4h x 10-14d
Vaginosis/Bacterial	- *Gardnerella vaginalis, Lactobacillia, Ureaplasma, S. viridans*	metronidazole 500 mg PO bid x 7d **OR** clindamycin 300 mg PO bid x 7d **Intravaginal gels:** metronidazole or clindamycin 5 g qhs x7d
Vaginitis/Trichomonal	- *Trichomonas vaginalis*	metronidazole 2 g PO x 1 dose **OR** 500 mg PO bid x 7d
Vaginitis/Gonorrheal	- *Neisseria gonorrhoeae*	ceftriaxone 250 mg IM x 1 dose
Vaginitis/Vulvovaginal candidiasis	- *Candida species*	OTC intravaginal agents **or** fluconazole 150 mg PO x 1 dose
Warts, anogenital	- HPV	Podofilox 0.5% topical soln bid 3 days in one week, rpt cycle for max of 4 wks Podophyllum resin 10-25% 1-2 times/wk Tri-/dichloroacetic acids 3-4 treatments q1-2wk Cervical warts must be managed in consultation with an expert

8.9 Heart

Infection site/diagnosis	Usual organisms	Primary treatment
Infective endocarditis/ native valve awaiting cultures, non-IV/drug user	- *S. viridans* - Other Streptococci species - *Enterococci* - *Staphylococci* species	penicillin G 20M U IV qd continuous or divided q4h. + oxacillin 2.0 g IV q4h + gentamicin 1.0 mg/kg IV q8h
Infective endocarditis/ native valve, IV drug abuse	- *S. aureus*	vancomycin 1g IV q12h **+/-** gentamicin 1 mg/kg IV q8h
Infective endocarditis/ native valve, culture positive: *S. viridans* and *S. bovis*	- *S. viridans* (most common cause of subacute IE, 50-60%) - *S. bovis* (assoc. with GI malignancy) - Group B *Strep* (pregnancy, older pts with underlying disease)	**PCN-susceptible:** Aqueous crystalline PCN G 12-18M U IV qd (cont. inf. or div 4-6 doses) x 4wks **OR** ceftriaxone 2 g IV/IM qd x 4wks PCN moderate resistance: Aqueous crystalline PCN G 24M U IV qd (cont. inf or div 4-6 doses) x 4wks **OR** ceftriaxone 2g IV/IM qd x 4wks **+** gentamicin 3 mg/kg IV/IM qd x 2wks **OR** vancomycin 30 mg/kg/d div 2 doses (max 2g/d) x 4wks
Infective endocarditis/ native valve, *S. aureus*	- *S. aureus* (associated with IV drug use, indwelling catheters, aggressive, high mortality) - *S. epidermidis*	**Oxacillin-susceptible:** nafcillin/oxacillin 12 g/d div 4-6 doses x 6wks **+/-** gentamicin 3 mg/kg/d IV/IM div 2-3 doses x 3-5d **If PCN allergy:** cefazolin 6 g/d div 3 doses x 6 wks **+/-** gentamicin **Oxacillin-resistant:** vancomycin 30mg/kg/d div 2 doses (max 2 g/d) x 6wks

Infection site/diagnosis	Usual organisms	Primary treatment
Infective endocarditis/ prosthatic valve, *S. aureus*	- As above	**Oxacillin-susceptible:** nafcillin/oxacillin 12g/d div 4-6 doses x 6wks + rifampin 900 mg/d IV/PO div 3 doses x 6wks + gentamicin 3 mg/kg/d IV/IM div 2-3 doses x 2wks **Oxacillin-resistant:** vancomycin 30 mg/kg/d div 2 doses (max 2g/d) x 6wks + rifampin 900 mg/d IV/PO div 3 doses x 6wks + gentamicin 3 mg/kg/d IV/IM div 2-3 doses x 2wks
Infective endocarditis/ native OR prosthetic valve, *Enterococcus*	- *Enterococcus faecium*	**Susceptible to PCN, genta, vanco:** ampicillin 12 g/d IV div 6 doses x 4-6wks + gentamicin 3 mg/kg/d IV/IM div 2-3 doses x 4-6wks **OR** aq. crystalline PCN 18-30M U IV cont inf. or div 6 doses + gentamicin **OR** vancomycin 30 mg/kg/d div 2 doses (max 2g/d) x 6wks + gentamicin 3mg/kg/d IV/IM div 3 doses x 6wks **PCN-resistant:** If beta lactamase-producing replace ampicillin with ampicillin-sulbactam 12 g/d IV div 4 doses x 6wks **If intrinsic PCN resistance** use vancomycin + gentamicin regimen **Gentamicin resistant:** Replace genta with streptomycin 15 mg/kg/d IV/IM div 2 doses x 4-6wks **VRE:** linezolid 1200 mg/d IV/PO div 2 doses x 8wks

Infection site/diagnosis	Usual organisms	Primary treatment
Infectious endocarditis/ native OR prosthetic valve, HACEK group organisms	- HACEK group (*Haemophilus species, Actinobacillus, Cardiobacterium, Eikenella, Kingella*)	ceftriaxone 2 g IV/IM qd x 4wks **OR** ampicillin-sulbactam 12 g/d IV div 4 doses x 4 wks **OR** ciprofloxacin 1000mg/d PO or 800 mg/d IV div 2 doses x 4wks
Infectious endocarditis/ native valve, culture negative	- HACEK - *T. whippelii* - *Q fever* - *Brucellosis* - *Bartonella* - Fungi	ampicillin-sulbactam 12 g/d IV div 4 doses x 4-6 wks + gentamicin 3 mg/kg/d IV/IM div 3 doses x 4-6wks + ciprofloxacin 1000 mg/d PO or 800 mg/d IV div 2 doses x 4-6wks **If PCN allergy** replace ampicillin-sulbactam with vancomycin 30 mg/kg/d div 2 doses (max 2g/d) x 4-6wks
Infectious endocarditis/ prosthetic valve, culture negative	- As above	vancomycin 30 mg/kg/d div 2 doses (max 2g/d) x 6wks + gentamicin 3 mg/kg/d IV/IM div 3 doses x 2wks + cefepime 6 g/d IV div 3 doses x6wks + rifampin 900 mg PO/IV div 3 doses x 6wks
Infectious endocarditis/ *Bartonella*	- *Bartonella quintana*	**Suspected, culture negative:** ceftriaxone 2 g IV/IM qd x 6wks + gentamicin 3 mg/kg/d IV/IM div 3 doses x 2wks +/- doxycycline 200 mg/d PO/IV div 2 doses x 6wks **Confirmed, culture positive:** doxycycline 200 mg/d PO/IV div 2 doses x 6wks + gentamicin 3 mg/kg/d IV/IM div 3 doses x 2wks

Infection site/diagnosis	Usual organisms	Primary treatment
Pericarditis/empiric initial treatment for purulent pericarditis	- Idiopathic (majority) - Viral - Bacterial - Mycoplasma - Fungal - Post radiation - Neoplastic - Trauma - Autoimmune - Drugs - Uremia - Hypothyroidism - etc.	**Regular resistance area:** oxacillin/nafcillin 2 g IV q6h (peds: 200 mg/kg/d IV div q6h, max: 2g q6h) + cefotaxime 2.5g IV q6h (peds: 200 mg/kg/d IV q6h, max: 2.5g q6h) **High PCN resistance area:** vancomycin 500mg IV q6h (peds: 60 mg/kg/d IV div q6h, max: 4g/d) + cefotaxime 2.5 g IV q6h (peds: 200mg/kg/d IV q6h, max: 2.5g q6h) **If surgery post-op, genitourinary infection source, immunocompromised:** Add to above gentamicin 3-6 mg/kg/d IV div q8-12h (peds: 2-2.25 mg/kg IV q8h) Antibiotics are rarely necessary in pericarditis; with a purulent effusion treat according to sensitivities
Rheumatic fever	- *Strep pyogenes* (Group A beta hemolytic)	**Carditis in RF:** prednisone 2 mg/kg/d PO x 1-2 weeks +/- aspirin **For pharyngitis:** Children: penicillin V 250 mg PO 2-3 times/day x 10 days Adults: penicillin V 500 mg PO 2-3 times/day x 10 days
See also surgical interventions of infectious endocarditis (→ 220).		

8.10 Joints

Infection site/diagnosis	Usual organisms	Primary treatment
Septic arthritis, monoarticular, in a sexually active patient	- *Neisseria gonorrhoeae* (75%)	ceftriaxone 1 g IV q24h. Continue IV therapy until 24-48 hours after improvement, then switch to oral abx to complete one week: cefixime 400 mg PO bid
Septic arthritis, monoarticular in a non-sexually active patient	- *S. aureus* (80%), - *Strep pneumo* + *Strep viridans* + Group B Strep (20%)	**Gram+ cocci in synovial fluid:** vancomycin 30 mg/kg/d IV div q12h x 14d followed by PO antibiotics **Gram- bacilli in synovial fluid:** ceftazidime 1-2 g IV q8h **or** ceftriaxone 2 g IV qd **or** cefotaxime 2 g IV q8h **If Pseudomonas aeruginosa** is considered to be a likely pathogen (eg, in IVDA) add gentamicin to ceftazidime
Septic arthritis in a prosthetic joint or after joint injection	- *S. aureus*	**Step 1:** Remove prosthesis and debride **Step 2:** IV antibiotics x 6 weeks **Step 3:** Monitoring for 2-4 weeks off abx, then aspirate joint **Step 4:** If no signs of infection, replace with new hardware. **Parenteral therapy for MSSA:** nafcillin or oxacillin 2g IV q4-6h x 6 weeks. **In MRSA:** vancomycin 30 mg/kg/d IV div q12h x 6 weeks.

8.11 Lung

Infection site/diagnosis	Usual organisms	Primary treatment
Empyema/empiric tx	- Gram+ : *S. aureus* *Strep pneumo* - Anaerobes: *Bacteroides* *Peptostreptococcus* - Gram- : *Klebsiella* *Pseudomonas* *Haemophilus*	Primary therapy is drainage + antibiotics. Empiric therapy while awaiting cultures (covers most anaerobes, MSSA, G+ cocci and G- bacilli): imipenem 0.5-1 g IV q6h.
Pneumonia/age > 18, non-smoker, community acquired	- *Strep pneumo* - *H. influenzae* - *M. pneumo*	azithromycin 500 mg PO x 1 dose, then 250 mg qd x 5d
Pneumonia/age > 18, community-acquired, hospitalized	- *Strep pneumo* - *H. influenzae* - *M. pneumo* - Gram- - *Legionella*	ceftriaxone 1-2 g IV qd **OR** ampicillin-sulbactam 1.5-3g IV q6h + azithromycin 500 mg PO x 1 dose then 250 mg qd **Alternative:** levofloxacin 500 mg PO/IV qd Treat for 7-14 days
Pneumonia/ hospitalized, requiring mechanical ventilation	- *Strep pneumo* - *S. aureus* - *H. influenza* - *Legionella* - *M. pneumoniae* - *P. aeruginosa* - other Gram neg	ceftriaxone 1 g IV q12h + azithromycin 500 mg qd. **If Pseudomonas is suspected:** Start piperacillin-tazobactam 4.5 g q6h **or** imipenem 500 mg IV q6h **or** ceftazidime 2 g q8h + levofloxacin 750 mg IV qd **IF MRSA is suspected:** vancomycin 15 mg/kg q12h adjusted for renal function can be added while waiting for culture results

Infection site/diagnosis	Usual organisms	Primary treatment
Pneumonia/aspiration pneumonia	- Anaerobes: *Peptostreptococcus* *Fusobacterium nucleatum* *Prevotella* *Bacteroides*	clindamycin 600 mg IV q8h **OR** amoxicillin-clavulanate 500-875 mg PO q12h + metronidazole 1 g IV x 1 dose then 500 mg IV/PO q6h

8.12 Pancreas

Infection site/diagnosis	Usual organisms	Primary treatment
Pancreatic abscess or infected pseudocyst	- *Enterobacteriaceae* - *Enterococci* - *S. aureus* - *S. epidermidis* - Anaerobes - *Candida*	Infected pseudocyst requires operative debridement and drainage; consider antibiotic coverage (ciprofloxacin + metronidazole, or imipenem)

8.13 Peritoneum

Infection site/diagnosis	Usual organisms	Primary treatment
Spontaneous bacterial peritonitis	- *Enterobacteriaceae* - *S. pneumoniae* - *Enterococci* - Anaerobes	Life-threatening disease: cefotaxime 2 g IV q8h

8.14 Pharynx

Infection site/diagnosis	Usual organisms	Primary treatment
Pharyngitis/Exudative or diffuse erythema	- Viral 50%, group - A,C,G Strep 15% - no pathogen isolated 30%	Criteria for diagnosis are: Tonsillar exudates, tender cervical lymphadenopathy, fever, absence of cough; diagnosed if 3 of 4 are positive. If criteria are met, perform rapid strep test with reflex culture. If positive begin: penicillin V 500 mg PO bid x 10d

8.15 Sinuses

Infection site/Diagnosis	Usual Organisms	Primary Treatment
Acute rhinosinusitis (Common cold)	- Viral (rhinovirus, parainfluenza, influenza, coronavirus, adenovirus, respiratory syncytial virus) - Bacterial - Rarely fungal	Treat only when bacterial sinusitis is suspected: amoxicillin-clavulanate 875-125 mg PO q12h **or** levofloxacin 500 mg PO qd x 7-10d

8.16 Skin

Infection site/Diagnosis	Usual Organisms	Primary Treatment
Bites/Dogs, cats, rats, other mammals	- Dogs: *Staph, Strep, Eikenella, Pasteurella, Proteus, C. canimorsus* - Cats: *Pasteurella, Actinomyces, Propionibacterium*	amoxicillin-clavulanate 500/125 mg PO tid or 875/125 mg PO bid (peds: 10-15mg/kg PO tid) **OR** amoxicillin 200-500 mg PO tid (peds: 30-50 mg/kg/d div tid, max: 500 mg/dose) + cephalexin 250-500mg PO tid (peds: 25-50mg/kg/d PO qid, max: 500mg/dose)
Bites/Human	- *Staph* - *Strep* - *Eikenella* - *Bacteroides* - *Corynebacterium* - *Peptostreptococcus*	**As in animal bites or alternatives:** ceftriaxone 1 g IV/IM qday (peds: 50 mg/kg/d IV/IM qday) + ampicillin-sulbactam 1.5-3 g IV/IM q6-8h (peds: <12yo not established, >12 adult dose) Consider *C. tetani* status and administer tetanus toxoid or IG as appropriate. Consider HBV and administer HBVIG and accelerated HBV vaccinations (0,1,2 mo) if high risk Consider HIV testing

Infection site/diagnosis	Usual organisms	Primary treatment
Bites/Black widow spider	- Not infectious	Antivenom Latrodectus mactans 1 vial in 50-250 ml NS, infuse 1ml/min over 15min, complete infusion in 1hr. Watch for allergic rxn in initial minutes! Consider supportive tx with opiates, benzos, diphenhydramine as needed
Bites/Brown recluse spider	- Not infectious	dapsone 50-100 mg PO qd x 6wks (caution in G6PD!) Cold compresses slow sphingomyelinase D activity (reduces necrosis) Consider steroid use to reduce inflam.

8.17 Urinary Tract

Infection site/diagnosis	Usual organisms	Primary treatment
Urinary tract infection/ acute uncomplicated	- *Enterobacteriaceae (E. coli)* - *S. saprophyticus* - *Enterococci*	TMP-SMX DS 2 mg/kg (one DS tablet has 160 mg of TMP) bid x 3d - usually 2 tabs BID **OR** ciprofloxacin 250mg PO bid x 3 days
Urinary tract infection/ recurrent (> 3 episodes/ year) in a young woman	- *E. coli* - *Proteus* - *S. saprophyticus*	ciprofloxacin 500mg PO bid x 7d **OR** amoxicillin-clavulanate 500/125mg PO tid x 14d **OR** TMP-SMX DS tab PO tid x 14d **OR** cefuroxime 500 mg PO bid x14d
Urinary tract infection-nosocomial, inpatient	- *E. coli* - *S. aureus* - *Pseudomonas* - *E. faecalis*	ciprofloxacin 500 mg PO bid x 14d **OR** TMP-SMX DS tab PO tid x 14d **OR** piperacillin-tazobactam 4/0.5 g IV q6h **OR** ceftazidime 500 mg IV/IM q8-12h Pseudomonas is common in indwelling catheter-related UTIs

Infection site/diagnosis	Usual organisms	Primary treatment
Urinary tract infection/ child <5 years old, uncomplicated	- *E. coli* (75-90%) - *Klebsiella* - *Proteus* - *GBS* (neonates) - *S. aureus* - *S. saprophyticus*	TMP-SMX 8-10 mg/kg/d PO div bid (not recomm in infants < 2mo) **OR** cefixime 8 mg/kg/d PO div q12-24h **OR** cefotaxime 100-200 mg/kg/d IV div q6-8h (neonate: div q8-12h, use lower dose) **OR** ampicillin 100-200 mg/kg/d IV/IM div q6h (neonate: 50-150 mg/kg/d div q8-12h) + gentamicin 7.5 mg/kg/d IV div q8h (neonate: 4 mg/kg/dose q24h)
Urinary tract infection/ child <5 years old, infected shunts		vancomycin 40 mg/kg/d IV div q6-8h (neonate: 15-20 mg/kg/d q8-12h) + ceftriaxone 50-75 mg/kg/d IV/IM div q12-24h + gentamicin (as above)
Pyelonephritis/ moderately ill, outpatient	- *Enterobacteriaceae (E. coli)* - *Enterococci*	ciprofloxacin 500 mg PO bid x 7d **OR** levofloxacin 250 mg PO qd x 7d
Pyelonephritis/ hospitalized	- *E. coli* - *Enterococci*	levofloxacin 500 mg IV qd x 14d **OR** ampicillin 1-2g IV q6h + gentamicin 1mg/kg IV q8h

8.18 Special Situations

Infection site/diagnosis	Usual organisms	Primary treatment
Neutropenic fever (empiric with ANC (absolute neutrophil count) < 500/mm^3)	- Aerobic gram-bacilli - Cephalosporin-resistant *S. viridans* - MRSA - Fungal	cefepime 2 g IV q8h **or** imipenem 500 mg IV q6h **if MRSA is suspected:** + vancomycin 1g IV q12h If no resolution after 4 days of broad spectrum antibiotics begin empiric fungal treatment, add: amphotericin B 3 mg/kg/d IV
Endocarditis Prophylaxis	-	Please see (→ 75)

8.19 Sepsis of Unknown Origin

Antibiotic Therapy in Sepsis of Unknown Origin – Pseudomonas Unlikely	
1 of the following:	
Cephalosporin 3rd/4th gen:	
ceftriaxone (Rocephin)	2 g IV daily
cefotaxime (Claforan)	2 g IV every 4 hours
OR	
β-lactam/β-lactamase inhibitor:	
piperacillin-tazobactam (Zosyn)	3.375 g IV every 6 hours x 7-10 days
ticarcillin-clavulanate (Timentin)	3.1 g IV every 4-6 hours (max 24 g/day)
OR	
Carbapenem:	
imipenem (Primaxin)	500-1000 mg IV every 6-8 hours (max 4 g/day or 50 mg/kg/day)
meropenem (Merrem)	1.5-3 g/day div every 8 hours
PLUS 1 of the following:	
vancomycin (Vancocin)	30-60 mg/kg/day IV div every 8-12 hours HAP, VAP: 15 mg/kg IV every 12 hours
OR	
linezolid (Zyvox)	600 mg IV every 12 hours
Adapted from Schmidt GA, Mandel Jess. Management of severe sepsis and septic shock. UpToDate Online v. 18.2. Accessed November 1st, 2010.	

Antibiotic Therapy in Sepsis of Unknown Origin – Pseudomonas Likely	
2 of the following:	
Antipseudomonal cephalosporin:	
ceftazidime (Fortaz, Tazicef)	30-50 mg/kg IV every 8 hours
cefepime (Maxipime)	1-2 g IV every 8-12 hours
OR	
Antipseudomonal β-lactam/β-lactamase inhibitor:	
piperacillin-taxobactam (Zosyn)	3.375 g IV every 6 hours x 7-10 days
ticarcillin-clavulanate (Timentin)	3.1 g IV every 4-6 hours (max 24 g/day)
OR	
Carbapenem:	
imipenem (Primaxin)	500-1000 mg IV every 6-8 hours (max 4 g/day or 50 mg/kg/day)
meropenem (Merrem)	1.5-3 g/day div every 8 hours
OR	
Antipseudomonal fluoroquinolone:	
ciprofloxacin (Cipro, Ciloxan, Cetraxal)	400 mg IV every 8-12 hours
OR	
Aminoglycocide:	
gentamicin	1-2.5 mg/kg/dose IV every 8-12 hours
amikacin	5-7.5 mg/kg/dose IV every 8 hours
OR	
Monobactam:	
aztreonam (Azectam, Cayston)	2 g IV every 6-8 hours (max 8 g/day)
PLUS 1 of the following:	
vancomycin (Vancocin)	30-60 mg/kg/day IV div every 8-12 hours HAP, VAP: 15 mg/kg IV every 12 hours
OR	
linezolid (Zyvox)	600 mg IV every 12 hours
Adapted from Schmidt GA, Mandel Jess. Management of severe sepsis and septic shock. UpToDate Online v. 18.2. Accessed November 1st, 2010.	

8.20 Pneumonia Severity Index – Risk Stratification

Step I in Risk Stratification

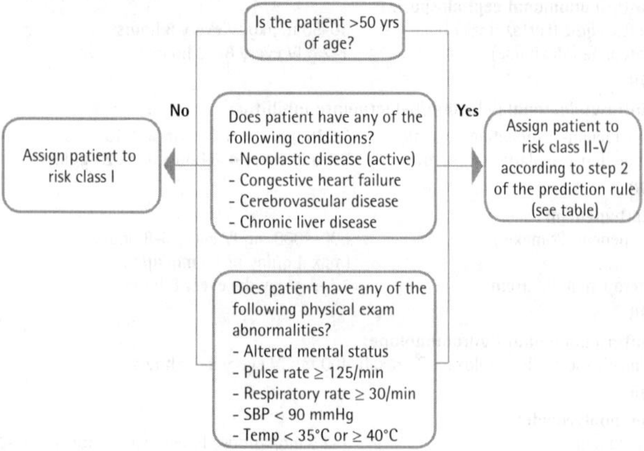

→ If patient is not in class I, proceed to step II.

Step II in Risk Stratification (Assignment to Classes II, III, IV, or V)	
Characteristic	**Points Assigned**
Demographic Factor	
Men	Age (yr)
Women	Age (yr) - 10
Nursing home Resident	+ 10
Coexisting illnesses	
Neoplastic disease	+ 30
Liver disease	+ 20
Congestive heart failure	+ 10
Cerebrovascular disease	+ 10
Renal Disease	+ 10
Physical examination findings	
Altered mental status	+ 20
Respiratory rate > 30/min	+ 20
Systolic BP < 90 mmHg	+ 20
Temperature < 35° C or > 40°C	+ 15
Pulse > 125/min	+ 10
Laboratory and radiographic findings	
Arterial pH < 7.35	+ 30
Blood urea nitrogen > 30 mg/dl (11 mmol/l)	+ 20
Sodium < 130 mmol/l	+ 20
Glucose > 250 mg/dl (14 mmol/l)	+ 10
Hematocrit < 30%	+ 10
Partial pressure of arterial oxygen < 60 mmHg	+ 10
Pleural Effusion	+ 10
Source: Fine MJ, Auble TE, Yealy DM, et al. N Engl J Med 1997; 336:243.	

Interpretation		
Pneumonia class	**Score**	**Management***
I	N/A	Outpatient therapy
II	≤ 70	Outpatient therapy
III	71 - 90	Brief observation and outpatient therapy
IV	91 - 130	Inpatient care
V	> 130	Inpatient care
*If patients are hypoxic in any class, they should be admitted for observation.		

8.21 Surgical Intervention for Infectious Endocarditis

Indications for surgery	- Moderate to severe CHF - Unstable prosthesis - Paravalvular extension - Persistent bacteremia despite optimal antibiotic treatment - Certain organisms (fungi, *P. aeruginosa*, *S. aureus*) - Relapse - Embolic events during 1st 2 weeks
Relative surgical indications	- Vegetations >10mm - Culture-negative prosthetic valve endocarditis (PVE) with unexplained fever >10d
Surgical timing	- Timing of surgery depends on optimization of hemodynamic status prior to surgery, not sterilization of blood cultures or duration of antibiotic therapy - Low risk of infecting new valve, some prefer bioprostheses

8.22 Bibliography

1) IDSA guidelines-Practice Guidelines for Management of Bacterial Meningitis

2) IDSA Practice Guidelines for Infectious Diarrhea

3) Clinical Practice Guidelines for Clostridium difficile Infection in Adults: 2010 Update by the Society for Healthcare Epidemiology of America (SHEA) and the Infectious Diseases Society of America (IDSA). Infection Control and Hospital Epidemiology. 2010; 31:431-455

4) Fenollar F, Puéchal X, Raoult Didier. Whipple's Disease. N Engl J Med. 2007; 356:55-66

5) CDC 2010 STD Treatment Guidelines on Genital Ulcers

6) IDSA/American Thoracic Society Consensus Guidelines on Management of CAP in Adults

8.23 5 Board-Style Questions

1) A 28-year-old woman is pregnant and found to have gonococcal urethritis on culture. What treatment should she receive, if any?

2) A surgical intern has a needle stick while drawing blood from an HIV+ patient. The needle was a hollow-bore "butterfly." There was blood from the patient on the needle when it punctured her glove. It is now 11pm. What should the intern do?

   a) Finish her shift, and first thing in the morning, when the personnel health office opens, go for evaluation, blood testing, and prophylaxis with HAART for 1 month.
   b) Hollow-bore needles do not require prophylaxis
   c) Report immediately to the ER for evaluation
   d) The chances of transmitting HIV are low enough in this case that no prophylaxis is necessary

3) An IV drug abuser is admitted with high temperature and a new heart murmur. What antibiotics should she be started on, if any, while awaiting culture results?

4) A 50-year-old man became ill while fixing up a house he recently purchased in Hawaii. The house was "a mess" and the man reports exposure to a mattress that was saturated with rat feces and urine. About 10 days after returning from Hawaii he reported the onset of fever, rigors, myalgias and headache. He reported to the nearest emergency department. What tests would confirm your suspected diagnosis in this patient?

5) A 55-year-old woman with diabetes mellitus type 2 who has been receiving immunosuppressive chemotherapy for breast cancer presents with acute sinusitis, fever, nasal stuffiness, and a purulent nasal discharge that has become bloody, and periorbital swelling. Nasal cultures are sent from the ER. ENT is consulted for endoscopic evaluation and for a possible biopsy. Based on the presentation of this patient, what treatment should be considered?

9 Internal Medicine

9.1 Preventive Medicine

9.1.1 US mortality (2009) vs worldwide mortality (2004) in all ages

US		World	
Rank	**Cause**	**Rank**	**Cause**
1	Heart disease	1	Heart disease
2	Cancer	2	Cerebrovascular disease
3	Chronic lower respiratory disease	3	Lower respiratory infections
4	Cerebrovascular disease	4	Chronic obstructive pulmonary disease
5	Accidents (unintentional injuries)	5	Diarrheal diseases
6	Alzheimer's disease	6	HIV/AIDS
7	Diabetes mellitus	7	Tuberculosis
8	Influenza and pneumonia	8	Trachea, bronchus, lung cancer
9	Nephritis, nephrotic syndrome	9	Road traffic accidents
10	Suicide	10	Prematurity and low birth weight
National Vital Statistics Report ,vol 59, number 4, March 2011, CDC		World Health Organization Fact sheet - The Top 10 Causes of Death 2004	

9.1.2 Levels of prevention

Primary prevention	Preventing disease from occurring (eg, fluoride in public water to prevent cavities).
Secondary prevention	Detection of disease at an early or asymptomatic stage where treatment can be effective (eg, Pap smears for cervical cancer).
Tertiary prevention	Prevention of complications or further progression of an established disease. (eg, ACE inhibitors for patients with congestive heart failure).

9.1.3 Screening tests

Characteristics of good screening tests	- High sensitivity - Specificity high enough to reduce the number of false positive tests - High positive predictive value
Ease and cost	Inexpensive and noninvasive
Safety	Must be safe, especially when screening a healthy population.
Acceptability/labeling	An uncomfortable test may be avoided

9.1.4 Exercise

Guidelines from the American Heart Association and the American College of Sports Medicine recommend either moderate intensity exercise for 30 minutes for a minimum of five days a week, or strenuous exercise for 20 minutes three days a week

Evidence Supporting Benefits of Exercise

Additional life expectancy[1]	- Moderate activity: 1.3 years - High activity: 3.5 years
Additional time without cardiac events[1]	- Moderate activity: 1.1 years - High activity: 3.2 years
VO_2 max[2]	Improved with hard intensity (65-75% maximal HR) + high frequency (5-7 days/week), hard intensity + low frequency (3-4 days/week), and moderate intensity (45-55% maximal HR) + high frequency. Greatest improvement seen in hard intensity + high frequency group
HDL-C[2]	Hard intensity + high frequency improved HDL compared with control group at 6 months
TC/HDL[2]	No statistically significant change

[1] Franco OH, de Laet C, Peeters A et al. Effects of physical activity on life expectancy with cardiovascular disease Archives of Internal Medicine 2005; 165:2355-2360.
[2] Duncan GE, Anton SD, Sydeman SJ et al. Prescribing exercise at varied levels of intensity and frequency, a randomized trial. Archives of Internal Medicine 2005; 165:2362-2369.
TC = Total cholesterol; HDL = High density lipoprotein; VO_2 max = Maximal oxygen consumption

9.1.5 Who needs a stress test before beginning an exercise program

Asymptomatic patients with diabetes or chronic kidney disease
Patients with multiple risk factors:
-Cigarette smoking -Hypertension (BP > 140/90 or on antihypertensive medication) -Low HDL cholesterol (< 40 mg/dl) -Family history of premature CHD (male 1st-degree relative <55, female <65) -Age (men >45, women >55)
Patients with electron beam CT results >75th percentile
Gibbons RJ, Balady GJ, Timothy Bricker J, et al. ACC/AHA 2002 guideline update for exercise testing: summary article. A report of the American College of Cardiology/American Heart Association Task Force on Practice Guidelines (Committee to Update the 1997 Exercise Testing Guidelines). Journal of the American College of Cardiology 2002; 40:1531.

9.2 Adult Vaccinations

9.2.1 Recommended annual vaccinations 2012

Vaccine	Age group (years)					
	19-21	22-26	27-49	50-59	60-64	>65
Influenza	1 dose annually					
Td/Tdap	Substitute 1 time-dose of Tdap for Td booster: then boost with Td every 10 years					Td/Tdap*
Varicella	2 doses					
HPV female	3 doses					
HPV male	3 doses					
Zoster					1 dose	
MMR	1 or 2 doses			1 dose		
PPSV	1 or 2 doses					1 dose
Meningococcal	1 or more doses					
Hepatitis A	2 doses					
Hepatitis B	3 doses					

Color Key

(light shading)	For all persons in this category who meet the age requirements and who lack evidence of immunity (eg, lack documentation of vaccination or have no evidence of previous infection)
(dark shading)	Recommended if some other risk factor is present (eg, based on medical, occupational, lifestyle, or other indications)
(white)	No recommendations

*In adults ≥65 years if contact with <12 month old child. Either Td or Tdap can be used if no infant contact.
Td/Tdap=tetanus, diphtheria, pertussis; HPV=human papilloma virus; PPSV=pneumococcal polysaccharide vaccine
For up-to-date adult immunization schedules from the CDC go to: http://www.cdc.gov/vaccines/schedules/downloads/adult/adult-schedule.pdf

Vaccines that might be indicated for adults based on medical and other indications					
Indication / Vaccine	Pregnancy	Imm. comp. conditions	HIV infection CD4 T cell count		Men who have sex with men (MSM)
			<200 cells/μL	≥200 cells/μL	
Influenza	1 dose TIV annually				1 dose TIV or AIV annually
Td/Tdap	Substitute 1 time dose of Tdap for Td booster; then boost with Td every 10 yrs				
Varicella	Contraindicated			2 doses	
HPV (female)	3 doses through age 26				
HPV (male)					
Zoster	Contraindicated			1 dose	
MMR	Contraindicated			1 or 2 doses	
PPSV		1 or 2 doses			
Meningococcal	1 or more doses				
HAV	2 doses				
HBV			3 doses		

Color key	
(light shading)	For all persons in this category who meet the age requirements and who lack documentation of vaccination or have no evidence of previous infection
(dark shading)	Recommended if some other risk factor is present (eg, on the basis of medical, occupational, lifestyle, or other indications)
(white)	No recommendations

Vaccines that might be indicated for adults based on medical and other indications (cont.)

Indication / Vaccine	Heart Deasease, CLD, Chronic alcoholism	Asplenia*	Chr. liver disease	RF, DM ESRD, on hemodialysis	Health care personnel
Influenza	1 dose TIV annually				1 dose TIV or LAIV annually
Td/Tdap	Substitute 1 time dose of Tdap for Td booster; then boost with Td every 10 yrs				
Varicella	2 doses				
HPV (female)	3 doses through age 26 yrs				
HPV (male)	3 doses through age 21 yrs				
Zoster	1 dose				
MMR	1 or 2 doses				
PPSV	1 or 2 doses				
Meningococcal	1 or more doses				
HAV	2 doses				
HBV	3 doses				

Color key

- (light) For all persons in this category who meet the age requirements and who lack documentation of vaccination or have no evidence of previous infection
- (dark) Recommended if some other risk factor is present (eg, on the basis of medical, occupational, lifestyle, or other indications)

Adult Vaccinations Footnotes

1) Administer a one-time dose of Tdap to adults aged less than 65 years who have not received Tdap previously or for whom vaccine status is unknown to replace one of the 10-year Td boosters, and as soon as feasible to all postpartum women, close contacts of infants younger than age 12 months and healthcare personnel with direct patient contact
2) All adults without evidence of immunity to varicella should receive 2 doses of varicella vaccine; special consideration should be given to those with some high-risk factor. The second dose should be given 4-8 weeks after the first dose
3) HPV vaccination is recommended for all women age $\leq$ 26 years who have not completed the vaccine series; a complete series consists of 3 doses; the second dose should be administered 1-2 months after first dose; the third dose should be administered 6 months after the first dose
4) A single dose of zoster vaccine is recommended for adults aged 60 years and older regardless of whether they report a previous episode of herpes zoster
5) Revaccination with PPV: one-time revac. after 5 years for persons with chronic renal failure or nephrotic syndrome; funct. or anatomic asplenia; immunosuppressive conditions. For persons aged $\geq$ 65 years, one-time revaccination if they were vaccinated $\geq$ 5 years previously and were aged < 65 years at the time of primary vaccination
6) Meningococcal conjugate vaccine is preferred for adults with risk factors and aged [55 years, although MPSV4 is an acceptable alternative. Revaccination after 5 years might be indicated for adults previously vaccinated with MPSV4 who remain at high risk for infection.
7) Hep A vaccine should be administered in a 2-dose schedule at either 0, 6-12 months or 0, 6-18 months. If the combined HepA and HepB vaccine is used, administer 3 doses at 0, 1 and 6 months

Approved by the Advisory Committee on Immunization Practices; the American College of Obstetricians and Gynecologists, the American Academy of Family Physicians and the American College of Physicians.
Source: US Centers for Disease Control

9.2.2 Contraindications to vaccines

Condition	Revaccination to be avoided
Allergy to eggs or egg protein	Avoid measles, mumps, influenza, and yellow fever vaccines. They are prepared in embryonated chicken eggs or culture and vaccines may contain residual egg protein
Allergy to neomycin or streptomycin	Avoid MMR vaccine because it contains trace amounts of neomycin
Immunocompromised host	Avoid live vaccines: oral polio, MMR, varicella zoster vaccine, yellow fever
Household members of immunocompromised host	Avoid oral polio. MMR is safe
Pregnant women	Avoid all live virus vaccines because of the potential risk to the fetus

Recent or current mild illness with or without a fever is not a contraindication for vaccination.

9.2.3 Influenza treatment and prophylaxis

Antiviral agent	Treatment	Prophylaxis*
Zanamivir (Relenza)	10 mg (2 inhalations) bid x 5 days	10 mg (2 inhalations) daily
Oseltamivir (Tamiflu)	75 mg po daily x 5 days **	75 mg po daily

* Duration of prophylaxis is 10 days after a household exposure, 7 days otherwise. For outbreaks in long term care facilities - min 2 weeks and continue up to 1 week after the most recent known case was identified

**Reduction in dose is recommended for Cr Cl <30

Source: CDC - Antiviral Agents for the Treatment and Chemoprophylaxis of Influenza - Recommendations of the ACIP. MMWR Rec and Reports Jan 2011, 60;1-24

9.3 Smoking

Risks of Cigarette Smoking: Estimated 5 million Premature Deaths Worldwide in 2000	
COPD	10-15% of smokers develop obstruction. Increased risk with alpha-1-antitrypsin deficiency
Lung cancer	Estimated 87% of lung cancers are caused by cigarettes, i.e. 162,500 deaths in 2006
Other cancer	Oral cavity, larynx, esophagus, bladder, kidney, pancreas, stomach, and cervix
Cardiovascular effects	2-4x greater incidence of coronary heart disease and sudden cardiac death Almost twofold risk of stroke compared with nonsmokers
Reproductive disorders	Infertility, premature menopause, decreased birth weight and length, increased risk of spontaneous abortions and complications (abruption, PROM, placenta previa)
Peptic ulcer disease	Major contributing factor
Osteoporosis	Accelerates bone loss and is a risk factor for hip fracture in women
Overall life expectancy	Heavy smoker at age 25 can expect a life expectancy at least 25% shorter than a nonsmoker

9.3.1 Smoking cessation recommendations

Strategy 1: Ask	Ask every patient at every visit about tobacco use
Strategy 2: Advise	Strongly urge all smokers to quit
Strategy 3: Assess	Ask every smoker if they are willing to quit at this time
Strategy 4: Assist	Help formulate a plan, encourage nicotine replacement or bupropion, provide advice and supplementary materials
Strategy 5: Arrange follow up	Schedule follow up in person or via telephone

Adapted from: Fiore et al. Treating Tobacco Use and Dependence. Quick Reference Guide for Clinicians. Rockville, MD: US Department of Health and Human Services. Public Health Service. October 2000.

9.4 Diet and Nutrition Health Effects

9.4.1 Preventive care screening in healthy adults (adapted from the U.S. Preventive Services Task Force)

Colorectal cancer	50 - 75 years old men and women
Breast cancer	Mammogram every 1- 2 years in all women over 40. BRCA testing in high risk women
Cervical cancer	Every 3 years until age 65 years
Osteoporosis	Bone mineral density test in women ≥ 65 and at risk women 60-64 years old
AAA	Abdominal US one time in men 65-75 years who have ever smoked
Dyslipidemia	Total and HDL cholesterol in men ≥ 35 years; men or women ≥ 20 years who have cardiovascular risk factors. Check q 5 yrs if normal
Diabetes	In patients with HTN

9.4.2 Dietary recommendations

Balanced calories	• Enjoy food, but eat less • Avoid oversized portions
Foods to increase	• Half of the plate should contain fruits and vegetables • Half the grains should be whole grains • Switch to fat-free or low fat (1%) milk
Foods to reduce	• **Sodium:** Choose foods with low sodium: limit intake to max 2,300 mg daily and to max 1,500 mg daily if age > 51 years, or person is African American or has hypertension, diabetes, or chronic kidney disease • **Saturated fats:** Replace with monounsaturated and polyunsaturated fatty acids (use oils to replace solid fats) • **Cholesterol:** Consume less than 300 mg per day of dietary cholesterol • **Sugar:** Drink water instead of sugary drinks • **Alcohol:** Limit alcohol to 1 drink per day for women and 2 drinks per day for men
Adapted from USDA and HHS 2010 Dietary Guidelines for Americans.	

9.5 Obesity

9.5.1 BMI scale

Body Mass Index (BMI) = Weight (Kg) / Height $(m)^2$	
Weight range	**BMI (kg/m^2)**
Normal	<25
Overweight	25-29.9
Obese	>30
Severe or morbid obesity	>40 (>35 in the presence of comorbidities)

Sample BMI Chart

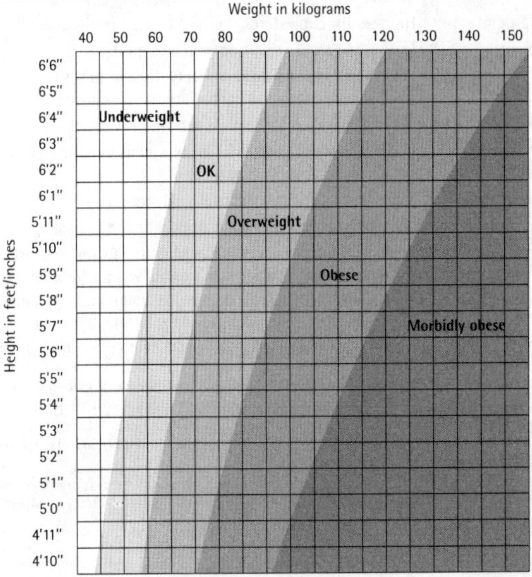

9.5.2 Health risk associated with obesity

Risk	Data
Mortality[1]	• Obese (BMI > 30 kg/m^2) at age 40 → life expectancy shortened by 6-7 years • Overweight (BMI 25 to 29.9 km/m^2) at age 40 → life expectancy shortened by approximately 3 years • Obese+smokers lived 13 to 14 years less than normal-weight nonsmokers
Hypertension[2]	Up to 50% prevalence of HTN in obese patients
Diabetes[3]	> 80% of cases of type II diabetes mellitus can be attributed to obesity
Dyslipidemia	High serum cholesterol, ↑LDL, ↑VLDL, ↑triglycerides, ↓HDL
Gout	Increased risk of hyperuricemia and gout
Heart disease	Increased risks of coronary artery disease, heart failure, atrial fibrillation/flutter, and cardiovascular all-cause mortality
Stroke	Increasing BMI is associated with increased risk of stroke
Hepatobiliary disease	Increased risk of cholelithiasis as well as hepatic steatosis and nonalcoholic fatty liver disease
Osteoarthritis	Most commonly in knees and ankle joints
Sleep apnea	Associated with significant morbidity and mortality
Cancer[4]	Both men and women with a BMI >40 had a higher risk of death from cancer than those with normal weight (relative risk 1.5-1.6). Cancers included: esophagus, colorectal, liver, gallbladder, pancreas, kidney, lymphoma, and multiple myeloma.

[1] Peeters A; Barendregt JJ, Willekens F. Obesity in adulthood and its consequences for life expectancy: a life-table analysis. Annals of Internal Medicine 2003 Jan 7;138(1):24-32.
[2] Sjostrom CD, Lissner L, Wedel H, Sjostrom L. Reduction in incidence of diabetes, hypertension and lipid disturbances after intentional weight loss induced by bariatric surgery: the SOS Intervention Study. Obes Res 1999; 7:477.
[3] Bray GA. Historical framework for the development of ideas about obesity. Handbook of obesity, Marcel Dekker, Inc, New York 1997.
[4] Calle EE, Rodriguez C, Walker-Thurmond K, Thun MJ. Overweight, obesity, and mortality from cancer in a prospectively studied cohort of U.S. adults. New England Journal of Medicine 2003; 348:1625.

9.5.3 Approach to treating obesity

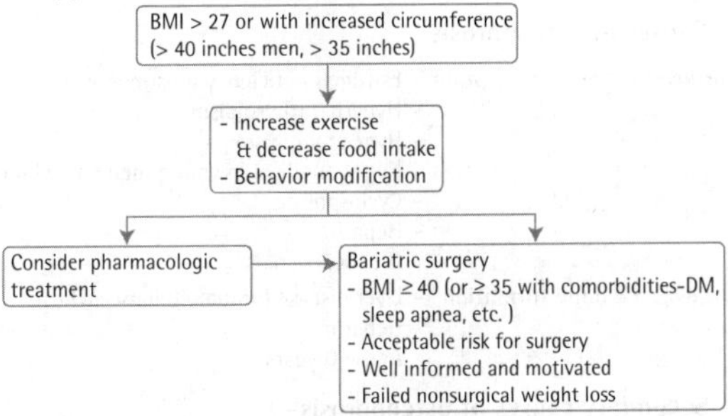

9.5.4 Drug therapy for treating obesity

Treatment should be undertaken when BMI ≥ 30 or ≥ 27 with comorbidities.

Medication	Side effects
orlistat (Xenical)	Intestinal borborygmi, cramps, flatus, fecal incontinence, oily spotting
benzphetamine (Didrex)	Hypertension, tachycardia, arrhythmias, palpitations, chest pain, T wave changes, CHF, stroke (should avoid in patients with CAD).
phendimetrazine (Bontril)	Hypertension, tachycardia, arrhythmias, CHF, or stroke (should avoid in patients with CAD).
diethylproprion (Tenuate)	Only approved for use <12 weeks due to potential for abuse
phentermine (Adipex)	Only approved for use <12 weeks due to potential for abuse

9.6 Osteoporosis

9.6.1 Causes of osteoporosis

High Turnover – ↑bone resorption	- Estrogen deficiency (postmenopausal) - Hyperparathyroidism - Hyperthyroidism - Hypogonadism in young men and women - Cyclosporine - Heparin - Glucocorticoids
Low Turnover – ↓bone formation	- Liver disease (primary biliary cirrhosis) - Heparin - Age>50 years

9.6.2 Secondary causes of osteoporosis

Endocrine disorders	- Hypogonadism - Hyperparathyroidism
Gastrointestinal disease	- Alcohol - Celiac disease - Severe liver disease - Inflammatory bowel disease
Marrow-related disorders	- Hemochromatosis - Multiple myeloma - Lymphoma
Organ transplantation	- Bone marrow - Solid organ
Genetic causes	- Hypophosphatasia - Osteogenesis imperfecta - Homocystinuria
Miscellaneous causes	- Ankylosing spondylitis - COPD - RA - Hemophilia

9.6.3 Bone density definitions (measured by DEXA scan)

Normal	Bone mineral density (BMD) within 1 standard deviation of the young adult reference mean
Osteopenia	1-2.5 standard deviations below the mean BMD
Osteoporosis	>2.5 standard deviations below the mean BMD
Severe (established) osteoporosis	Osteoporosis + one or more fragility fractures

9.6.4 Management of osteoporosis

Nonpharmacologic therapy	- Diet, exercise, and smoking/alcohol cessation - Calcium + vitamin D supplementation
Pharmacologic therapy	- Bisphosphonates (alendronate, risedronate) are first-line treatment - Selective estrogen receptor modulators (raloxifene) - PTH (teriparatide) - Calcitonin - Estrogens

9.7 4 Board-Style Questions

1) A 16-year-old ballerina reports long-standing chest pain. Pain is worse with eating. Examination reveals erosion of the dental enamel and red lesions over the MCP joints of the left hand. What is the cause of this patient's chest pain?

2) A 58-year-old man was started on lovastatin approximately 4 weeks ago. He now presents to your office with myalgias and weakness in the lower extremities. What should be done for this patient?

3) A patient with AIDS presents to your office after exposure to someone with measles. What should be done for this patient?

4) A 72-year-old woman presents with sudden vision loss in the left eye. ESR is 103. What is the next step in this patient's management?

10 Women's Health and Pregnancy

10.1 Pregnancy

10.1.1 Pregnancy definitions

1st trimester	From first day of last menstrual period through week 12
2nd trimester	From 13th to the 27th week of gestation
3rd trimester	From 28th week of gestation to delivery

10.1.2 Obstetric notation

A woman's obstetric history is indicated by the GP (gravida/para) shorthand notation. The complete notation is illustrated in the table below using G4P3113 as an example:

G	4	4 total prior pregnancies
P	3	3 live births
	1	1 preterm birth
	1	1 miscarriage
	3	3 living children
This is also often expressed as using the GPA notation where G=total pregnancies, P=live births, and A=abortions/miscarriages; eg, G4P3A1=4 pregnancies, 3 live births, 1 miscariage		

10.1.3 Gestational milestones

Weeks	Findings
1	Beta-HCG positive
12	Uterine fundus palpable at the pubic symphysis Doppler ultrasound of fetal heart rate
16	First fetal movements
17-20	Fetoscope hears fetal heart rate
18	Baby's sex can be determined by ultrasound
20	Uterine fundus palpable at umbilicus
38-42	Infant is full-term

10.1.4 Prenatal care

Keys to prenatal social and demographic assessment	- Names of patient, partner, emergency contact - Marital status - Age - Home address - Telephone numbers for day, night, emergency - Education	- Occupation - Partner's name and occupation - Pediatrician - Primary care physician - Hospital for delivery - Religion (Jehovah's witness?)
Keys to prenatal assessment of past obstetric history	- Date of delivery - Gestational age at delivery - Location of delivery - Sex of child - Birth weight - Mode of delivery - Type of anesthesia	- Length of labor - Outcome (miscarriage, stillbirth, ectopic, etc.) - Details (eg, type of cesarean section scar, forceps, etc.) - Complications (maternal, fetal, child)
Menstrual history	- Last menstrual period (definite or uncertain?) - Last normal menstrual period	- Cycle length - Method and compliance with contraception - Age of menarche
Current pregnancy history	- Medications - Alcohol/cigarette/illicit drug use - Vaginal bleeding - Nausea, vomiting, weight loss	- Infections - Exposure to toxic substances or radiation
Key prenatal labs	- Blood type and antibody screen - Rhesus type - Hematocrit or hemoglobin - PAP smear if due - Rubella status (immune or nonimmune)	- Syphilis screen - Urinary infection screen - Hepatitis B surface antigen - HIV counseling and testing - Chlamydia - Thyroid function

Prenatal assessment of gestational age	**1. Naegele's Rule:** Expected date of delivery (EDD) = Add one year to last menstrual period (LMP), subtract three months from that date, then add 7 days. EDD = LMP + 1 YR - 3 MO + 7 DAYS	
	2. Physical exam	
	Week of pregnancy	**Size of pregnant uterus**
	6-8	Small pear
	8-10	Orange
	10-12	Grapefruit
	12	Palpable above pubic symphysis
	16	Fundus palpable midway between pubic symphysis and umbilicus
	3. Sonographic assessment of fetal age	
	Gestational age (wks)	**Parameter used in assessment**
	4-6	Mean sac diameter
	7-14	Crown-rump length
	14-20	Biparietal diameter (BPD), head circumference (HC), femur length (FL)
	Hadlock formula Used to estimate fetal weight; usually automatically calculated by ultrasound machine: $\log_{10} BW = 1.4787 + 0.001837 (BPD)^2 + 0.0458 (AC) + 0.158 (FL) - 0.003343 (AC \times FL)$ AC: abdominal circumference; BW: body weight (fetus)	
Anatomical signs of fetal maturity	**Week of pregnancy (wks)**	**Finding**
	32-35	Femoral epiphyseal and proximal tibial ossification centers well visualized
		Proximal humeral epiphysis correlates with lung maturity

10.1.5 Gestational diabetes

Criteria for GDM diagnosis based on glucose tolerance testing	
1-Step Method	**2-step Method**
100 g OGTT (need 2/4 positive tests)	**Step 1**
Fasting ≥95 mg/dL 1 hour ≥180 mg/dL 2 hour ≥155 mg/dL 3 hour ≥140 mg/dL, or	50 gram OGTT Fasting ≥95 mg/dL 1 hour ≥130 mg/dL if 1 abnormal, then perform step 2 **Step 2**
If 75 gram (need 2/3 positive tests)	100 gram OGTT
Fasting ≥95 mg/dL 1 hour ≥180 mg/dL 2 hour ≥155 mg/dL	Fasting ≥95 mg/dL 1 hour ≥180 mg/dL 2 hour ≥155 mg/dL 3 hour ≥140 mg/dL

Glycemic thresholds for pregnancy	
ADA	**ACOG**
Fasting ≤95 mg/dL	Fasting ≤95 mg/dL
1 hour postprandial ≤140 mg/dL 2 hour postprandial ≤120 mg/dL	1 hour postprandial ≤130 mg/dL

10.1.6 HELLP syndrome criteria

Hemolysis	Microangiopathic hemolytic anemia with characteristic schistocytes (also called helmet cells) on blood smear Other signs suggestive of hemolysis include an elevated indirect bilirubin and a low serum haptoglobin concentration (≤25 mg/dL).
Elevated Liver enzymes	Serum AST ≥70 IU/L.* Total bilirubin ≥1.2 mg/dL
Low platelets	Platelet count ≤100,000 cells/microL

ALT may be used instead of, or in addition to, AST levels, but an advantage of AST is that it reflects both hepatocellular necrosis and red cell hemolysis.
Adapted from Sibai BM, Ramadan MK, et al. Maternal morbidity and mortality in 442 pregnancies with hemolysis, elevated liver enzymes, and low platelets (HELLP syndrome). Am J Obstet Gynecol. 1993;169(4):1000.

10.1.7 Preeclampsia and eclampsia

Criteria for the diagnosis of preeclampsia	
Systolic blood pressure	$\geq$ 140 mmHg **OR**
Diastolic blood pressure	$\geq$ 90 mmHg[1] **AND**
Proteinuria	$\geq$0.3 grams of protein in a 24-hour urine specimen[2]

The elevation in blood pressure should be sustained, which is generally regarded as 2 measurements at least 6 hours, but no more than 7 days apart.

Eclampsia = preeclampsia + seizures

[1] Diastolic blood pressure is determined based upon the fifth Korotkoff sound (disappearance) with patient sitting.
[2] A random urine protein determination of 30 mg/dl or 1+ on dipstick is suggestive, but not diagnostic, of the presence of this criterion.

10.1.8 Maternal serum markers in fetal syndromes

Maternal serum marker pattern in selected fetal syndromes						
	Second trimester markers				First trimester markers	
Genetic disorder	AFP	uE3	hCG	Inh A	PAPP-A	beta hCG
Down syndrome	↓	↓	↑	↑	↓	↑
Trisomy 18	↓	↓↓	↓↓	↔	↓↓	↓↓
Trisomy 13	↔	↔	↔	↔	↓↓	↓
turner syndrome with hydrops	↓	↓	↑	↑	↓↑	↓↑
Turner syndrome without hydrops	↓	↓	↓	↓	↓↑	↓↑
Triploidy (paternal)	↔	↓	↑	↑	↓↑	↑↑
Triploidy (maternal)	↔	↓	↓	↓	↓↑	↓↓
Smith-Lemli-Opitz syndrome	↓	↓↓	↓	NR	NR	NR

Second trimester markers: AFP (alpha-fetoprotein); uE3 (unconjugated estriol); hCG (human chorionic gonadotropin); inh A (inhibin A).
First trimester marker: PAPP-A (pregnancy-associate plasma protein A); beta hCG (beta human chorionic gonadotropin.)
↑: increased; ↓: decreased; ↔ : unaffected; ↓↑: variable; NR : not reported

10.1.9 Drug use in pregnancy

Categories for Drug Use in Pregnancy	
Category	**Description**
A	Adequate, well-controlled studies in pregnant women have not shown an increased risk of fetal abnormalities.
B	Animal studies have revealed no evidence of harm to the fetus, however, there are no adequate and well-controlled studies in pregnant women. or Animal studies have shown an adverse effect, but adequate and well-controlled studies in pregnant women have failed to demonstrate a risk to the fetus.
C	Animal studies have shown an adverse effect and there are no adequate and well-controlled studies in pregnant women. or No animal studies have been conducted and there are no adequate and well-controlled studies in pregnant women.
D	Adequate, well-controlled or observational studies, in pregnant women have demonstrated a risk to the fetus. However, the benefits of therapy may outweigh the potential risk.
X	Adequate, well-controlled or observational studies, in animals or pregnant women have demonstrated positive evidence of fetal abnormalities. The use of the product is contraindicated in women who are or may become pregnant.

Relatively Safe Drugs Probably safe in pregnancy (no medications are 100% safe)	
Symptoms	**Medication**
Allergy	Benadryl(B)
Asthma	albuterol (C), metaproterenol (C), cromolyn (B), beclomethasone inhaled (C), budesonide inhaled (B)
Cold/flu	acetaminophen(C), Sudafed, Robitussin DM
Constipation	Metamucil, Fibercon, Colace, Milk of Magnesia, Senokot
Diarrhea	(for 24h only, after the 12th week of pregnancy) Imodium
Antibiotic creams	Cacitracin, Neosporin

Headache	acetaminophen (Tylenol)
Heartburn	Maalox, Mylanta, Tums
Hemorrhoids	Preparation H, Anusol, Tucks
Nausea/vomiting	Emetrol, vitamin B5 100mg PO daily
Rashes	Hydrocortisone cream/ointment, Benadryl cream, Caladryl lotion/cream, Aveeno oatmeal bath
Thyroid disease	Synthroid
Yeast infection	Monistat, Terazol (these are class C, be careful using the applicator)

Busse WW. NAEPP Expert Panel Report. Journal of Allergy and Clinical Immunology 2005; 115:34.

Known Teratogens

These are known teratogenic drugs and environmental factors that should be avoided during pregnancy

- ACE inhibitors (benazepril, captopril, enalapril etc.)
- Androgenic hormones
- Busulfan
- Chlorobiphenyls
- Cigarette smoking
- Cocaine
- Warfarin (Coumadin)
- Cyclophosphamide
- DES (diethylstilbestrol)
- Etretinate
- Fluconazole (high doses)
- Iodides
- Isotretinoin (Accutane)
- Lithium
- Mercury, organic
- Methimazole
- Methotrexate
- Misoprostol
- Penicillamine
- Phenytoin
- Tetracyclines
- Thalidomide
- Toluene (abuse)
- Valproic acid

10.2 Algorithms

10.2.1 Abnormal vaginal bleeding

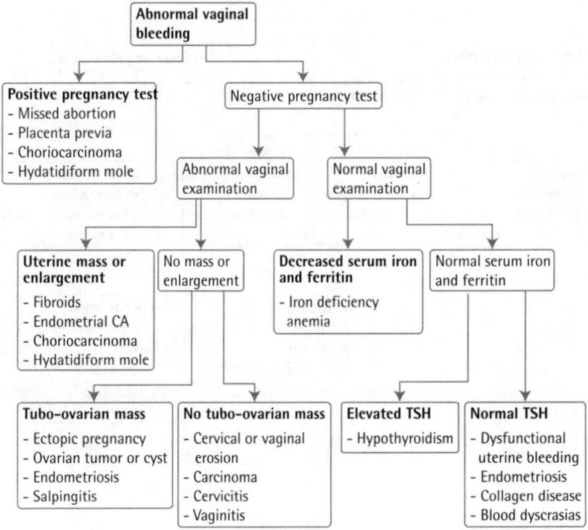

10.2.2 Vaginal discharge

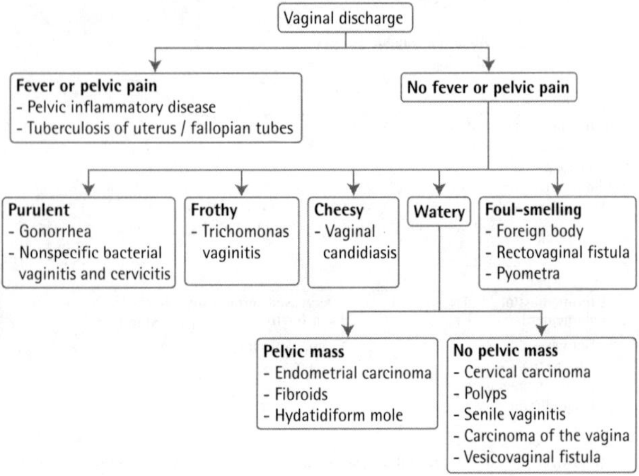

10.2.3 Breast mass

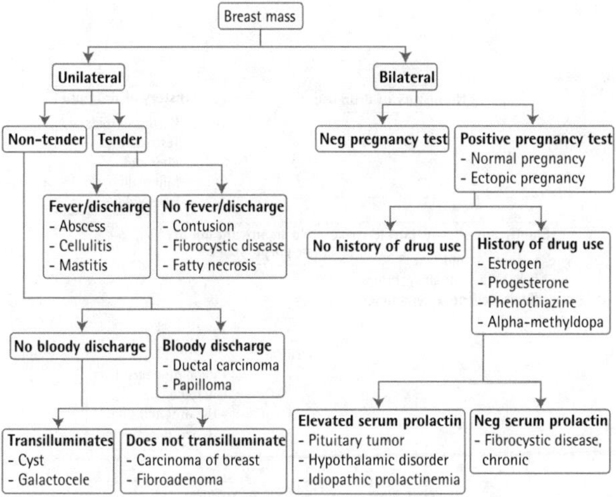

10.2.4 Hirsutism

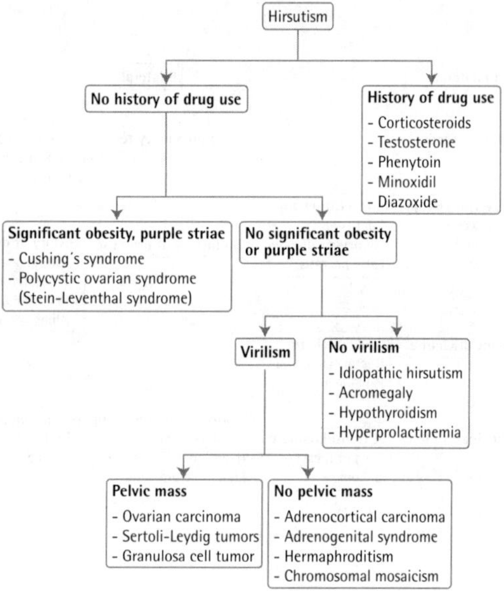

5 Board-Style Questions

1) It is discovered during the third trimester of pregnancy that a mother's serum has HBsAg (+). What should be done in this situation?

2) How is osteoporosis defined?
   a) An increased turnover or calcium in newly formed bone.
   b) Bone mineral density T-score of 2.5 standard deviations below the mean for normal healthy adults aged 30-40.
   c) Bone mineral density Z-score of 2.5 standard deviations below the mean for aged match adults.
   d) A decrease in both bone mass and matrix in trabecular and cortical bone.

3) What is the test of choice to diagnose osteoporosis?
   a) Single-photon absorptiometry
   b) Double-photon absorptiometry
   c) Dual-energy x-ray absorptiometry (DEXA)
   d) Quantitative computed tomography (CT) scan
   e) Plain x-ray of the thoracic spine

4) Carcinoma of the cervix is usually associated with which of the following viruses?
   a) Herpes simplex virus (HSV) type 1
   b) HSV type 2
   c) Human papillomavirus (HPV)
   d) Human parvovirus
   e) Adenovirus

5) A 22-year-old woman presents with a 2-week history of worsening pelvic pain and scant vaginal bleeding. She is sexually active and uses no contraception. There is no vaginal discharge. She has regular menstrual periods, but missed her last period, three weeks ago. What is the most important diagnosis to EXCLUDE?
   a) Incomplete abortion
   b) Threatened abortion
   c) Ruptured corpus luteum cyst
   d) Pelvic inflammatory disease (PID)
   e) Ectopic pregnancy

11 Nephrology

11.1 Acute Renal Failure

Acute Renal Failure (ARF) - General Breakdown

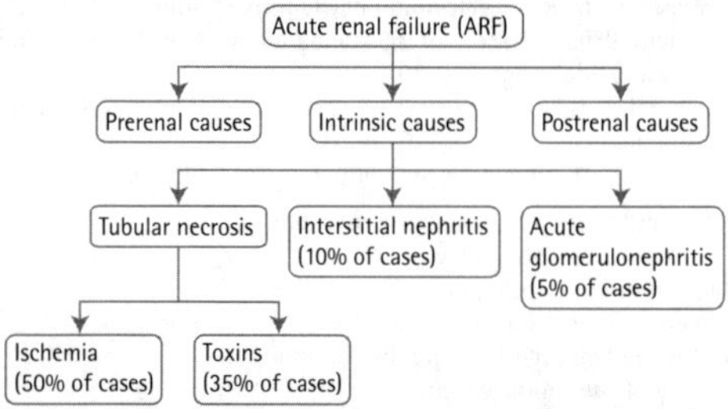

Thadhani R, Pascual M, Bonventre JV. Acute renal failure. N Engl J Med. 1996 May 30;334(22):1448-60.

ARF - Workup

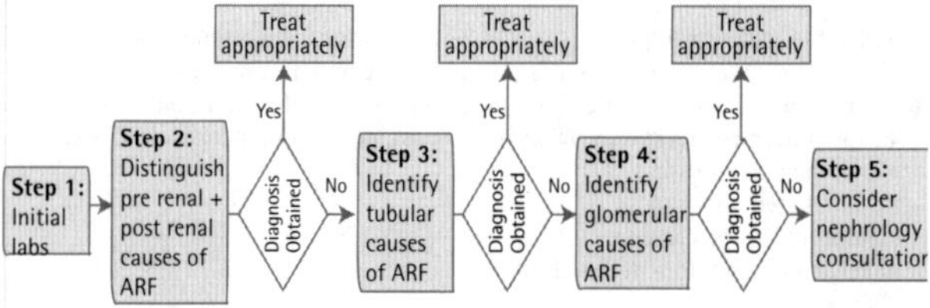

11.1.1 Step 1: Initial tests

- Check vital signs
- Physical exam
- Metabolic panel for BUN and creatinine
- Urinalysis
- Monitor urine output

11.1.2 Step 2: Distinguish prerenal, intrinsic, and postrenal azotemia

Test	Prerenal	Intrinsic	Postrenal
Vital signs	Hypotensive, tachycardic, ↑Wt.	Normal	Normal
Physical exam	↓ Skin turgor, dry mucous membranes, ↓axillary sweat, ↑thirst	Normal	Distended bladder, enlarged prostate gland
BUN/Cr ratio	> 20	10 - 20	10 - 20
Urine spec. grav	> 1.020	~ 1.010	> 1.010 early, < 1.010 late
UOsm (mOsm/kg)	> 350	~ 300	Variable
UNa (mEq/L)	< 20	> 30	< 20 early, > 40 late
FeNa %	< 1	> 2-3	< 1 early, > 3 late
Common causes	Decreased renal perfusion, fluid deficits, CHF, cirrhosis, sepsis	See steps 3 and 4	Prostatic enlargement, urolithiasis, retroperitoneal disease, meds-induced crystalluria (acyclovir, sulfonamides, methotrexate, protease inhibitors, eg, indinavir)
Prompt treatment	Replace volume deficits, do not give diuretics!	See steps 3 and 4	Ultrasound or CT to evaluate for obstructive uropathy Consider urology consultation early

11.1.3 Step 3: Identify tubular causes of ARF

	Acute tubular necrosis (ATN)	Glomerulonephritis	Acute interstitial nephritis (AIN)
Urine findings	Dark granular casts, renal epithelial cells/ casts	RBCs, dysmorphic RBC > 20%, RBC casts, WBCs, WBC casts, proteinuria, smoky-colored urine	+/-Urine eosinophils, WBC, WBC casts, hyaline casts, +/-serum eosinophils (consider cholesterol emboli syndrome)
Causes	**Ischemic:** Hypotension, **Toxic:** Medications (aminoglycosides), heme pigments, cocaine rhabdomyolysis, myeloma light chain proteins, uric acid crystals	Lupus, hepatitis, vasculitis, pulmonary renal syndromes	Medications (see AIN-causing medication table)

Modified from: Albright RC. Acute renal failure: A Practical Update, Mayo Clinic Proceedings 2001;76:67-74

Medications that can cause acute interstitial nephritis (AIN)	
Category	**Examples**
Antibiotics	Penicillins, cephalosporins, sulfonamides, rifampin, ciprofloxacin
Diuretics	Thiazides, furosemide
Pain meds	NSAIDS (aspirin, ibuprofen, etc)
H2 blockers	Cimetidine, PPIs
Uric acid	Allopurinol
Seizure	Phenytoin
Herbal	"Slimming teas" or Han Fang Ji (aristolochic acid)

11.1.4 Step 4: Distinguish the glomerular diseases

	Nephrotic syndrome	Nephritic syndrome
Character	> 3.5 g of proteinuria/day, anasarca, lipiduria with hyperlipidemia, ↓albumin, hypercoagulable state	Smokey-brown urine, ↓ GFR, oliguria, hypertension and edema
Microscopy	Oval fat bodies	RBC casts
Associated disorders	**Age < 15 years**	
	- Minimal change disease - Focal glomerulosclerosis - Mesangial proliferative glomerulonephritis	- Postinfectious glomerulonephritis - IgA nephropathy - Thin basement membrane disease - Hereditary nephritis - Henoch-Schönlein purpura - Mesangial proliferative glomerulonephritis (GN) - Membranoproliferative GN
	Age 15–40 years	
	- Focal glomerulosclerosis - Minimal change disease - Membranous nephropathy (including lupus) - Diabetic nephropathy - Preeclampsia - Postinfectious glomerulonephritis - HIV	- IgA nephropathy - Thin basement membrane disease - Lupus - Hereditary nephritis - Mesangial proliferative glomerulonephritis - Postinfectious glomerulonephritis - Rapidly progressive glomerulonephritis (RPGN) - Fibrillary glomerulonephritis - Membranoproliferative GN
	Age > 40 years	
	- Focal glomerulosclerosis, - Minimal change disease - Membranous nephropathy (including lupus) - Diabetic nephropathy - Preeclampsia - Postinfectious glomerulonephritis - HIV	- IgA nephropathy - Rapidly progressive glomerulonephritis (RPGN) - Vasculitis - Fibrillary glomerulonephritis - Postinfectious glomerulonephritis

11.2 Urinary Cast Analysis

Type of casts	Associated disorders
Hyaline	Concentrated urine, pyelonephritis, CRI
RBC	Glomerulonephritis, seen in athletes
WBC	Acute pyelonephritis or glomerular disorder
Epithelial cell	ATN, acute glomerulonephritis
Granular	Nonspecific, advanced renal disease
Waxy	Nonspecific, advanced renal disease
Fatty	Nonspecific, nephritic syndrome, hypothyroidism
Fatty casts, "Maltese cross" on polarized light	Nephritic syndrome
Broad	Nonspecific, chronic renal disease

11.3 Renal Ultrasound Interpretation

Focus	Finding	Possible cause
Kidney size	< 9 cm	Suggests chronic renal disease
	> 2 cm size difference	Unilateral renal artery stenosis
Hydronephrosis	Dilated renal pelvis	Obstructive nephropathy (acute or chronic)
Cysts	Multiple bilateral cortical cysts	Autosomal-dominant polycystic kidney disease; associated with cerebral aneurysms

11.4 Urinary Stones

Stones should always be suspected when the patient presents with symptoms such as intense acute pain and/or obstruction.

Stone Type	Shape	Associated disorders	Treatment
Calcium phosphate or Calcium oxalate	Envelope, dumbbell, or needle (oxalate)	**Urine:** ↑ calcium, ↑ oxalate, ↑ urate, ↓ citrate **Diet:** low fluid intake, ↓ calcium, ↓ potassium, ↑ sodium, ↑ sucrose, ↑ protein	**Diet:** ↑ fluid intake > 2L/d Low-Na diet **Thiazide diuretics** for hypercalciuria GI workup for oxalate stones
Magnesium ammonium phosphate (Struvite)	"Coffin lid"	Urease-producing organisms: *Proteus*, *Klebsiella*, or *Staph saprophyticus*	+/- **antibiotics**; stone removal by **percutaneous nephrolithotomy** is the first line of treatment
Uric Acid	Rhombic plates	Gout, hyperuricemia from tumor lysis, metabolic syndrome, hyperuricosuria	**Diet:** ↑ fluid intake >2L/d Low-Na diet **Allopurinol** 100 mg/d PO qd if serum uric acid is increased. Alkalinization of urine with **potassium bicarbonate** or potassium citrate 60-80 mEq/d
Cystine	Hexagonal	Cystinuria	**Diet:** ↑ fluid intake >2L/d Low-Na diet Urine alkalinization with **potassium citrate** or potassium bicarbonate 3-4 mEq/d div tid

11.5 Hematuria

11.5.1 Hematuria types

Definitions and Types

- **Microscopic hematuria:** Three or more red blood cells per high-power microscopic field in urinary sediment from two of three properly collected urinalysis specimens
- **Gross hematuria:** Overtly bloody, smoky or tea-colored urine
- **Three general categories:** Renal, prerenal, postrenal

Distinguishing Extraglomerular from Glomerular Hematuria

	Extraglomerular	Glomerular
Color (if macroscopic)	Red or pink	Red, smoky brown, or "Coca-Cola"
Clots	May be present	Absent
Proteinuria	<500 mg/day	May be >500 mg/day
RBC morphology	Normal	Some RBCs are dysmorphic
RBC casts	Absent	May be present

11.5.2 Differential diagnosis

Common Causes of Dark Urine

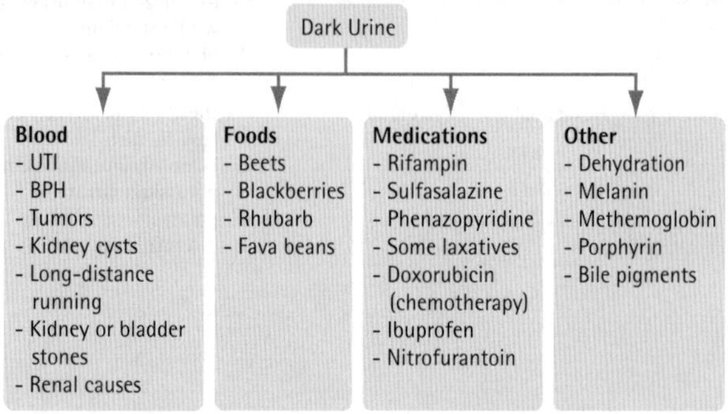

Hematuria Causes by Organ

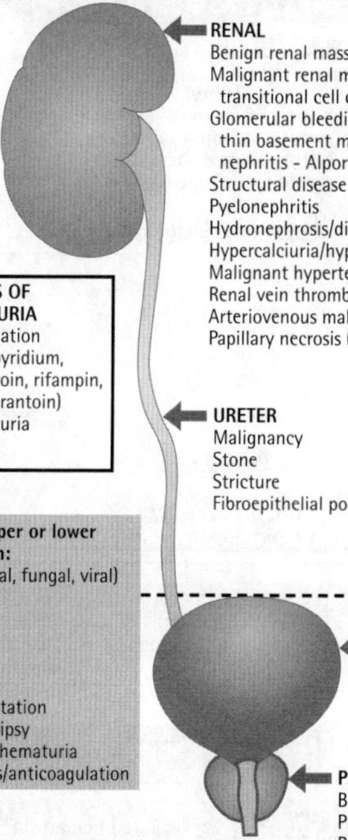

RENAL
- Benign renal mass
- Malignant renal mass (renal cell carcinoma, transitional cell carcinoma)
- Glomerular bleeding (IgA nephropathy, thin basement membrane disease, hereditary nephritis - Alport's syndrome)
- Structural disease (PKD)
- Pyelonephritis
- Hydronephrosis/distension
- Hypercalciuria/hyperuricosuria
- Malignant hypertension
- Renal vein thrombus/renal artery embolism
- Arteriovenous malformation
- Papillary necrosis (sickle-cell disease)

MIMICS OF HEMATURIA
- Menstruation
- Drugs (pyridium, phenytoin, rifampin, nitrofurantoin)
- Pigmenturia
- Beeturia

URETER
- Malignancy
- Stone
- Stricture
- Fibroepithelial polyp

Renal and/or upper or lower collecting system:
- Infection (bacterial, fungal, viral)
- Malignancy
- Urolithiasis
- Tuberculosis
- Shistosomiasis
- Trauma
- Recent instrumentation including lithotripsy
- Exercise-induced hematuria
- Bleeding diathesis/anticoagulation

Upper collecting system

Lower collecting system

BLADDER
- Malignancy (transitional cell carcinoma, squamous cell carcinoma)
- Radiation
- Cystitis

PROSTATE/URETHRA
- Benign prostatic hyperplasia
- Prostate cancer
- Prostatic procedures (biopsy, transurethral resection of the prostate)
- Traumatic catheterization
- Urethritis
- Urethral diverticulum

11.5.3 Clinical evaluation

Clinical Evaluation for Hematuria in Low-Risk Patients

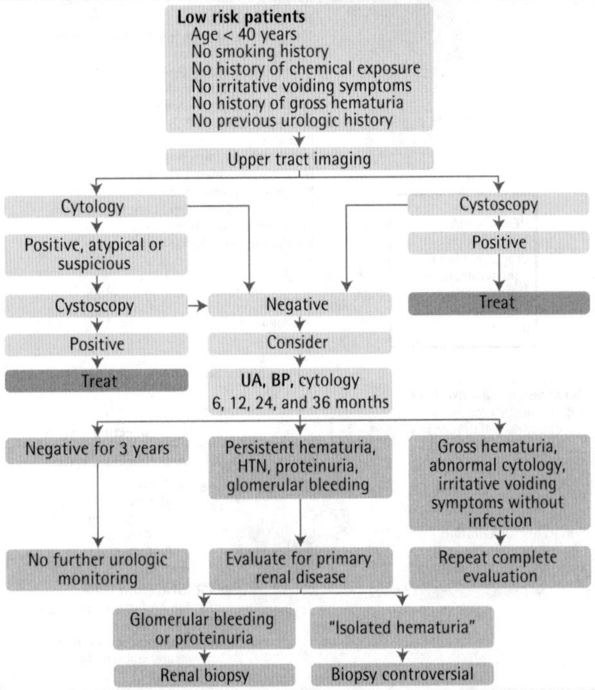

BP=blood pressure, HTN=hypertension, UA=urinalysis

Adpated from Grossfeld GD, et al. Evaluation of asymptomatic microscopic hematuria in adults: The American Urological Association best practice policy recommendations. Urology. 2001;57:599-610.

Clinical Evaluation for Hematuria in High-Risk Patients

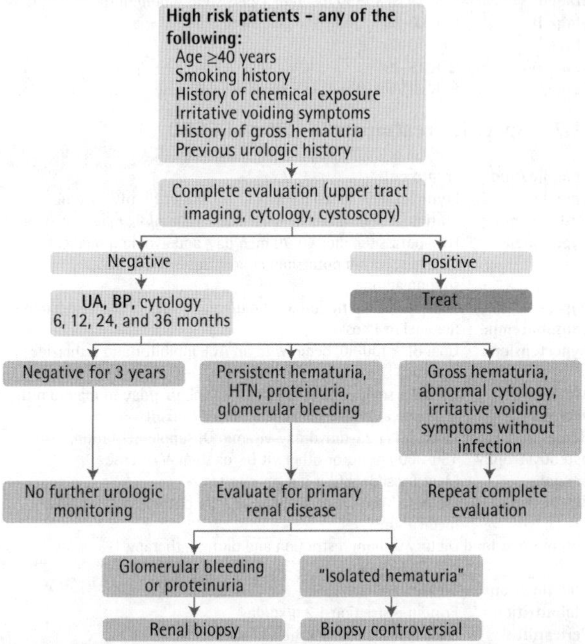

BP=blood pressure, HTN=hypertension, UA=urinalysis
Adpated from Grossfeld GD, et al. Evaluation of asymptomatic microscopic hematuria in adults: The American Urological Association best practice policy recommendations. Urology. 2001;57:599-610.

11.6 Classification of Chronic Renal Disease

Stage I	Normal GFR (>90 mL/min) + persistent albuminuria
Stage II	GFR 60-89 mL/min and persistent albuminuria
Stage III	GFR 30-59
Stage IV	GFR 15-29
Stage V	GFR <15 mL/min or end stage renal disease

11.7 Specific Treatments in CRI and ESRD

Renal Insufficiency: GFR Normal - 15mL/min	
Complication	**Treatment**
Anemia	Erythropoietin based on weight for target Hb of ~11 g/dL
Dyslipidemia	Statins (atorvastatin) to lower LDL <100mg/dL; maybe <70 mg/dL
Hyperkalemia	Low-potassium diet 40-70 mEq/day, and avoiding medications that raise serum potassium concentrations: NSAIDS, spironolactone
Hyper-phosphatemia	Phosphorus restriction 5-10 mg/kg/day with phosphate binders Renagel or Phoslo
Hypertension	Goal BP <130/80, begin with an ACE inhibitor and a thiazide diuretic
Metabolic acidosis	Consider sodium bicarbonate 0.5-1 mEq/kg/day to maintain the serum bicarbonate concentration >22 mEq/L
Renal osteodystrophy	Calcitriol (1,25-dihydroxy-vitamin D) supplementation, 150-300 pg/mL, or other vit D, for stage V disease
Sexual dysfunction	Men: Try sildenafil if not on nitrates Women: Maximizing dialysis, and discontinuing offending medications
Volume overload	Dietary sodium restriction and diuretic therapy 1-3 g/day
End Stage Renal Disease (ESRD): GFR < 15 mL/min	
Complication	**Treatment**
Malnutrition	Protein restriction 1.2 g/kg/day
Pericarditis	Dialysis leads to resolution of symptoms
Thyroid dysfunction	Evaluation of thyroid function tests, many symptoms of hypothyroidism and uremia overlap
Uremic bleeding	If symptomatic, consider dDAVP, dialysis, FFP, platelet transfusion, estrogen or PRBC transfusion
Uremic neuropathy	Dialysis leads to resolution of symptoms

11.8 Six Indications for Acute Dialysis

1. Severe electrolyte abnormalities (K^+, Na^+, Ca^{2+})
2. Volume overload
3. Severe acid-base imbalance
4. Pronounced azotemia (BUN >100) is a relative indication
5. Symptomatic uremia (pericarditis, encephalopathy, bleeding, pruritus, nausea, vomiting)
6. Toxins

11.9 Renal Tubular Acidosis (RTA)

	Type I (distal)	Type II (proximal)	Type IV (↓ R-A)*
Defect	Inability to excrete H^+ ions in dist. tub.	$HCO3^-$ lost in the proximal tubule	Defective NH_4 production
Urine pH	> 5.5	< 5.5	< 5.5
Serum K^+	Low	Low	High
Fanconi's syndr.	-	+	-
Nephrolithiasis	+	-	-
Treatment	Bicarbonate tabs 3-5 mEq/kg/d	Hydrochlorothiazide and Na^+ restriction	Lasix, Florinef, Kayexalate
Example causes	amphotericin	acetazolamide	Diabetes

* R-A = Renin-Aldosterone; Type IV RTA is the most common

11.10 Glomerular Arteriole Drug Action

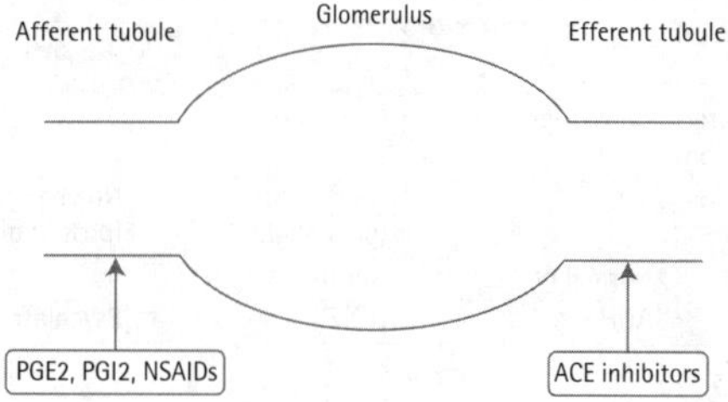

11.11 Antihypertensive Drug Action Sites in the Nephron

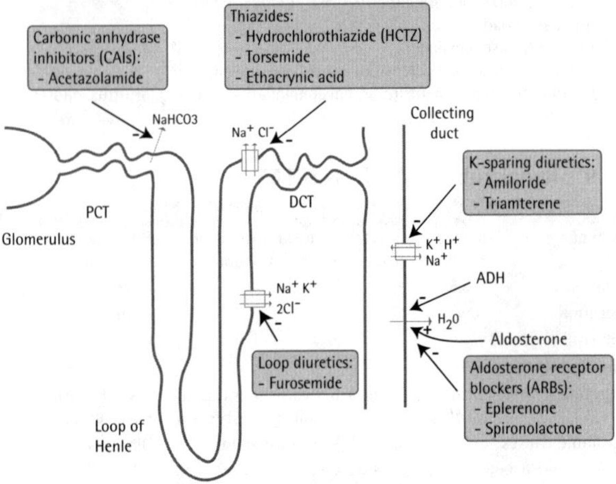

11.12 Three Common Causes of Dilute Urine

Test	Central DI	Nephrogenic DI	Psychogenic Polydypsia
Urine Osm after H_2O deprivation	No change	No change	↑
Urine Osm after vasopressin	↑ ↑	No change (poss. slight ↑)	No change (poss. slight ↑)
Serum Na^+	Normal or ↑	Normal or ↑	↓
Treatment	ADH	HCTZ	Psychiatry consult

11.13 5 Board-Style Questions

1) A patient recently passed a renal stone that was found to be calcium oxalate. She asks you if she should restrict her intake of calcium. What is your response?
2) A 72-year-old man with anemia is found to have Fanconi's syndrome with bicarbonaturia as well as phosphaturia and uricosuria. The patient is taking no medications. What diagnosis should be considered in this patient with type II RTA?
3) A 42-year-old woman from Indonesia presents with "coca-cola"-colored urine. She is found to have 1.4 grams of protein/24 hrs. She reports a recent URI beginning 3 days ago. What is the likely cause?
4) What are the initial treatment options for an 8-year-old child who presents with abdominal pain, arthralgias, and labs revealing a BUN of 25 and creatinine of 1.4? She is also noted to have a rash with palpable purpura on the lower extremities. RBC casts are visualized in the urine, and serum IgA is high.
5) A 28-year-old man presents with hemoptysis and hematuria. He is found to be in acute renal failure. Renal biopsy reveals a linear pattern on immunofluorescence. What additional test would confirm the diagnosis?

12 Neurology

12.1 CNS Neuroanatomy

Vascular Territories of the Cerebral Hemispheres

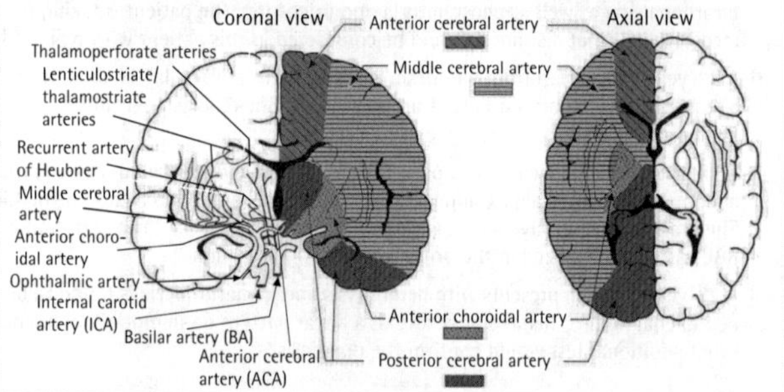

Cerebral Veins

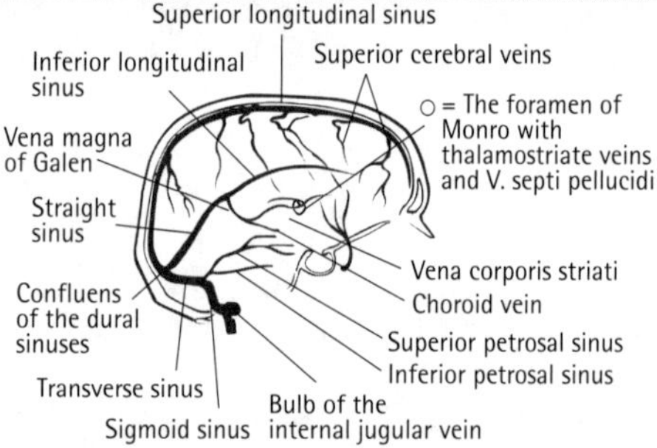

Cerebral Arteries

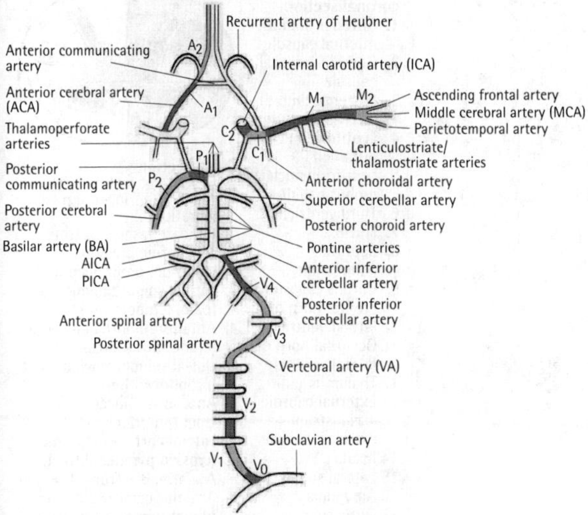

Segments of the intracranial arteries:

M - Middle cerebral artery (MCA)
A - Anterior cerebral artery (ACA)
P - Posterior cerebral artery (PCA)
C - Internal carotid artery (ICA
V - Vertebral artery (VA)

Neuroanatomy of the Brain

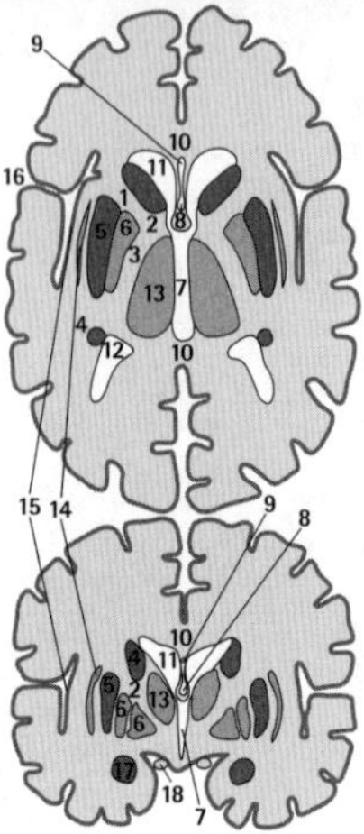

Horizontal section, coronal section

1. Anterior limb of internal capsule
2. Genu of internal capsule
3. Posterior limb of internal capsule
4. Lentiform nuclei, putamen
5. Lentiform nuclei, globus pallidus
6. Third ventricle
7. Fornix
8. Septum pellucidum
9. Corpus callosum
10. Frontal horn of lateral ventricle
11. Occipital horn of lateral ventricle
12. Thalamus
13. External capsule + claustrum + extreme capsule
14. Insula
15. Lateral sulcus
16. Amygdala
17. Optic tract

Spinal Cord

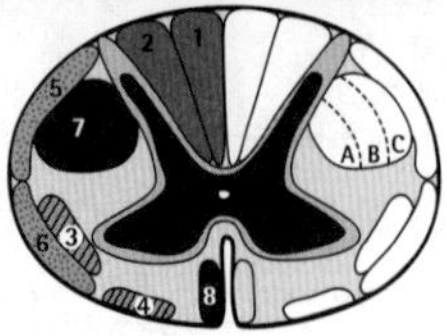

Cross-section

1. Gracile fasciculus (fine touch, proprioception, vibration)
2. Cuneate fasciculus (fine touch, fine pressure, vibration, proprioception)
3. Lateral spinothalamic tract (pain, temperature)
4. Anterior spinothalamic tract (crude touch, pressure)
5. Dorsal spinocerebellar tract (proprioception)
6. Anterior spinocerebellar tract (proprioception)
7. Lateral corticospinal tract (crossed pyramidal tract, A = arm, B = trunk, C = leg)
8. Anterior corticospinal tract (direct pyramidal tract)

12.2 Four-Minute Neurologic Exam

Mental status	- Assess arousal - Check orientation (person, place, time) - Language: name an object, repeat a phrase, follow a command - Recall: remember 3 things for 3 minutes; where were you born?
Cranial nerves	- **I**: not usually tested; strong odor (soap, tobacco) may be used - **II**: pupillary reaction to light, fundoscopic exam, visual acuity - **III**, IV, VI: extra ocular movements - **V**: light touch perception over face bilaterally, temporal and masseter muscle strength, corneal reflex usually not done - **VII**: symmetrical smile and eyebrow raising, blow out cheeks - **VIII**: test hearing by rubbing fingers together next to pt. ear; Weber (lateralization), Rinne (air vs. bone conduction); balance - **IX, X**: gag reflex, palate elevation, listen for hoarseness - **XI**: shoulder shrug - **XII**: stick tongue out
Motor	- Tone (rigid/flaccid) - Power (0-5): Test upper extremity hand grip, forearm flexion/ extension; lower extremity hip flexion, knee flexion/extension, ankle dorsi/plantar flexion
Reflexes	- Biceps (C5/6) - Triceps (C7/8) - Knee jerk (L3/4) - Ankle jerk (S1/2) - Babinski
Sensory	- Light touch - Pin prick - Temperature - Vibration
Coordination	- Finger-to-nose and heel-to-shin - Rapid alternating movements of hand and foot - Romberg test, gait (tandem, on toes, on heels) - Pronator drift

Modified per Goldberg.

12.3 Motor System Evaluation

Bulk/Tone	Inspect for muscle atrophy or hypertrophy. Check passive movements in upper and lower extremities. - Central lesions are characterized by spasticity - Peripheral lesions have normal or reduced tone	
Power/ motor strength	**0**: no contraction **1**: trace contraction **2**: weak contraction, less than force of gravity **3**: movement stronger than gravity	**4**: movement against some resistance **5**: normal, movement against full resistance
Reflexes	Deep tendon reflexes and plantar response:	
	0: absent **1+**: reduced (hypoactive) **2+**: normal	**3+**: increased (hyperactive) **4+**: clonus
	Damage to the motor pathway causes an abnormal extensor plantar response → Babinski sign	
Involuntary movements	- Hyperkinetic DO → abnormal involuntary movements - Bradykinetic DO → inability to properly initiate voluntary movement - Tremor, myoclonus, chorea, athetosis, ballismus, tics	
Gait abnormalities	- **Spastic gait:** Stiff, foot-dragging walk in which affected leg stiffly rotates away and then towards the body. DDx: CVA, CNS tumor, abscess, trauma, MS - **Waddling gait:** Distinctive duck-like walk. DDx: Hip dysplasia, muscular dystrophy (gluteus medius m. weakness), spinal muscle atrophy, superior gluteal n. dysfunction. - **Steppage gait:** Foot drop where foot hangs, forcing patient to step higher with affected foot in order to prevent toes from dragging. DDx: Peroneal n. dysfunction, Guillain-Barré, MS, herniated disk, poliomyelitis, polyneuropathy - **Propulsive (shuffling) gait:** Stooped, rigid posture, head and neck bent forward. DDx: Drugs, CO poisoning, Parkinson's disease - **Scissors gait:** Legs flexed slightly at the hips and knees, giving the appearance of crouching, with the knees and thighs hitting or crossing in a scissors-like movement. DDx: CVA, cervical spondylosis, MS, pernicious anemia, spinal cord tumor	

12.4 Mini Mental State Test

Date orientation		**Repeating a phrase**	
Year (1), season (1), date (1), day of week (1), month (1)	5	Ask the patient to say "no ifs, ands, or buts." (1 pt. if successful on first try)	1
Place orientation		**Verbal commands**	
State (1), county (1), town (1), building (1), floor / room (1)	5	Give patient a plain piece of paper and say: "Take this paper in your right hand, fold it in half, and put it on the floor." (1pt. for each correct action)	3
Register 3 Objects		**Written commands**	
Name 3 objects slowly and clearly. Ask the patient to repeat them. (1 pt. for each item correctly repeated)	3	Show patient a piece of paper with "**CLOSE YOUR EYES**" printed on it. (1 pt. if the patient's eyes close)	1
Serial sevens		**Writing**	
Ask patient to count backwards from 100 by 7 five times, OR ask to spell "world" backwards. (1 pt. for each correct answer or letter)	5	Ask patient to write a sentence. (1 pt. if sentence has a subject, a verb, and makes sense)	1
Recall 3 objects		**Drawing**	
Ask patient to recall the objects mentioned above. (1 pt. for each item correctly remembered)	3	Ask patient to copy a pair of intersecting pentagons onto a piece of paper. (1 pt. for 10 corners and 2 intersecting lines)	1
Naming		**Scoring (max.)**	**30**
Point to your watch and ask the patient what it is. Repeat with a pencil.	2	24-30: within normal limits ≤ 23: cognitive impairment (further formal testing recommended)	
Mod. per Folstein			

12.5 Glasgow Coma Scale

Clinical description		Grade
Somnolence: sleepy, easy to wake		
Stupor: hypnoidal, hard to wake		
Best motor response	Localizing response to pain	5
	Withdraws from pain	4
	Flexor response to pain	3
	Extensor posturing to pain	2
	No response to pain	1
Best verbal response	Oriented	5
	Confused conversation	4
	Inappropriate speech	3
	Incomprehensible speech	2
	None	1
Eye opening	Spontaneous eye opening	4
	Eye opening in response to speech	3
	Eye opening in response to pain	2
	No eye opening	1

GCS > 8 = somnolent		
>12	Mild	
12-9	Moderate	
GCS < 8 = unconscious		
Somnolence: sleepy, easy to wake		
Stupor: hypnoidal, hard to wake		
8-7	Coma grade I	**Light coma**
6-5	Coma grade II	
4	Coma grade III	**Deep coma**
3	Coma grade IV	

Some centers score GCS out of 14 (not 15), omitting "withdrawal from pain".

12.6 NIH stroke scale (NIHSS)

	Description	Grade
1a. Level of Consciousness (LOC)	Alert	0
	Not alert but arousable by minor stimulation	1
	Not alert and needs repeated stimulation or is obtunded	2
	Reflex response	3
1b. LOC questions – ask month/age	Answers both questions correctly	0
	One question correct	1
	Neither question correct	2
1c. LOC commands – open/close eyes, grip/release nonparetic hand	Performs both tasks correctly	0
	One task correctly	1
	Neither task correctly	2
2. Best gaze – horizontal extraocular movements	Normal	0
	Partial gaze palsy	1
	Forced deviation	2
3. Visual Field – by confrontation, finger counting or visual threat	No visual loss	0
	Partial hemianopia	1
	Complete hemianopia	2
	Bilateral hemianopia	3
4. Facial Palsy – symmetry of grimace	Normal symmetrical movements	0
	Minor paralysis	1
	Partial paralysis	2
	Complete paralysis	3
5. Motor Arm – extend arms palm down, 90 degree if sitting or 45 degree if supine; drift scored if arm falls before 10 seconds	No drift	0
	Drift but does not hit bed	1
	Some effort against gravity	2
	No effort against gravity	3
	No movement	4

6. Motor Leg - raise leg to 30 degree supine for 5 seconds	No drift	0
	Drift but leg does not hit bed	1
	Some effort against gravity	2
	No effort against gravity	3
	No movement	4
7. Limb Ataxia - test finger to nose and heel to shin	Absent	0
	Present in one limb	1
	Present in two limbs	2
8. Sensory - sensation or grimace to pinprick or withdrawal from noxious stimuli	Normal, no sensory loss	0
	Mild/moderate	1
	Severe loss	2
9. Best Language - describe picture, read items	No aphasia	0
	Mild/moderate	1
	Severe	2
	Mute global aphasia	3
10. Dysarthria - read list of words	Normal	0
	Mild/moderate	1
	Severe	2
11. Extinction and Inattention - touch patient's both hands and show fingers in both visual fields	No abnormality	0
	Visual, tactile, auditory or personal inattention/extinction	1
	Profound deficit	2

The level of stroke severity as measured by the NIH stroke scale scoring system:	
No stroke	0
Minor stroke	1-4
Moderate stroke	5-15
Moderate/severe stroke	15-20
Severe stroke	21-42

Note: strokes with scores greater than 4 points may be treated with tPA.

- G/E outcome is the approximate percentage of patients with good or excellent outcomes at 3 months.
- Lacunar Strokes have reduced NIHSS score and increased probability of excellent recovery at 3 months as compared to nonlacunar (OR = 3.1).

Source: Adams HP, et al. Baseline NIHSS score strongly predicts outcome after stroke. *Neurology* 1999 Jul 13; 53(1):126-31

12.7 Brain Death

Checklist for determination of brain death (all must be checked)	
Prerequisites	- Coma, irreversible and cause known - Neuroimaging explains coma - CNS depressant drug effect absent (if indicated toxicology screen; if barbiturates given, serum level <10 µg/mL) - No evidence of residual paralytics (electrical stimulation if paralytics used). - Absence of severe acid-base, electrolyte, endocrine abnormality - Normothermia or mild hypothermia (core temperature >36°C) - Systolic blood pressure >100 mm Hg - No spontaneous respirations
Examination	- Pupils nonreactive to bright light - Corneal reflex absent - Oculocephalic reflex absent (tested only if C-spine integrity ensured) - Oculovestibular reflex absent - No facial movement to noxious stimuli at supraorbital nerve, temporomandibular joint - Gag reflex absent - Cough reflex absent to tracheal suctioning - Absence of motor response to noxious stimuli in all 4 limbs (spinally mediated reflexes are permissible)
Adapted from 2010 Brain Death Guidelines	

12.8 Apnea Testing

All must be checked:
- Patient is hemodynamically stable - Ventilator adjusted to provide normocarbia ($PaCO_2$ 34-45 mm Hg) - Patient preoxygenated with 100% FiO_2 for >10 minutes to PaO_2 >200 mm Hg - Patient well-oxygenated with a PEEP of 5 cm of water - Provide oxygen via a suction catheter to the level of the carina at 6 L/min or attach T-piece with CPAP at 10 cm H_2O - Disconnect ventilator - Spontaneous respirations absent - Arterial blood gas drawn at 8-10 minutes, patient reconnected to ventilator - PCO_2 > 60 mmHg, or 20 mmHg rise from normal baseline value **OR:** - Apnea test aborted
Ancillary testing (only 1 needs to be performed; to be ordered only if clinical examination cannot be fully performed due to patient factors, or if apnea testing inconclusive or aborted)
- Cerebral angiogram - Cerebral scintigraphy (HMPAO SPECT Tc 99m scan) - EEG - Transcranial Doppler Ultrasound (TCD) - Time of death (DD/MM/YY) ____ - Name of physician and signature _____
Source: Eelco F.M. Wijdicks, Panayiotis N. Varelas, Gary S. Gronseth, et al. Evidence-based guideline update: Determining brain death in adults : Report of the Quality Standards Subcommittee of the American Academy of Neurology. Neurology 2010;74;1911. http://www.neurology.org/content/74/23/1911.full.pdf+html

12.9 Cerebrospinal Fluid (CSF)

	Normal levels	Acute bacterial meningitis	Acute viral meningitis	TB meningitis*	Subarachnoid hemorrhage	Traumatic tap
WBC count/µl	< 5	1000s	100s	100s	few	variable
RBC count/µl	0	0	0	0	100s	100-1000s
WBC differential**	L/M = 7:3	N > L	L > N	various leukocytes	+/- some neutrophils	subtract 1 WBC for every 1000 RBCs
Total protein mg/dl	23-38	typically 100-500	typically normal	typically 100-200	may be elevated	increase 1mg per 100 RBCs
Glucose ratio (CSF/plasma)	typically > 0.5	< 0.3	> 0.6	< 0.5	normal, >0.5	normal, >0.5
Others	ICP: 6-22 cm H_2O	-	PCR of HSV DNA	PCR of TB DNA	xanthochromia present	no xanthochromia

*With treated bacterial meningitis, immunodepression or aseptic meningitis, fewer cells are possible
**L = lymphocytes, N = neutrophils, M = monocytes

12.10 Lumbar Puncture

Tube	Send it to	Fluid qty.	What to send
1	Hematology	2 ml	Cell count with WBC diff and xanthochromia
2	Chemistry	5-6 ml	Protein, Glucose (oligoclonal bands, IgG synthetic rate)
3	Micro	5-6 ml	Gram stain, Bacterial Cx, Fungal Cx and smear, India Ink, Crypto, Toxo, VDRL, AFB, Viral Cx (PCR for HSV, EBV, JC)
4	Hematology	2 ml	Cell count with WBC diff
5	Extra/Freezer	10 ml	"Didya" tube (did ya send it for ...?). Save for frozen cytology 10-15 ml

12.11 Dermatomes

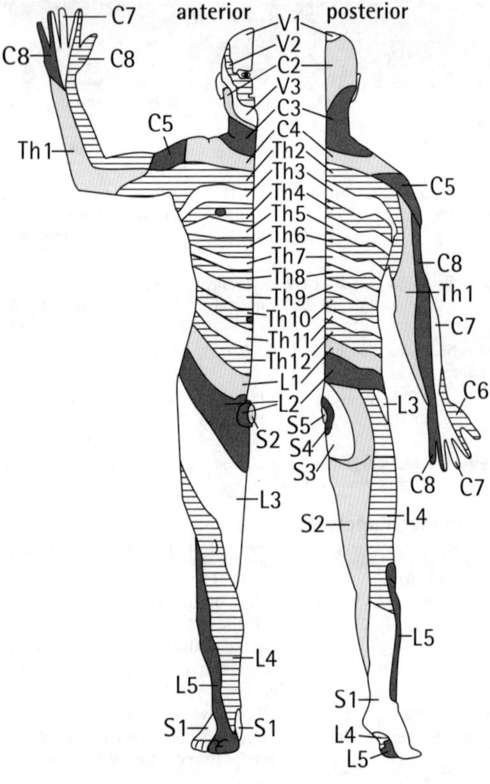

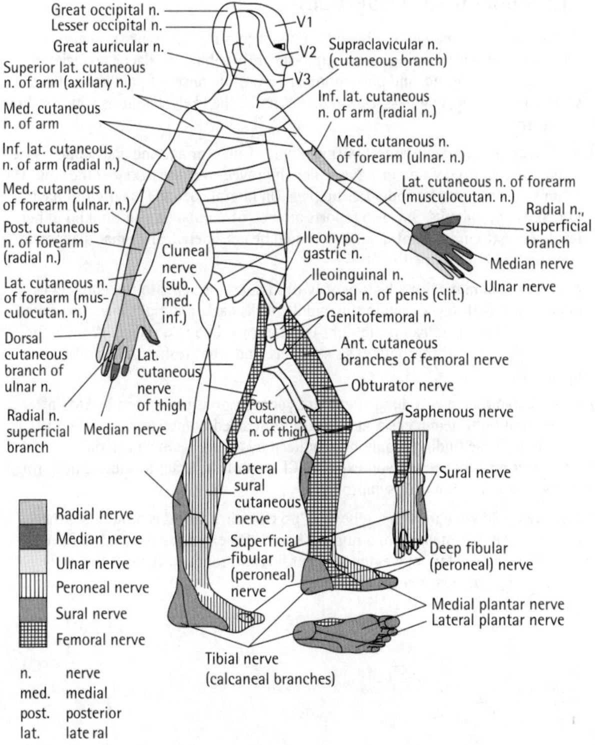
Great occipital n.
Lesser occipital n.
Great auricular n.
Superior lat. cutaneous n. of arm (axillary n.)
Med. cutaneous n. of arm
Inf. lat. cutaneous n. of arm (radial n.)
Med. cutaneous n. of forearm (ulnar. n.)
Post. cutaneous n. of forearm (radial n.)
Lat. cutaneous n. of forearm (musculocutan. n.)
Dorsal cutaneous branch of ulnar n.
Radial n. superficial branch
Median nerve
V1
V2
V3
Supraclavicular n. (cutaneous branch)
Inf. lat. cutaneous n. of arm (radial n.)
Med. cutaneous n. of forearm (ulnar. n.)
Lat. cutaneous n. of forearm (musculocutan. n.)
Radial n., superficial branch
Median nerve
Ulnar nerve
Cluneal nerve (sub., med. inf.)
Ileohypogastric n.
Ileoinguinal n.
Dorsal n. of penis (clit.)
Genitofemoral n.
Ant. cutaneous branches of femoral nerve
Obturator nerve
Lat. cutaneous nerve of thigh
Post. cutaneous n. of thigh
Saphenous nerve
Lateral sural cutaneous nerve
Sural nerve
Superficial fibular (peroneal) nerve
Deep fibular (peroneal) nerve
Medial plantar nerve
Lateral plantar nerve
Tibial nerve (calcaneal branches)
Radial nerve
Median nerve
Ulnar nerve
Peroneal nerve
Sural nerve
Femoral nerve
n. nerve
med. medial
post. posterior
lat. late ral

12.12 5 Board-Style Questions

1) A 40-year-old woman with a history of headaches reports to her primary care physician's office reporting severe right-sided throbbing headache, associated with nausea, vomiting, and photophobia. Before the onset of pain she noticed seeing a flickering, colorless, zigzag line. What is the likely diagnosis and first-line treatment?

2) A 28-year-old woman presents with diplopia. One year ago she had sudden onset of pain and blurred vision in 1 eye which improved over the next 2-3 months. On exam she is not able to abduct either eye. On lateral gaze she is noted to have horizontal nystagmus. She also reports an area of numbness and tingling in her left lower extremity. What diagnosis should be considered, and what diagnostic test should be performed?

3) A 51-year-old man with a history of IV drug abuse presents to the emergency department with fever, pain in the middle of his back, and right lower extremity weakness. Plantar reflex on the right is extensor (+Babinski reflex). What is the most likely cause of this patient's symptoms, and what tests would confirm the diagnosis?

4) A 74-year-old man with long standing hypertension is brought in by EMS after developing right hemiparesis, along with right sided numbness and difficulty speaking. These findings could be produced by a CVA in which arterial distribution? What would you expect a CT scan of the brain to show if performed within the first 3 hours of symptoms?

5) A 78-year-old woman with a reported "psychiatric history" is brought to the emergency department from a nursing home. On exam she is noted to have repetitive, involuntary movements of her lips and tongue. What is the likely cause, and what treatment is effective?

13 Oncology

13.1 Cancer Screening

Screening recommendations are based on Cancer Screening in the United States, 2011: A Review of Current American Cancer Society Guidelines and Issues in Cancer Screening. CA Cancer J Clin 2011;61:8-30.

Cancer Related Checkup: Men and women age >20 years, on the occasion of a periodic health examination, the cancer-related checkup should include examination for cancers of the thyroid, testicles, ovaries, lymph nodes, oral cavity, and skin; sexual practices; and environmental and occupational exposures.

13.1.1 Breast cancer screening

- Breast Self-Examination (BSE): Beginning in early 20's.
- Clinical Breast Exam (CBE): Should be part of a periodic health exam, at least **every three years** for women in their **20s and 30s**, and **every year** for women **>40**
- Mammography: Begin annual mammograms at age 40.

13.1.2 Cervical cancer screening

- PAP Test: Screening should begin approximately three years after a women begins having vaginal intercourse, but no later than age 21.
- Screening should be done **every year** with conventional **Pap tests** or every two years using liquid-based tests.
- At or after age 30, women who have had three normal test results in a row may get screened every 2-3 years, or every 3 years with an HPV DNA test plus cervical cytology.
- Women 70 and older who have had three or more consecutive normal Pap tests and no abnormal Pap tests in the last 10 years and women who have had a total hysterectomy may choose to stop cervical cancer screening.

13.1.3 Colorectal cancer screening

- Fecal occult blood test (FOBT) or Fecal immunochemical test (FIT): Annual, starting age 50.
- Stool DNA Test: Interval uncertain, starting age 50.
- Flexible sigmoidoscopy (FSIG): Every 5 years, starting at age 50.
- FOBT or FIT with FSIG: Annual FOBT or FIT, and FSIG every 5 years starting age 50.
- Double-contrast barium enema (DCBE): Every 5 years, starting at age 50.
- Colonoscopy: Every 10 years, starting at age 50.

13.1.4 Endometrial cancer screening

- At menopause, women at average risk should be informed about risks and symptoms of endometrial cancer and strongly encouraged to report any unexpected bleeding or spotting to their physicians.

13.1.5 Prostate cancer screening

- Prostate-specific antigen (PSA) and digital rectal examination (DRE): Men who have at least 10 year life expectancy should have an opportunity to make an informed decision with their health care provider about whether to be screened for prostate cancer, after receiving information about the benefits, risks, and uncertainties associated with prostate cancer screening.
- Men at **high risk:** African-American men and men with a family history (brother or father diagnosed with prostate cancer before age 65) should begin testing at **age 45.**

13.2 ECOG Performance Status Scale

Grade	Definition
0	Patient is fully active, able to carry out all pre-disease performance without restriction.
1	Patient is restricted in physical activity, but ambulatory and able to carry out work of a light or sedentary nature, eg, light house work, office work.
2	Patient is ambulatory and capable of all self-care but unable to carry out any work activities. Up and about > 50% of waking hours.
3	Patient is capable of only limited self-care, confined to bed or chair more than 50% of waking hours.
4	Patient is completely disabled, and cannot carry on any self-care. Totally confined to bed or chair.

* ECOG: Eastern Cooperative Oncology Group

13.3 Key Oncologic Definitions

Terminology	Definition
Complete response (CR)	Disappearance of all target lesions. Any pathological lymph nodes must have reduction in short axis to <10 mm. This does not mean the cancer has been cured.
Partial response (PR)	At lest a 30% decrease in the sum of diameters of target lesions, taking as reference the baseline sum diameters.
Stable disease (SD)	Neither sufficient shrinkage to qualify for PR nor sufficient increase to qualify for PD.
Progressive disease (PD)	> 20% increase in the sum of diameters of target lesions.
Progression-free survival (PFS)	The length of time during and after treatment that the cancer does not grow. Progression-free survival includes the amount of time patients have experienced a CR+PR+SD.
Overall survival (OS)	The percentage of subjects in a study who have survived for a defined period of time. Usually reported as time since diagnosis or initial treatment. Often reported as a five-year survival rate.
Stage	The extent of a cancer in the body. Staging is usually based on the size of the tumor, presence of lymph nodes that contain cancer, and whether the cancer has spread from the original site to other parts of the body.
Grade	Pathologic characteristics of the particular tumor cells, based on how abnormal the cancer cells look under a microscope and how quickly the tumor is likely to grow and spread.
Induction therapy	Initial treatment such as chemotherapy, radiation, or hormone therapy used to reduce a cancer. Also called first-line therapy.
Consolidation therapy	Treatment that is given after cancer has disappeared following the initial therapy.
Maintenance therapy	Treatment that is given to help keep cancer from coming back after it has disappeared following the initial therapy.
Adjuvant therapy	Additional cancer treatment given after the primary treatment to lower the risk that the cancer will come back.
Neoadjuvant therapy	Treatment given as a first step to shrink a tumor before the main treatment, which is usually surgery, is given.

Ref: Revised Recist guideline (version 1.1) European J of cancer 2009 45:228-247.
National Cancer Institute: Dictionary of Cancer Terms: accessed on 3/19/11.

13.4 Classifications

13.4.1 Breast cancer

TNM classification	
Primary Tumor (T)	
Tx	Primary tumor cannot be assessed
T0	No evidence of primary tumor
Tis	Carcinoma in situ
Tis DCIS	Ductal carcinoma in situ
Tis LCIS	Lobular carcinoma in situ
Tis Paget's	Paget's disease of the nipple NOT associated with invasive carcinoma and/or carcinoma in situ (DCIS/LCIS) in the underlying breast. Breast carcinoma associated with Paget's disease are categorized based on the size and characteristics of the parenchymal disease, although the presence of Paget's disease should still be noted
T1	Tumor ≤20 mm in greatest dimmension
T1mi	Tumor ≤1 mm
T1a	Tumor >1 mm but ≤5 mm
T1b	Tumor >5 mm and ≤10 mm
T1c	Tumor >10 mm and ≤20 mm
T2	Tumor >20 mm and ≤50 mm
T3	Tumor >50 mm
T4	Tumor of any size with distinct extension to the chest wall/skin (ulceration/nodules)
T4a	Extension to the chest wall, not including only pectoralis muscle adherence/invasion
T4b	Ulceration and/or ipsilateral satellite nodules and/or edema (including peau d'orange) of the skin, which do not meet criteria for inflmmaatory ca
T4c	Both T4a and T4b
T4d	Inflammatory carcinoma

Regional Lymph Nodes (N)	
Nx	Regional nodes can not be assessed
N0	No regional lymph node metastasis
N1	Metastasis to movable ipsilateral level I/II axillary lymph node(s)
N2	Metastasis to ipsilat. axillary lymph node(s) fixed or matted, or in clinically detected ipsilat. internal mammary nodes in the absence of evident axillary node metastases
N2a	Metastases in ipsilat. level I/II axillary lymph nodes fixed to one another (matted) or to other structures
N2b	Metastases only in clinically detected ipsilat. internal mammary nodes and in absence of clinically evident level I/II axillary lymph node metastates
N3	Metastasis in ipsilat. infraclavicular (level III axillary) lymph node(s) with or without level I, II axillary node involvement; or in clinically detected ipsilateral internal mammary lymph node(s) with clinicallyevident level I, II axillary lymph node metastases; or metastases in ipsilateral supraclavicular lymph node(s) with or without axillary or internal mammary lymph node involvement
N3a	Metastases in ipsilateral infraclavicular lymph nodes
N3b	Metastases in ipsilateral internal mammary lymph node(s) and axillary lymph nodes
N3c	Metastasis in ipsilateral supraclavicular lymph node(s)
Distant Metastasis (M)	
Mo	No clinical or radiographic evidence of distant metastases
cMo(i+)	No clinical or radiographic evidence of distant metastases, but deposits of molecularly or microscopically detected tumor cells in circulating blood, bone marrow, or other nonregional nodal tissue ≤0.2 mm in a patient w/o symptoms or signs of metastases
M1	Distant detectable metastases as determined by classic clinical and radiographic means and/or histologically proven >0.2 mm

Stage	TNM	5y Surv	Therapy Generalizations*
0	Tis, N0, M0	98%	DCIS- lumpectomy and radiation therapy vs modified radical mastectomy. Tamoxifen is used to prevent a second malignancy in either breast
I	T1, N0, M0	96%	Individualized therapy generally consisting of breast conserving surgery plus radiation vs mastectomy Chemotherapy including an anthracycline containing regimen, eg, dose dense (every 2 wks) doxorubicin + cyclophosphamide (AC) followed by paclitaxel (P) Adjuvant chemotherapy is recommended to reduce the risk of recurrent breast cancer. In premenopausal women tamoxifen is used for 5 years in those with ER+ disease In postmenopausal women, an aromatase inhibitor is used for at least 5 years in those with ER+ disease In patients with HER2+ disease, trastuzumab should be given for 1 year
IIA	T0, N1, M0 T1, N1, M0 T2, N0, M0	82%	
IIB	T2, N1, M0 T3, N0, M0		
IIIA	T0, N2, M0 T1, N2, M0 T2, N2, M0 T3, N2, M0	53%	
IIIB	T4, Any N, M0		
IIIC	Any T, N3, M0		
IV	Any T, Any N, M1	17%	**Hormonal therapy:** Pts with ER or PR positive disease **Chemotherapy:** Single agent chemotherapy may be used sequentially, eg, capecitabine; HER2+ pts should also receive trastuzumab

TNM staging adapted from the AJCC Cancer Staging Manual 7th ed. New York, NY; Springer Verlag; 2010.
*Therapy information adapted from Siedman H et al. Ca J Clin. 1987;37(5):258-290.

Prognosis

10-year relative survival in breast cancer

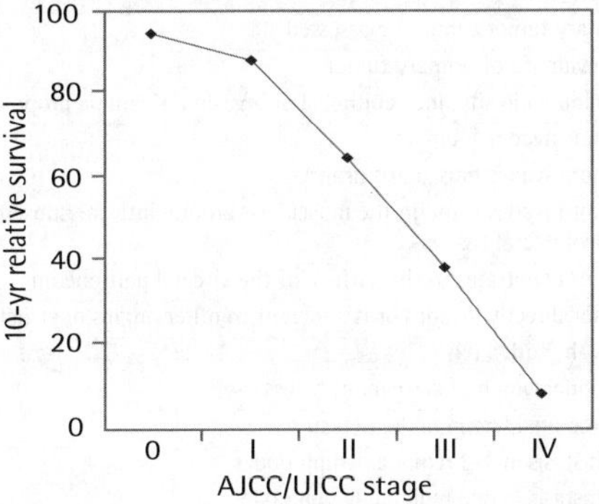

AJCC/UICC (TNM) breast cancer stage. CA Cancer J Clin 2006;56:37-47

13.4.2 Colorectal cancer

TNM Classification	
Primary Tumor (T)	
TX	Primary tumor cannot be assessed
T0	No evidence of primary tumor
Tis	Carcinoma in situ, intraepithelial or invasion of lamina propria
T1	Tumor invades submucosa
T2	Tumor invades muscularis propria
T3	Tumor invades through the muscularis propria into the subserosa, into pericolorectal tissues
T4a	Tumor penetrates to the surface of the visceral peritoneum
T4b	Tumor directly invades or is adherent to other organs or structures
Regional Lymph Nodes (N)	
NX	Regional lymph nodes cannot be assessed
N0	No regional lymph node metastasis
N1	Metastasis in 1-3 regional lymph nodes
N1a	Metastasis in one regional lymph node
N1b	Metastasis in 2-3 regional lymph nodes
N1c	Tumor deposit(s) in the subserosa, mesentery, or nonperitonealized pericolic or perirectal tissues without regional nodal metastasis
N2	Metastasis in 4 or more regional lymph nodes
N2a	Metastasis in 4-6 regional lymph nodes
N2b	Metastasis in seven or more regional lymph nodes
Distant Metastasis (M)	
M0	No distant metastasis
M1a	Metastasis confined to one organ or site (eg, liver, lung, ovary, nonregional node)
M1b	Metastasis in more than one organ/site or the peritoneum

Stage	TNM	Dukes stage	5y Surv Colon/ Rectal	Therapy Generalizations*
0	Tis, N0, M0	–		
I	T1-2, N0, M0	A	> 90% / > 90%	Surgical resection alone
IIA	T3, N0, M0	B	75-85% / 70-85%	Colon: Chemotherapy may be considered for high risk stage II patients: inadequately sampled nodes (<12), T4 lesion, perforation, or poorly differentiated histology
IIB	T4a, N0, M0	B		
IIC	T4b, N0, M0	B		
IIIA	T1-2, N1/N1c, M0 T1, N2a, M0	C	59% / 55%	Systemic adjuvant chemotherapy after surgery with 5-fluorouracil/ leucovorin, oxaliplatin (FOLFOX) or 5-fluorouracil/leucovorin, capecitabine can replace infusional 5-FU *for rectal cancer preoperative chemoradiation is standard for patients with T3 or regional node involvement
IIIB	T3-4a, N1/N1c, M0 T2-T3, N2a, M0 T1-T2, N2b, M0	C	42% / 35%	
IIIC	T4a, N2a, M0 T3-T4a, N2b, M0 T4b, N1-N2, M0	C	27% / 24%	
IV	Any T, any N, M1a or M1b	-	< 5% / < 5%	FOLFOX with bevacizumab, FOLFIRI + Cetuximab (KRAS wild type only)

Reproduced from American Joint Committee on Cancer (AJCC), Chicago Illinois. The original source for this material is the AJCC Cacner Staging manual 7th edition (2010) published by Springer-Verlag, New York, www.springeronline.com

Note: cTNM is the clinical classification. pTNM is the pathologic classification. The y prefix is used after neoadjuvant pretreatment (ypTNM).

13.4.3 Non-small cell lung cancer

TNM Classification	
Primary Tumor (T)	
Tx	Primary tumor cannot be assessed, or tumor proven by the presence of malignant cells in sputum or bronchial washings but not visualized by imaging or bronchoscopy
T0	No evidence of primary tumor
Tis	Carcinoma in situ

T1	Tumor ≤3 cm, surrounded by lung or visceral pleura, without bronchoscopic evidence of invasion more proximal than the lobar bronchus (ie, not in the main bronchus)
T1a	Tumor ≤2 cm in greatest dimension
T1b	Tumor >2 cm but ≤3 cm in greatest dimension
T2	Tumor >3 cm but ≤7 cm with any of the following: - Involves main bronchus, ≥2 cm distal to the carina - Invades visceral pleura - Associated with atelectasis or obstructive pneumonitis that extends to the hilar region but does not involve the entire lung
T2a	Tumor >3 cm but ≤5 cm in greatest dimension
T2b	Tumor >5 cm but ≤7 cm in greatest dimension
T3	Tumor >7 cm or one that directly invades any of the following: - Parietal pleural chest wall (including superior sulcus tumors) - Diaphragm - Phrenic nerve - Mediastinal pleura - Parietal pericardium or - Tumor in the main bronchus <2 cm distal to the carina but without involvement of the carina; or associated atelectasis or obstructive pneumonitis of the entire lung or separate tumor nodule(s) in the same lobe
T4	Tumor of any size that invades any of the following - Mediastinum - Heart - Great vessels - Trachea - Recurrent laryngeal nerve - Esophagus - Vertebral body - Carina - Separate tumor nodule(s) in a different ipsilateral lobe

Regional Lymph Nodes (N)	
Nx	Regional lymph nodes cannot be assessed
N0	No regional lymph node metastases
N1	Metastasis to ipsilateral peribronchial and/or ipsilateral hilar lymph nodes and intrapulmonary nodes, including involvement by direct extension
N2	Metastases to an ipsilateral mediastinal and/or subcarinal lymph node(s)
N3	Metastasis in contralateral mediastinal, contralateral hilar, ipsilateral or contralateral scalene, or supraclavicular lymph node(s)
Distant Metastasis (M)	
M0	No distant metastasis
M1	Distant metastasis present
M1a	Separate tumor nodule(s) in a contralateral lobe tumor with pleural nodules or malignant pleural (or pericardial) effusion
M1b	Distant metastasis

Adapted from the AJCC Cancer Staging Manual 7th ed. New York, NY; Springer Verlag; 2010.

Staging

Stage	TNM	5-yr Surv	Therapy Generalizations
Occult carcinoma	TX, N0, M0	-	-
0	Tis, N0,M0	-	-
IA	T1a, N0, M0	56%	Surgery alone
	T1b, N0, M0		
IB	T2a, N0, M0	56%	Surgery +/- chemotherapy
IIA	T2b, N0, M0	32%	Surgery + chemotherapy +/- radiotherapy
	T1a, N1, M0		
	T1b, N1, M0		
	T2a, N1, M0		
IIB	T2b, N1, M0	32%	Surgery + chemotherapy +/- radiotherapy
	T3, N0, M0		

IIIA	T1a, N2, M0	9%	Chemotherapy +/- radiotherapy
	T1b, N2, M0		
	T2a, N2, M0		
	T2b, N2, M0		
	T3, N1, M0		
	T3, N2, M0		
	T4, N0, M0		
	T4, N1, M0		
IIIB	T1a, N3, M0	9%	Chemotherapy +/- radiotherapy
	T1b, N3, M0		
	T2a, N3, M0		
	T2b, N3, M0		
	T3, N3, M0		
	T4, N2, M0		
	T4, N3M0		
IV	Any T, Any N, M1a	2%	Chemotherapy
	Any T, Any N, M1b		

Adapted from the AJCC Cancer Staging Manual 7th ed. New York, NY; Springer Verlag; 2010.

13.4.4 Small cell lung cancer

Two-stage Definition of Small Cell Carcinoma (SCC)	
Limited-stage disease	Disease confined to the ipsilateral hemithorax, which can be safely encompassed within a tolerable radiation field.
Extensive-stage disease	Disease beyond ipsilateral hemithorax, which may include malignant pleural or pericardial effusion or hematogenous metastases.

TNM Description

Stage	TNM	5-yr survival	% of cases	Treatment
Limited stage	I - IIIB	15 - 25%	30	Chemo+XRT
Extensive stage	IV	1 %	70	Chemo

13.4.5 Ovarian cancer

TNM Classification	
TNM	**Description**
T1	Limited to ovaries (one or both)
T1a	Limited to one ovary, capsule intact
T1b	Limited to both ovaries, capsule intact
T1c	One or both ovaries with any of the following: Ruptured capsule, tumor on ovarian surface, malignant cells in ascites or peritoneal washings.
T2	Involves one or both ovaries with pelvic extension
T2a	Extension or implants on uterus and/or tubes
T2b	Extension to other pelvic tissues
T2c	Pelvic extension with malignant cells in ascites or peritoneal washings
T3	Involves one or both ovaries with microscopically confirmed peritoneal metastasis and/or regional LN metastasis
T3a	Microscopic peritoneal metastasis beyond pelvis
T3b	Macroscopic peritoneal metastasis beyond pelvis 2 cm or less in greatest dimension
T3c	Peritoneal metastasis beyond pelvis more than 2cm in greatest dimension and/or regional LN metastasis
T4	Distant metastasis (excludes peritoneal metastasis)
N0	No regional lymph node metastasis
N1	Regional lymph node metastasis
M0	No distant metastasis
M1	Distant metastasis

Stage			
Stage	**TNM**	**5-yr survival**	**Treatment**
IA	T1a, N0, M0	92.7%	Surgery
IB	T1b, N0, M0	85.4%	
IC	T1c, N0, M0	84.7%	Surgery + Chemo
IIA	T2a, N0, M0	78.6%	
IIB	T2b, N0, M0	72.4%	
IIC	T2c, N0, M0	64.4%	
IIIA	T3a, N0, M0	50.8%	
IIIB	T3b, N0, M0	42.4%	Surgery + Chemo
IIIC	T3c, N0, M0	31.5%	
	Any T, N1, M0		
IV	Any T, AnyN, M1	17.5%	

*American College of Surgeons, National Cancer Database.

13.5 Cancer of Occult Primary Origin

Definition	Histologically proven metastatic malignant tumors whose primary site cannot be identified during pretreatment evaluation.
Prevalence total	5%-10% of all cancer diagnoses.
Prevalence postmortem	On postmortem exam the primary tumor is not identified in 20%-50% of patients.
Life expectancy	Life expectancy after diagnosis is 6-9 months.
Treatment	Even if the primary is identified, the treatment is usually palliative.

13.5.1 Workup for cancer of occult primary

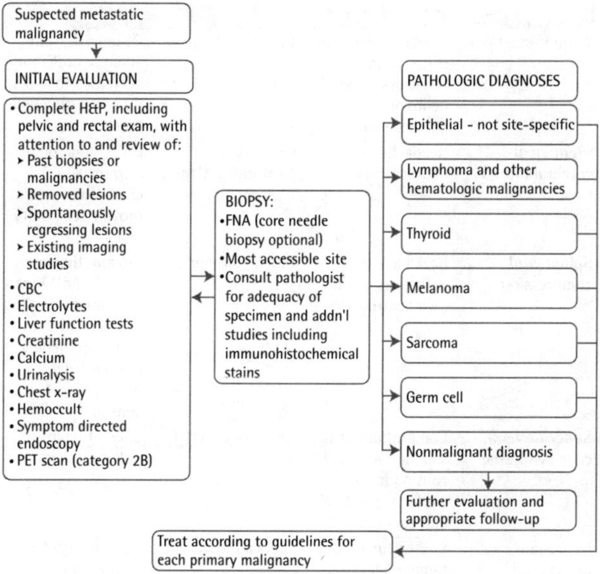
Suspected metastatic malignancy
INITIAL EVALUATION
• Complete H&P, including pelvic and rectal exam, with attention to and review of:
➤ Past biopsies or malignancies
➤ Removed lesions
➤ Spontaneously regressing lesions
➤ Existing imaging studies
• CBC
• Electrolytes
• Liver function tests
• Creatinine
• Calcium
• Urinalysis
• Chest x-ray
• Hemoccult
• Symptom directed endoscopy
• PET scan (category 2B)
BIOPSY:
•FNA (core needle biopsy optional)
•Most accessible site
•Consult pathologist for adequacy of specimen and addn'l studies including immunohistochemical stains
PATHOLOGIC DIAGNOSES
Epithelial - not site-specific
Lymphoma and other hematologic malignancies
Thyroid
Melanoma
Sarcoma
Germ cell
Nonmalignant diagnosis
Further evaluation and appropriate follow-up
Treat according to guidelines for each primary malignancy

13.6 Eight Oncologic Emergencies

Condition	Possible findings	Confirmatory test	Tx./intervention
Brain metastasis	Headache, mental status changes, weakness, focal neurologic deficits, papilledema	CT with contrast or MRI	**Dexamethasone** 10mg IV or PO then decreased to 4-6mg PO q6h with whole brain irradiation
Meningeal carcinomatosis	Headache or cranial neuropathies	CSF cytology (performed **after** a CT scan)	Local radiation or intrathecal chemotherapy may provide temporary relief
Spinal cord compression	Back pain, focal deficits esp. in the lower extremities	MRI of the spine	**Dexamethasone** 10mg IV or PO then decreased to 4-6mg PO q6h with radiation therapy. Also emergent neurosurgical consult
Superior vena cava syndrome	Compression of the superior vena cava causing facial swelling, chest pain, and cough	Chest x-ray or CT scan	Chemotherapy or radiation therapy
Malignant pericardial effusion	Chest pain, dyspnea, tamponade	Echocardiogram	Pericardiocentesis with window procedure or pericardial stripping. Alternatively, sclerosis with bleomycin
Malignant pulmonary effusion	Chest pain, dyspnea	Chest x-ray with decubital views	Thoracentesis and sclerotherapy or pleurectomy

Condition	Possible findings	Confirmatory test	Tx./intervention
Malignant ascites	Abdominal distension	Ultrasound or CT scan	Systemic therapy and therapeutic paracentesis
Bone metastasis	May result in spontaneous fracture	X-ray	Prophylactic surgical pinning and radiation therapy. Bisphosphonates may decrease pain and bone loss

13.7 Paraneoplastic Syndromes

Syndrome	Key findings	Treatment
Hypercalcemia	Associated with squamous cell histology. Caused by metastasis to the bone, ectopic production of parathyroid hormone-related peptide, ↑ vitamin D metabolites	1) IV fluids 2) **zolendranate** 4mg IV over 15 min or **pamidronate** 60-90mg IV over 4 h 3) **calcitonin** 4 units/kg IV q 12 x 4 doses Other: Lasix, prednisone 20-40 mg po QD, and dialysis
SIADH	↓ serum Na^+, ↓ serum Osm, euvolemic, urine Osm inappropriately elevated. Not related to hypothyroidism, thiazide or adrenal insufficiency	Fluid restriction ~1L/day 3% saline Tolvaptan (not yet approved)
Anorexia/cachexia	↓ body weight, ↓ muscle mass, ↓ adipose tissue caused by cytokines such as TNF-α, IL-6, IL-1β. Unlike starvation, weight loss in cancer arises in both muscle and fat	**Megestrol acetate** (Megace ES) 625/5ml po QD

Dermatomyositis	Symmetric proximal muscle weakness, typical rash, ↑ serum muscle enzymes, typical changes on EMG, typical muscle biopsy finding	**Prednisone** 0.5-1.5 mg/kg/d
Lambert-Eaton syndrome	Proximal muscle weakness with ↓ deep tendon reflexes. Confirmed by the presence of antibodies to voltage-gated calcium channel	Treatment of primary malignancy may improve the symptoms
Erythrocytosis	↑ production of erythropoietin causing a Hb >16.5 g/dL in women and >18.5 g/dL in men	Removal of Epo-secreting tumor or phlebotomy
Granulocytosis (leukemoid rxn)	WBC count >50,000/μL not caused by leukemia	Usually no intervention is necessary for WBC <100k
Thrombocytosis	Platelet count >600,000/μL. Evaluate for bleeding or iron deficiency leading to reactive thrombocytosis	Consider platelet apheresis for platelet counts >800,000/μL, also consider platelet lowering agent such as hydroxyurea
Thromboembolic disease	Occurs in 11% of patients with cancer. Caused by various procoagulants in the tumor (tissue factor, cancer procoagulant, TNF, IL-1)	Anticoagulation, preferred agent is low molecular weight heparin
Fever	Associated with IL-6 and IL-1 elevations	Ibuprofen 400 mg PO qid, Tylenol 650 mg PO bid

13.8 Basic Concepts of Chemotherapy

The cell cycle is a series of steps that both normal cells and cancer cells go through in order to grow and reproduce to form new cells. There are 5 phases in the cell cycle, designated by letters and numbers:

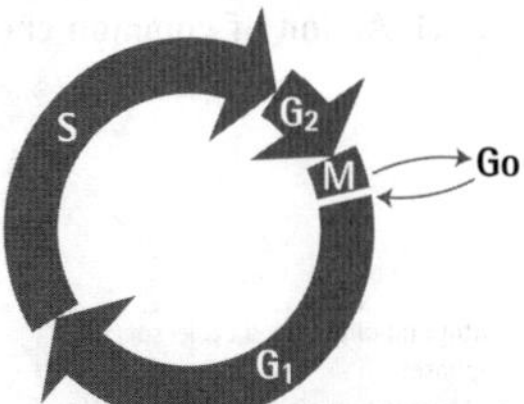

Phase	Description
G0 phase resting	Cells have not yet started to divide. Cells spend much of their lives in this phase. Depending on the type of cell, it can last for a few hours to a few years. When the cell is signaled to reproduce, it moves into the G1 phase.
G1 phase	During this phase, the cell starts making more proteins to get ready to divide. This phase lasts about 18 to 30 hours.
S phase	In the S phase, the chromosomes containing the genetic code (DNA) are copied so that both of the new cells formed will have the right amount of DNA. This phase lasts about 18 to 20 hours.
G2 phase	The G2 phase occurs just before the cell starts splitting into two cells. It lasts from 2 to 10 hours.
M phase Mitosis	In this phase, which lasts only 30 to 60 minutes, the cell actually splits into 2 new cells.

Many chemotherapy drugs work only on actively reproducing cells (not on cells in the resting phase, G0). Some of these drugs specifically attack cells in a particular phase of the cell cycle (the M or S phases, for example). Understanding how these drugs function helps oncologists predict which drugs are likely to work well together. Although chemotherapy drugs attack reproducing cells, they cannot tell the difference between reproducing cells of normal tissues (that are replacing worn-out normal cells) and cancer cells. The damage to normal cells can result in side effects. Proper administration of chemotherapy involves balancing between destroying the cancer cells (in order to cure or control the disease) and sparing the normal cells (to lessen undesirable side effects).

13.9 Chemotherapeutic Agents

13.9.1 Action of common chemotherapeutic agents

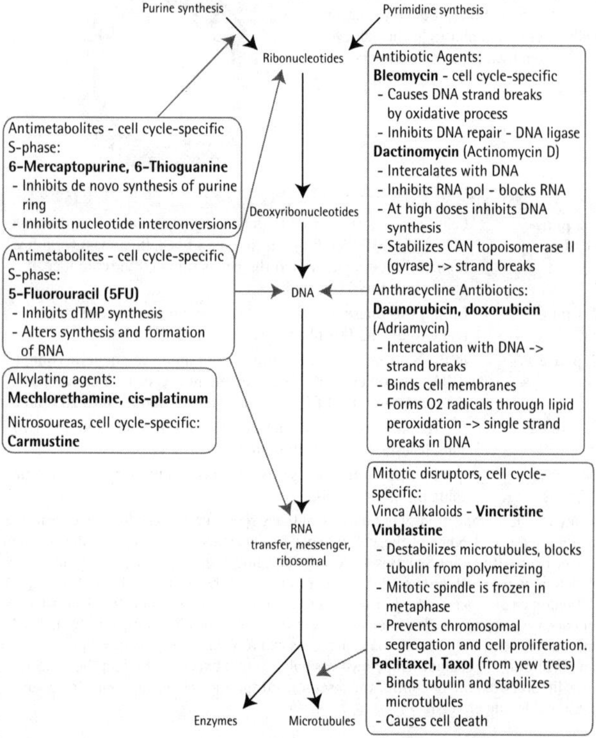

Purine synthesis
Pyrimidine synthesis
Ribonucleotides
Deoxyribonucleotides
DNA
RNA
transfer, messenger,
ribosomal
Enzymes
Microtubules
Antimetabolites - cell cycle-specific
S-phase:
6-Mercaptopurine, 6-Thioguanine
- Inhibits de novo synthesis of purine ring
- Inhibits nucleotide interconversions
Antimetabolites - cell cycle-specific
S-phase:
5-Fluorouracil (5FU)
- Inhibits dTMP synthesis
- Alters synthesis and formation of RNA
Alkylating agents:
Mechlorethamine, cis-platinum
Nitrosoureas, cell cycle-specific:
Carmustine
Antibiotic Agents:
Bleomycin - cell cycle-specific
- Causes DNA strand breaks by oxidative process
- Inhibits DNA repair - DNA ligase
Dactinomycin (Actinomycin D)
- Intercalates with DNA
- Inhibits RNA pol - blocks RNA
- At high doses inhibits DNA synthesis
- Stabilizes CAN topoisomerase II (gyrase) -> strand breaks
Anthracycline Antibiotics:
Daunorubicin, doxorubicin
(Adriamycin)
- Intercalation with DNA -> strand breaks
- Binds cell membranes
- Forms O2 radicals through lipid peroxidation -> single strand breaks in DNA
Mitotic disruptors, cell cycle-specific:
Vinca Alkaloids - Vincristine
Vinblastine
- Destabilizes microtubules, blocks tubulin from polymerizing
- Mitotic spindle is frozen in metaphase
- Prevents chromosomal segregation and cell proliferation.
Paclitaxel, Taxol (from yew trees)
- Binds tubulin and stabilizes microtubules
- Causes cell death

13.9.2 Common chemotherapy medications

Generic name	Trade name	Class	Major toxicities
5-fluorouracil	generic	Antimetabolite	Myelosuppression, hand-foot syndrome, chest pain with elevated cardiac enzymes (full cardiac workup is necessary)
6-mercaptopurine	Purinethol	Antimetabolite	Myelosuppression, hepatotoxicity
bleomycin	generic	Tumor antibiotic	Erythroderma, irreversible pulmonary fibrosis, allergic reaction
capecitabine	Xeloda	Antimetabolite	Diarrhea, hand-foot syndrome, myelosuppression
carboplatin	Paraplatin	Platinum	Myelosuppression, anaphylaxis, abdominal pain
chlorambucil	Leukeran	Alkylating agent	Myelosuppression, interstitial pneumonia, pulmonary fibrosis
cisplatin	Platinol AQ	Platinum	Nephrotoxicity, hearing loss, neuropathy, severe nausea/vomiting, myelosuppression
cladribine	Leustatin	Antimetabolite	Myelosuppression
cyclophosphamide	Cytoxan	Alkylating agent	Myelosuppression, potentially fatal acute hemorrhagic cystitis, alopecia, sterility, nausea/vomiting
cytarabine	generic	Antimetabolite	Myelosuppression, cerebellar dysfunction
decarbazine	generic	Alkylating agent	Nausea/vomiting, flu-like symptoms
daunorubicin	Daunoxome	Tumor antibiotic	Myelosuppression, cardiotoxicity, discoloration of urine

Generic name	Trade name	Class	Major toxicities
docetaxel	Taxotere	Plant alkaloid	Myelosuppression, fluid retention, neuropathy
doxorubicin	Adriamycin	Tumor antibiotic	Myelosuppression, cardiotoxicity, discoloration of urine
doxorubicin liposomal	Doxil	Tumor antibiotic	Myelosuppression, cardiotoxicity, peripheral edema, plantar palmar erythrodysesthesia
etoposide	generic	Plant alkaloid	Myelosuppression, diarrhea
fludarabine	Fludara	Antimetabolite	Myelosuppression, neurotoxicity, edema, weakness, cough
gemcitabine	Gemzar	Antimetabolite	Myelosuppression, peripheral edema, rash, nausea/vomiting
hydroxyurea	Hydrea	Other	Myelosuppression, atrophic skin
idarubicin	Idamycin	Tumor antibiotic	Myelosuppression, cardiotoxicity, discoloration of urine
ifosfamide	Ifex	Alkylating agent	Nausea/vomiting, myelosuppression, encephalopathy, hemorrhagic cystitis-(↓incidence with mesna)
irinotecan	Camptosar	Plant alkaloid	Diarrhea, myelosuppression
melphalan	Alkeran	Alkylating agent	Myelosuppression, mucositis
methotrexate	Trexall	Antimetabolite	Dermatitis, interstitial nephritis, pneumonitis, hepatitis, crystalline nephropathy, folic acid deficiency

Generic name	Trade name	Class	Major toxicities
mitomycin-C	generic	Tumor antibiotic	Myelosuppression, hemolytic uremic syndrome
oxaliplatin	Eloxatin	Platinum	Myelosuppression, neuropathy, intolerance to cold, cold liquids, uncommon pulmonary fibrosis
paclitaxel	Taxol	Plant alkaloid	Myelosuppression, neuropathy, anaphylactoid reactions, arthralgias, arrhythmias
paclitaxel nanoparticle	Abraxane	Plant alkaloid	Myelosuppression, neuropathy, anaphylactoid reactions, arthralgias, arrhythmias
pemetrexed	Alimta	Antimetabolite	Myelosuppression, Vit B12/ Folate deficiency, fatigue, rash
temozolomide	Temodar	Alkylating agent	Myelosuppression
topotecan	Hycamtin	Plant alkaloid	Myelosuppression, nausea/ vomiting
vinblastine	generic	Plant alkaloid	Myelosuppression, peripheral & autonomic neuropathy, SIADH
vincristine	generic	Plant alkaloid	Myelosuppression, peripheral & autonomic neuropathy, SIADH
vinorelbine	Navelbine	Plant alkaloid	Myelosuppression, anemia, pain at infusion site, neuropathy, fatigue

13.9.3 10 Key chemotherapeutic toxicities you should know!

Drug	Toxicity
doxorubicin (Adriamycin)	Cardiotoxicity, red urine color
bleomycin	Irreversible pulmonary fibrosis, allergic reaction
cyclophosphamide	Potentially fatal acute hemorrhagic cystitis, alopecia, sterility, bladder cancer
5-FU (fluorouracil)	Chest pain with elevated cardiac enzymes (full cardiac workup is necessary) hand-foot syndrome
mitomycin-C	Myelosuppression, hemolytic-uremic syndrome (HUS)
vincristine & vinblastine	Peripheral & autonomic neuropathy, SIADH
cisplatin	Nephrotoxicity, hearing loss, neuropathy, severe nausea/ vomiting
methotrexate	Interstitial pneumonitis, hepatitis, crystal nephropathy, folic acid deficiency
ifosfamide	Hemorrhagic cystitis, neurologic toxicity
paclitaxel	Anaphylactoid reactions, myelosuppression, arthralgias

13.9.4 Commonly used therapeutic monoclonal antibodies in oncology

M-Ab name	Trade name	Target	Indication
rituximab	Rituxan	CD20 antigen, found on B cells	Non-Hodgkin lymphoma
trastuzumab	Herceptin	HER2/Neu protein	Breast cancer
gemtuzumab ozogamicin	Mylotarg	CD33, found on most leukemia cells	Acute myelogenous leukemia (AML)
alemtuzumab	Campath	CD52 antigen found on B cells and T cells	Chronic lymphocytic leukemia (CLL)
ibritumomab tiuxetan	Zevalin	CD20 antigen, found on B cells	Non-Hodgkin lymphoma
tositumomab	Bexxar	CD20 antigen, found on B cells	Non-Hodgkin lymphoma
cetuximab	Erbitux	EGFR protein	Colorectal cancer and head and neck cancers
bevacizumab	Avastin	VEGF protein, for angiogenesis	Colorectal cancer
panitumumab	Vectibix	EGFR	Colorectal cancer

13.9.5 A few common regimens

Name	Agents	Indication
R-CHOP	Rituximab, cyclophosphamide, doxorubicin, vincristine, prednisone	Non-Hodgkin Lymphoma
ABVD	Doxorubicin, bleomycin, vinblastine, dacarbazine	Hodgkin's disease
AC → T	Doxorubicin, cyclophosphamide, then dose-dense paclitaxel	Breast cancer
FOLFOX	Oxaliplatin, leucovorin, fluorouracil	Colon cancer
FOLFIRI	Irinotecan, leucovorin, fluorouracil	Colon cancer
CMF	Cyclophosphamide, methotrexate, fluorouracil	Breast cancer

13.10 Palliative Care

Six-Step Protocol for Breaking Bad News - SPIKES	
Setting	Establish the right setting. Allocate adequate time for the encounter. Ensure the patient's privacy. Review your communication plan before entering the room.
Perception	Find out the patient's perception and understanding of his or her condition. Pay attention to the patient's words. Make a mental note of the discrepancies between medical facts and the patient's perspective.
Invitation	Obtain a clear invitation by the patient to give the information: "How would you like me to handle the information that we will obtain from these tests?" or "Are you the sort of person who wants all the details on their condition?"
Knowledge	Use of the patient's current understanding of his/her condition as a starting point to provide knowledge and medical facts. Use the same level of language as the patient uses. Give the information in small chunks. Check for patient understanding at each step.
Empathy	Be empathetic: "This must be very hard for you." Recognize that crying and anger are normal responses when receiving bad news. Provide realistic hope: "You will receive the best available treatment."
Strategy	Explain your treatment strategy. Encourage the patient's participation in decision-making. Summarize main points, answer questions. Negotiate next contact.
Baile WF, Buckman R, Lenzi R et al. The Oncologist 2000;5:302-311	

13.11 5 Board-Style Questions

1) A 52-year-old man is evaluated in the hospital for fever. He is found to have endocarditis, and blood cultures identify Streptococcus bovis. What non-cardiac diagnostic procedure should be performed?
2) A 58-year-old postmenopausal woman with estrogen receptor-positive breast cancer underwent lumpectomy and chemotherapy two years ago. he was started on Tamoxifen 1.5 years ago and now reports episodes of "menstrual bleeding." What diagnosis should be considered?
3) Which cancers have been associated with Epstein-Barr virus infection?
4) A 52-year-old woman smoker presents with edema of the upper extremities and face, dyspnea, and is noted to have neck vein distention on physical examination. Endobronchial biopsy the same day reveals small cell lung cancer. It is determined to be limited stage. What treatment(s) should be considered for this patient?
5) A 62-year-old man is found to have a prostate nodule. His PSA is 2.3 (upper limit of normal is 4.0). What should be done for this patient?

14 Pain Management

The recommendations in this chapter were adapted from the American Cancer Society Pain Management Guidelines for 2005.

14.1 Basic Principles of Pain Management

Ask	Always remember to ask the patient about the presence of pain and be willing to accept the patient's report of pain.
Assess	Perform a comprehensive pain assessment, including: - Onset, duration, and location. - Quality (sharp, dull, diffuse, throbbing, etc). - Intensity (1-10 scale, for example). - Aggravating and alleviating factors (what makes it better or worse). - Effect on function and quality of life. - Patient's goal for pain control. - Response to prior treatments if condition is chronic. - History and physical exam.
Treat	- With older adults, start low, go slow, but go!! - Avoid intramuscular route, the oral route is preferred. - Treat persistent pain with regularly scheduled medications. - Two drugs of the same class (eg, NSAIDs) should not generally be given concurrently. The exception is that a long-acting opioid may be prescribed along with a short-term opioid (see breakthrough pain section). - Avoid meperidine and propoxyphene.
Monitor	- Assess and reassess pain frequently. - Most opioid agonists have no ceiling dose for analgesia; titrate to relief and assess for side effects. - Assess, anticipate, and manage opioid side effects aggressively. - Discuss goals and plans with patient and family.
Addiction	Addiction rarely occurs unless there is a history of substance abuse. Watch for red flags: 1) Compulsive use 2) Loss of control 3) Use despite harm

14.2 Management of Breakthrough Pain

General guidelines	- Use **long-acting** opioids around the clock for **baseline** management of persistent pain. - Use **short-acting** opioids PRN (rescue) for **breakthrough** pain. - Consider using the same drug for both baseline and rescue doses whenever possible (eg, long-acting morphine + short-acting morphine).
Rescue dosing	- The rescue dose is 10%-15% of the 24h total daily dose. - Oral rescue doses should be available every 1-2h; parenteral doses every 15-30 minutes.
Adjustment	- If the patient is consistently taking ≥**3** rescue doses daily, consider increasing the baseline around-the-clock dose. - Recalculate the rescue dose whenever the baseline dose is changed.
Example	If a patient's baseline coverage is MS Contin 200 mg q12h, what would the rescue dose be? 1. Calculate total daily dose: 200 mg x 2 = 400 mg morphine/day 2. Establish rescue dose: 10%-15% of 400 mg = 40-60 mg short-acting morphine 3. Oral rescue dose therefore is: morphine 40-60 mg PO q1-2h 4. Parenteral rescue dose (based on continuous infusion): Calculate based on 25%-50% of hourly dose

14.3 Nonopioid Analgesics

Drug	Average dose	Side effects	Comments
acetaminophen (Tylenol)	500-1000mg q4-6h (max: 4 g/d, 3g/d if liver dysfunction or elderly)	Minimal	Liver toxicity in overdose
Non Steroidal Anti-Inflammatory Drugs (NSAIDs) - Use with caution in the elderly!!			
aspirin	500-1000mg q4-6h (max: 4 g/d)	see footnote *	Caution with hepatic/ renal disease
choline magnesium trisalicylate (Trilisate)	500-1000 mg q8-12h (max: 3 g/d)	Lower incidence of GI bleeding, minimal antiplatelet activity	Caution with hepatic/ renal disease
ibuprofen (Motrin, Advil, etc)	200-400 mg q4-6h (max: 2400 mg/d)	see footnote *	Caution with hepatic/ renal disease
naproxen (Naprosyn)	500 mg initial then 250 mg q6-8h (max: 1500 mg/d)	see footnote *	Caution with hepatic/ renal disease
nabumetone (Relafen)	500-750 mg q8-12h (max: 2 g/d)	see footnote *	Caution with hepatic/ renal disease
ketorolac (Toradol)	30 mg IV initial, then 15-30 mg q6h (max: 150 mg/d day 1, 120 mg/ d thereafter)	see footnote *	In elderly, 30mg starting dose, 15mg thereafter. Use restricted to 5d max. Caution with hepatic/ renal disease
celecoxib (Celebrex)	100-200 mg q12h (max: 200-400 mg/d)	Lower incidence of adverse GI effects	Contraindicated in sulfonamide allergy. No platelet effects. Risk of cardiovascular events. Use lowest possible dose
Other			
Drug	**Average dose**	**Side effects**	**Comments**
tramadol (Ultram)	25-50mg q4-6h (max: 400 mg/d, 300 mg/d in the elderly)	Headache, confusion, sedation	Atypical opioid with addn'l nonopioid effects. Available combined with non-opioids. Lowers seizure threshold

* Common NSAID side effects: GI ulceration and bleeding, decreased platelet aggregation, renal toxicity

14.4 Opiod Equianalgesic Chart

Opioid	Parenteral	Oral	Starting dose for opioid-naive[1]	PROM[2]
Simple Opioids - No Ceiling Dose				
morphine	10 mg	30 mg	15 mg for both sustained and immediate release	1
hydromorphone (Dilaudid)	1.5 mg	7.5 mg	4 mg	3.5-7.5
oxycodone	N/A	20 mg	10 mg sustained release 5 mg immediate release	2
fentanyl	0.1 mg	N/A	25 µg/h patch is equal to approx. 50 mg of oral morphine qd	150
methadone	5 mg	10 mg	3-5 mg PO for long term use (can accumulate due to long half life) Consult pain specialist before prescribing	3
Combination Opioid Drugs - With Ceiling Dose				
hydrocodone + aspirin, acetaminophen, or ibuprofen (Vicodin, Lortab, Vicoprofen)	N/A	30 mg	5, 7.5, or 10 mg hydrocodone with aspirin, acetaminophen, or ibuprofen (4 g/d ceiling dose with acetaminophen)	1
oxycodone + acetaminophen (Percocet, Tylox)	N/A	20 mg	5 mg oxycodone with 325 or 500 mg acetaminophen (4 g/d ceiling dose with acetaminophen)	2

1. Equianalgesic doses are approximate and must be adjusted based on individual patient response.
2. PROM = potency relative to oral morphine (approximate)

Also Remember!
2 Tylenol 3 tabs ~ 1 Percocet ~ 5 mg PO morphine ~ 2 mg IV morphine
(Tylenol 3 = codeine + acetaminophen)

14.5 Converting Doses in Opioid Switches

Example:

Change patient's current morphine regimen of 30 mg PO q4h to hydromorphone.

1. Calculate 24-hour dose of current opioid (morphine):
   30 mg x 24h/4h = 30 mg x 6 = 180 mg/day
2. Locate equivalency entry from table (hydromorphone - morphine):
   7.5 mg hydromorphone = 30 mg morphine
3. Set up equation to solve for new opioid (hydromorphone) daily dose:

   $$\frac{180\ \text{mg}}{30\ \text{mg}} = \frac{X}{7.5\ \text{mg}}$$

   and solve for X:
   $X = 7.5 * 180/30 = 45$ mg/d
4. Divide new daily dose by number of doses to find per dose amount:
   45 mg / 6 doses = 7.5 mg q4h
5. Reduce calculated dose of new opioid (hydromorphone) by 25%-50% to account for incomplete cross tolerance. Titrate up as needed.

14.6 Fentanyl Transdermal System - Duragesic Patch

The Duragesic patch is indicated for patients with demonstrated opioid tolerance whose pain cannot be managed by other opioid or combination regimens. **Use extreme caution in opioid-naive patients!** Opioid tolerance means patients who have been taking one of the following daily oral doses for **at least 1 week**: 60 mg morphine, 30 mg oxycodone, 8 mg hydromorphone, or an equivalent equianalgesic dose of another opioid.

The Duragesic patch is designed to deliver a continuous **25 µg/h per 10 cm^2** which is approximately equivalent to a dose of 50 mg morphine qd.	Dose (µg/h)	Size (cm^2)	Fentanyl content (mg)
	12	5	1.25
	25	10	2.5
	50	20	5
	75	30	7.5
	100	40	10
Duragesic Fentanyl Transdermal System drug package insert, ©2005 Janssen			

14.7 Management of Opioid Adverse Effects

Adverse effect	Management considerations
Constipation	Begin bowel regimen when opioid therapy is initiated. Include a mild stimulant laxative (eg, senna, cascara) + stool softener (eg, Colace) at bedtime or in divided doses as routine prophylaxis.
Sedation	Tolerance typically develops. Hold sedatives/anxiolytics, dose reduction. Consider stimulants such as caffeine, methylphenidate or dextroamphetamine.
Nausea/vomiting	Dose reduction, opioid rotation. Consider metoclopramide, prochlorperazine, scopolamine patch.
Pruritus	Dose reduction, opioid rotation. Consider an antihistamine (eg, diphenhydramine).
Hallucinations	Dose reduction, opioid rotation. Consider neuroleptics (eg, haloperidol, risperidone).
Confusion/ delirium	Dose reduction, opioid rotation, neuroleptic therapy (eg, haloperidol, risperidone).
Myoclonic jerking	Dose reduction, opioid rotation. Consider clonazepam, baclofen.
Respiratory depression	Sedation precedes respiratory depression. Hold opioid! Give low dose naloxone - dilute 0.4 mg (1 ml of a 0.4 mg/ml amp of naloxone) in 9 ml of normal saline (NS) for final concentration of 0.04 mg/ml.

14.8 Adjuvant Antidepressants

Drug	1° Indication	Dose range*	Comments
Tricyclics (TCAs)			
amitriptyline (Elavil)	Neuropathic pain	Start: 25 mg PO qhs (10 mg or less in elderly) Range: 75-150mg qhs	Side effects include dry mouth, drowsiness, dizziness, constipation, urinary retention, confusion. Titrate dose every few days to minimize SEs. Avoid in elderly and use caution in pts with cardiovascular disease.
nortriptylene (Pamelor)	Neuropathic pain	Same as above	Lower SEs than amitriptyline. Titrate dose.
desipramine (Norpramin)	Neuropathic pain	Same as above	Lower SEs than amitriptyline. Titrate dose.
Selective Serotonin and Norepinephrine Reuptake Inhibitors (SSNRIs)			
duloxetine (Cymbalta)	Diabetic peripheral neuropathy	Start: 30 mg PO qd Range: 30-60 mg qd sustained release	Do not use with MAOIs. Consider lower starting dose if tolerability is a concern.
Anticonvulsants			
gabapentin (Neurontin)	Neuropathic pain	Start: 100-300 mg PO tid, increase by 100 mg tid q3d Range: 300-3600mg/d div 3 doses	Adjust in renal dysfunction. First choice as anticonvulsant. Can cause drowsiness. No drug-drug interactions (DDIs).
carbamazepine (Tegretol)	Neuropathic pain	Start: 100 mg PO bid Range: 400-800 mg/d, max: 1600 mg/d	Requires serum level monitoring. Multiple DDIs
lamotrigine (Lamictal)	Neuropathic pain	Start: 25-50 mg/d Range: 200-600mg/d	Reports of serious skin rashes.

Drug	1° Indication	Dose range*	Comments
Corticosteroids			
dexamethasone (Decadron)	Spinal cord compression, bony metastases	Start: 4-8 mg PO q8-12h or 10-20 mg IV q6h	High-dose therapy should not exceed 72h. May improve appetite.
prednisone	Spinal cord compression, bony metastases	5-10 mg PO qd-bid	For cancer pain, continue treatment until side effects outweigh benefit.
Local Anesthetic			
lidocaine topical (Lidoderm patch)	Post-herpetic neuralgia	1-3 patches over painful area(s)	Patch may be cut to fit painful area(s). Place only on intact skin.
Other			
baclofen (Lioresal)	Muscle spasticity	5-10 mg PO tid-qid Range: 80-120 mg PO qd	Use caution in renal insufficiency.

* The dose ranges are for use in the drug's primary indication, however, doses in the lower range should be used for the treatment of depression.

15 Pediatrics

15.1 Vitals Signs by Age

Age	Baseline HR		BP (50th %ile)	RR
	Min	Max	(mm Hg)	(/min)
First wk	95	160	75/55	30–50
1 – 4 wk	105	180	80/50	30–50
1 – 6 mo	110	180	90/50	30–50
6 – 12 mo	110	170	90/55	20–40
1 – 3 yrs	100	150	100/60	20–30
3 – 8 yrs	65	130	105/70	20–25
8 – 12 yrs	60	110	115/75	16-22
12 - 15 yrs	60	110	125/80	14–20

15.2 Apgar Score

Criteria	0 Points	1 Point	2 Points
A = Appearance	entire body blue	blue extremities	entire body pink
P = Pulse	absent	<100/min	>100/min
G = Grimace (response to suction)	no response	grimace	cough, sneeze, or cry
A = Activity (muscle tone)	atonic	decreased, some extremity flexion	active motion
R = Respiratory effort	absent	slow, irregular	good, crying
Scoring at 1 and 5 minutes after birth.			
Interpretation: 8 points: mild risk; 6-8 points: newborn is impaired; <6 points: newborn's life is severely threatened, transfer immediately to NICU			

15.3 Primitive Reflexes

Reflexes	Present until	Reflexes	Present until
Sucking reflex	3 mo	Galant reflex	3-6 mo
Rooting reflex	3 mo	Asym tonic neck (ATNR)	4-9 mo
Palmar reflex	3 mo	Tonic labyrinthine	6-9 mo
Plantar reflex	9 mo	Moro reflex	3-6 mo
Babinski reflex	4-6 mo		

15.4 Recommended 3-Year Well Child Visit Schedule

Visit number	Interval
1	1-2 days after discharge from nursery
2	7-14 days
3	1 month
4	2 months
5	4 months
6	6 months
7	9 months
8	12 months
9	15 months
10	18 months - do developmental screening*
(10.5)	21 months if developmental concerns**
11	24 months
12	30 months
13	36 months
14 and greater	between 4 and 18 yrs of age yearly

The following topics should be addressed at every well child visit, as appropriate:

- Nutrition
- Gates on swimming pools
- Knee braces/pads for sports
- Seat belts and car seats
- Helmets for bicycles/skateboards
- Home/kitchen safety

* New AAP recommendations recommend screening tests such as the Parents´ Evaluation of Developmental Status (PEDS), and the Checklist for Autism in Toddlers (M-CHAT).

** Optional visit if there is concern regarding developmental problems

15.5 Developmental Milestones

Age	Language	Gross motor	Visual-motor/ Problem-solving	Social/adaptive
1 mo	Alerts to sounds	Raises head slightly from prone	Follows to midline, has tight grasp, visually fixes	Regards face
2 mo	Smiles socially (after being stroked or talked to)	Holds head in midline, lifts chest off table	No longer clenches fist tightly, follows object past midline	Recognizes parent
4 mo	Laughs, orients to voice	Rolls front to back, supports on wrists and shifts weight	Reaches with arms in unison, brings hands to midline	Enjoys looking around environment
6 mo	Says: "Ah-goo", razzes, orients to bell (localizes laterally)	Sits unsupported, puts feet in mouth in supine position	Unilateral reach, uses raking grasp	Recognizes strangers
9 mo	"Mama", "Dada" indiscriminately, waves bye-bye, understands 'no'	Pivots when sitting, pulls to stand, cruises	Uses pincer grasp, probes with forefinger, holds bottle, throws objects	Starts to explore environment, plays gesture games (eg, patty-cake)
12 mo	Uses 2 words other than "dada/mama"	Walks alone	Uses mature pincer grasp, releases voluntarily, marks paper with pencil	Imitates actions, comes when called, cooperates with dressing
18 mo	Uses 2 word combinations	Runs, throws objects from standing without falling	Scribbles spontaneously, builds tower of 3 blocks, turns 2-3 pages at a time	Copies parent in tasks (sweeping, dusting), plays in company of other children

2 yr	Uses pronouns (I, you, me) inappropriately, follows 2-step commands	Walks up and down steps without help	Imitates stroke with pencil, builds tower of 7 blocks, turns pages one at a time, removes shoes, pants, etc.	Parallel play
3 yr	Uses minimum 250 words, 3-word sentences, uses plurals, past tense, knows all pronouns, understands concept of "2"	Can alternate feet when going up steps, pedals tricycle	Copies a circle, undresses completely, dresses partially, dries hands if reminded	Group play, shares toys, takes turns, plays well with others, knows full name, age, sex
4 yr	Knows colors, says song or poem from memory, asks questions	Hops, skips, alternates feet going down steps	Copies a square, buttons clothing, dresses self completely, catches ball	Tells "tall tales", plays cooperatively with a group of children
5 yr	Prints first name, asks what a word means	Skips alternating feet, jumps over low obstacles	Copies triangle, ties shoes, spreads with knife	Plays competitive games, abides by rules, likes to help in household tasks

Capute AJ, Palmer FB, Shapiro BK et al. Clinical linguistic and auditory milestone scale: prediction of cognition in infancy. Dev med child neruol 1986; 28: 762.
Capute AJ, Accardo PJ. Linguistic and auditory milestones during the first two years of life. Clinical Paediatrics 1978; 17:847.

15.6 Tanner Stages of Pubertal Changes

Stage	Pubic Hair	Girls - Breast	Boys - Penis	Boys - Testes
I	None	Prepubertal	Prepubertal	Prepubertal
II	Sparse, long, slightly pigmented; **F:** medial border labia, age 10.5-13	Age 10-12 Breast buds, areolae enlarge	Age 10-12.5 Slight enlargement	Age 10-12.5 Scrotum enlarges, reddens, and rugae appear; testes enlarge
	M: at base of penis, age 11-13			
III	Coarse hair spreads over pubis	Age 11-13 Elevation of breast contour; coarse hair spreads over pubis	Age 12-14 Penis lengthens	Age 12-14 Further growth
	F: 11-13			
	M: 13-15			
IV	Adult hair but not spread to inguinal crease	Age 12-14.5 Areola and papilla form 2° mound	Age 13-15 Larger glans and breadth increases	Age 13-15 Larger, scrotum darkens
	F: 12-14			
	M: 13-15			
V	Adult hair distribution that spreads to medial thigh	Age 13.5- 17 Adult: nipple projects, areola part of general breast contour	Age 14-16 Adult size	Age 14-16 Adult size
	F: 13-15			
	M: 14-16			

Significant clinical note: African-American girls may mature earlier than Caucasian girls

15.7 Failure to Thrive - Differential Diagnoses

Differential Diagnosis	History	Workup
GERD	Spitting, vomiting	Upper GI, pH probe, esophagoscopy
Malabsorption (Cystic fibrosis, celiac disease, lactase deficiency)	Abdominal distention, cramping, diarrhea	D-xylose, stool fat, TTG-tissue transglutaminase or biopsy, sweat chloride*
Parasitosis, TB, inadequate access to cooking facilities and refrigeration	Foreign travel, homeless, living in shelter	Stool for O&P, duodenal biopsy, string test, PPD
Adenoid hypertrophy	Snoring, periodic breathing during sleep, restless sleep, noisy or mouth breathing	Lateral neck film
Chronic aspiration, cystic fibrosis	Symptoms of asthma, bronchitis	Chest film, sweat chloride (> 60% diagnostic)
Diabetes	Polyuria, polydypsia, polyphagia	Blood glucose
HIV or other immune deficiency	Frequent minor infections	Serologic tests, immunoglobulins, PPD with anergy

*Source: North American Society for Pediatric Gastroenterology, Hepatology and Nutrition Celiac Disease Clinical Guidelines

15.8 Recommended Childhood Immunization Schedule 2012

Age	Months										Years			
Vaccine	Birth	1	2	4	6	12	15	18	19–23	2–3	4–6	7–10	11–12	13–18
Hepatitis B	HepB 1	Hep B 2				Hep B 3						Ages for catch up		
Rotavirus			RV	RV	RV									
Diphtheria, tetanus, pertussis[2]			DTaP	DTaP	DTaP		DTaP				DTaP		Tdap	
H. influenzae type B			Hib	Hib	Hib	Hib								
Pneumococcal			PCV	PCV	PCV	PCV				PPSV		For high risk groups		
Inactivated polio			IPV	IPV		IPV					IPV4	Ages for catch up		
Influenza							Influenza yearly							
Measles, mumps, rubella						MMR					MMR	Ages for catch up		
Varicella						Varicella					Varicella	Ages for catch up		
Hepatitis A						HepA x 2 doses				HepA				
Meningococcal										MCV 4		MCV 4 high risk group	MCV4	MCV4 for catch up
HPV													HPVx3 (females)	HPV
Legend		Regularly scheduled			Range of recomm. ages for all children			Catch-up vaccinations			High-risk groups			

Source: http://www.cdc.gov/vaccines/recs/schedules/child-schedule.htm
http://www.cdc.gov/vaccines/recs/schedules/downloads/child/0-6yrs-schedule-pr.pdf
http://www.cdc.gov/vaccines/recs/schedules/downloads/child/7-18yrs-schedule-pr.pdf

15.9 Childhood Rash Differentials

Disease	Rash	Location	Mucosa	Addn'l Comments
Measles	Erythematous, maculopapular rash	Starts on face, extends to body	Koplik spots	**2 phases** **1:** high fever x 3d **2:** followed by cough, coryza, conjunctivitis
Rubella (German measles)	Erythematous maculopapular rash	Starts on face, extends to body	Palate papules (Forchheimer sign)	Low fever, post.-auric/cerv., occ. LAD, arthritis, eye pain
Varicella	Papules→blisters → crusts (dew drop on rose petal)	Trunk more than face/limbs; lesions in all stages	Mucosal spots	Low fever, post-inf. enceph., cerebel. ataxia, GBS, pneumonia
Scarlet fever	Pinpoint rash, blanches on pressure	Starts axillae & groin → trunk/neck	Tonsillitis, strawberry tongue	Group A strep, tx with penicillin x 10d
Roseola (exanthema subitum)	Fine pink rash	Mainly truncal	None	Febrile convulsions, LAD
5th disease (erythema infectiosum)	Lacy reticular maculopapular rash	"Slapped cheek"→ trunk→limbs	None	-
Kawasaki syndrome	Extremity erythema and edema, scarlet fever-like	Generalized	Strawberry tongue, erythema, cracked lips, nonpurulent conjunctivitis	High fever for 5d, cerv. LAD, coronary art. aneurysm, sterile pyuria, early: thrombocytopenia, late: thrombocytosis, desquamation; ↑ AST & ALT

15.10 Neonatal Hyperbilirubinemia

15.10.1 Hyperbilirubinemia differentials

	Indirect hyperbilirubinemia		Direct hyperbilirubinemia
Conjugated bilirubin ↓	Physiological icterus, Crigler-Najjar syndr., Gilbert syndr., hypothyroid, drugs, hormones	Intrahepatic cholestase	Neonatal cholestase, infection (CMV, rubella, hepatitis, toxoplasmosis), alpha-1 anti-trypsin deficiency, intrahepatic biliary hypoplasia, galactosemia, tyrosinemia, parenteral nutrition
Hemolysis ↑	Blood group incompatibility, hemolytic anemia, infection	Extrahepatic biliary atresia	Extrahepatic biliary atresia, choledochal cyst, cystic fibrosis
Erythrocyte ↑	Polycythemia, excessive bruising		
Enteral bilirubin resorption ↑	Intestinal obstruction, biliary atresia, ↓ caloric intake, hyper-bilirubinemia in breastfed children		

15.10.2Guidelines for phototherapy

Age	Guidelines for phototherapy	Guidelines for plasma exchange *	Guidelines for plasma exchange
25–48 h	> 15 mg/dl	> 20 mg/dl	> 25 mg/dl
49–72 h	> 18 mg/dl	> 25 mg/dl	> 30 mg/dl
> 72 h	> 20 mg/dl	> 25 mg/dl	> 30 mg/dl

* If bilirubin level does not decrease 1-2 mg/dl after 4-6 h phototherapy
These guidelines do not apply to premature infants!

15.10.3 Bhutani nomogram

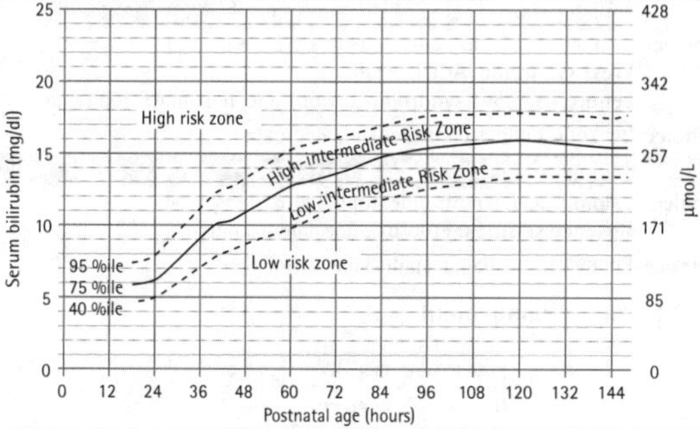

When using this nomogram, remember that "risk" refers to the risk of a subsequent bilirubin level in that infant > 95%ile for age.

Bhutani VK, Johnson L, Sivieri EM. Predictive ability of a predischarge hour-specific serum bilirubin for subsequent significant hyperbilirubinemia in healthy term and near-term newborns. Pediatrics. 1999 Jan;103(1):6-14.

15.11 Pediatric Neurology

15.11.1 Febrile seizures

	Benign	Complicated
Age at 1st seizure	6 mo – 5 yrs	<6 mo or >5 yrs
Clinical	Primary generalized	Focal-motor
Postictal	No pathological findings in EEG	Paralysis EEG: focal changes, hypersynchronous activity
Duration	<15 min	>15 min
Episodes	only 1 or 2	>4; >2 in 24 h
Prognosis	2% chronic epilepsy	10% chronic epilepsy
Therapy	Drugs not indicated. Treat underlying DO. May use **diazepam rectal** 0.5mg/kg/dose PRN.	Further workup required. Consider anticonvulsants. Neurology consult recommended.

15.11.2 Pediatric epilepsy therapy

Focal Epilepsy (Juvenile Myoclonic)	
1st choice	Valproic acid, lamotrigine, topiramate, zonisamide, levetiracetam **West syndrome**: ACTH, vigabatrin **Lennox-Gastaut syndrome**: lamotrigine, felbamate, topiramate
2nd choice	Benzodiazapines (clonazepam), valproate
Generalized Epilepsy (Tonic-Clonic)	
1st choice	Valproic acid, lamotrigine, topiramate, zonisimide **Absence seizures:** ethosuximide, lamotrigine
2nd choice	Phenytoin, carbamazepine, vigabatrin

15.11.3 Seizure management

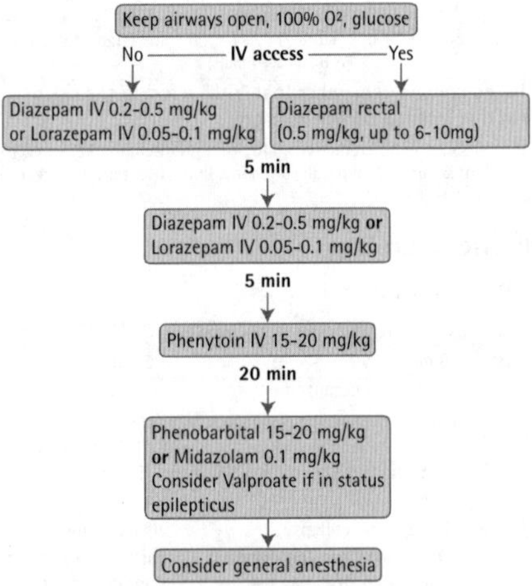

15.12 Pediatric Infectious Diseases

15.12.1 Pneumonia

Age	Organisms	Suggested empiric treatment
< 6 wk	*Group B Strep* *C. trachomatis* *Staph. aureus* *Listeria*	**ampicillin** 150 mg/kg/d IV div q8h **+ cefotaxime** 150 mg/kg/d IV div q8h **or + gentamicin** 3-5 mg/kg/d IV x 10-21d **For chlamydia:** **erythromycin** 50 mg/kg/d div q6h PO x 14d (assoc. with pyloric stenosis); alt: **azithromycin** 20 mg/kg PO qd x 3d
6 wk – 6 mo	RSV, *Pneumococcus* *H. influenzae* *Group A Strep* *C. trachomatis* *Staph. aureus* *B. pertussis*	**cefotaxime** 150 mg/kg/d IV div q8h **or ceftriaxone** 50-75 mg/kg/d IV div q12-24h (max: 2g/d) **or amoxicillin** 80-100 mg/kg/d PO div q12h x 7-10d Consider alt. empiric tx for **pneumococcal resistance:** **cefotaxime** 200-300 mg/kg/d + possible **vancomycin** (esp. in white-out) 40 mg/kg/d div q6-8h
6 mo – 5 yrs	RSV, Parainfluenza Influenza Adenovirus, *Pneumococcus*	**azithromycin** PO 10 mg/kg qd day 1, then 5 mg/kg qd day 2-5 **or amoxicillin** 80-100 mg/kg/d PO div q12h x 7-10d **or clindamycin** 10-30 mg/kg/d PO div q6-8h InflA+B: **oseltamivir**
> 5 yrs	*M. pneumoniae* *Pneumococcus* Adenovirus	**amoxicillin or macrolide** PO (**azithromycin** 10 mg/kg PO qd day 1, then 5 mg/kg qd day 2-5, **erythromycin** 30-50mg/kg/d PO div q6-8h) **or doxycycline** init: 2.2 mg/kg/dose PO/IV bid x 1d, then 2.2-4.4 mg/kg/dose qd-bid PO/IV

Source: CDC and American Academy of Pediatrics. Summary of Influenza Antiviral Treatment Recommendations for 2010-2011 Season - US. http://www.cdc.gov/flu/professionals/antivirals/antiviralrec2010.htm

15.12.2 Meningitis

Age	Organisms	Suggested empiric treatment
< 6 wk	*Strep. agalactiae* *Gram B Strep* *E. coli* *Listeria* *N. gonorrheae*	**ampicillin** 200-400 mg/kg/d div q4-6h **+ cefotaxime** 200 mg/kg/d IV div q6h **or + gentamicin** 4 mg/kg/d div q12-24h x 4-21 days Gonorrheal: **ceftriaxone** 25-50 mg/kg/d IV qd x 7 days
> 6 wk	*H. influenzae* *S. pneumoniae* *N. meningitidis*	**cefotaxime** 200 mg/kg/d div q6h **or ceftriaxone** 100 mg/kg/d IV div q12-24h (max: 2g/d)
> 24 mo	*N. meningitidis* *S. pneumoniae* *H. influenzae*	**or cefepime** 150 mg/kg/d IV div qh8 (>2mo olds) **+ Vancomycin** 60 mg/kg IV q6h **+ dexamethasone*** 0.15 mg/kg IV q6h x 2 days
Post-exposure prophylaxis, unknown agent		
rifampin <1mo: 10 mg/kg PO q12h; >1mo: 20 mg/kg PO q12h (max. 600 mg/d) for 2 days; Alternatively, use single dose **ceftriaxone** 125 mg IM		

*Administer dexamethasone 10 min before antibiotics; dexamethasone is recommended in children >6 weeks of age with Hib meningitis, but its use is controversial in pneumococcal meningitis.
Sources: 2010 STD guidelines children from CDC IDSA website guidelines on meningitis: http://cid.oxfordjournals.org/content/39/9/1267.full.pdf+html

15.12.3 Urinary tract infections

Age	Organisms	Symptoms	Suggested empiric treatment
New-born	**Most common:** *E. coli* *Klebsiella* *Proteus* *S. aureus* *S. saprophyticus* **Neonates:** *Group B Strep* **Complicated:** *Enterococcus* *Pseudomonas*	Poor feeding, pale skin, irritability, sepsis	**ampicillin** 100 mg/kg/d IV div q8h **+ cefotaxime** 150 mg/kg/d IV div q6-8h **or + gentamicin** 3–5 mg/kg/d IV qday
Infant < 6 mo		Fever, diarrhea, vomiting, meningismus	**ampicillin** 100 mg/kg/d IV div q8h **+ cefotaxime** 150 mg/kg/d IV div q6-8h **or + gentamicin** 2.5 mg/kg/d div q8h
6mo - Toddler		Dysuria, fever, loin tenderness, abdominal pain, 2° enuresis	**TMP-SMX** 8-10 mg/kg/d PO div q12h **or cephalexin** 25-100 mg/kg/d PO div q6h **or amoxicillin-clavulonic acid** 20-40mg/kg/d PO div q8h **or cefpodoxime** 10 mg/kg/d div q12h
Child > 6 yrs		Polyuria, foul-smelling urine	

Suggested test	Urinalysis (nitrites, leukocyte esterase, sediment, electrolytes), culture, renal and urinary tract U/S, poss. reflux study, voiding cystourethrogram (VCUG), ^{99m}Tc DMSA scan **U/S + VCUG** is recommended in the following 3 groups: - All male children with 1st UTI - Female children <5 yrs with 1st UTI - All children with recurrent UTIs or suspected pyelonephritis
Antibiotic prophylaxis	Indications: VUR, obstruction, recurrent UTIs (controversial); Treatments: **methenamine mandelate** 75 mg/kg/d PO div q12h **or TMP-SMX** 2-10 mg/kg/d PO qhs **or nitrofurantoin** 1-2 mg/kg/d PO qhs

15.12.4 Management of fever of unknown origin (FUO)

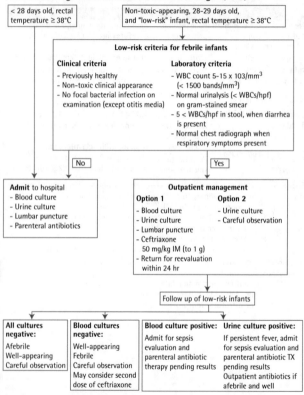

< 28 days old, rectal temperature ≥ 38°C

Non-toxic-appearing, 28-29 days old, and "low-risk" infant, rectal temperature ≥ 38°C

Low-risk criteria for febrile infants

Clinical criteria
- Previously healthy
- Non-toxic clinical appearance
- No focal bacterial infection on examination (except otitis media)

Laboratory criteria
- WBC count 5-15 x 103/mm^3 (< 1500 bands/mm^3)
- Normal urinalysis (< WBCs/hpf) on gram-stained smear
- 5 < WBCs/hpf in stool, when diarrhea is present
- Normal chest radiograph when respiratory symptoms present

No

Admit to hospital
- Blood culture
- Urine culture
- Lumbar puncture
- Parenteral antibiotics

Yes

Outpatient management

Option 1
- Blood culture
- Urine culture
- Lumbar puncture
- Ceftriaxone 50 mg/kg IM (to 1 g)
- Return for reevaluation within 24 hr

Option 2
- Urine culture
- Careful observation

Follow up of low-risk infants

All cultures negative:
Afebrile
Well-appearing
Careful observation

Blood cultures negative:
Well-appearing
Febrile
Careful observation
May consider second dose of ceftriaxone

Blood culture positive:
Admit for sepsis evaluation and parenteral antibiotic therapy pending results

Urine culture positive:
If persistent fever, admit for sepsis evaluation and parenteral antibiotic TX pending results
Outpatient antibiotics if afebrile and well

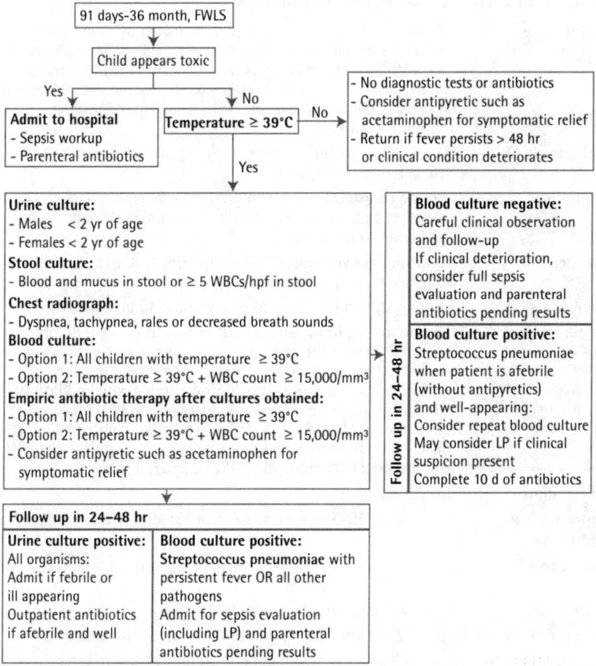
91 days-36 month, FWLS
Child appears toxic
Yes
No
Admit to hospital
- Sepsis workup
- Parenteral antibiotics
Temperature ≥ 39°C
No
- No diagnostic tests or antibiotics
- Consider antipyretic such as acetaminophen for symptomatic relief
- Return if fever persists > 48 hr or clinical condition deteriorates
Yes
Urine culture:
- Males < 2 yr of age
- Females < 2 yr of age
Stool culture:
- Blood and mucus in stool or ≥ 5 WBCs/hpf in stool
Chest radiograph:
- Dyspnea, tachypnea, rales or decreased breath sounds
Blood culture:
- Option 1: All children with temperature ≥ 39°C
- Option 2: Temperature ≥ 39°C + WBC count ≥ 15,000/mm³
Empiric antibiotic therapy after cultures obtained:
- Option 1: All children with temperature ≥ 39°C
- Option 2: Temperature ≥ 39°C + WBC count ≥ 15,000/mm³
- Consider antipyretic such as acetaminophen for symptomatic relief
Follow up in 24–48 hr
Blood culture negative:
Careful clinical observation and follow-up
If clinical deterioration, consider full sepsis evaluation and parenteral antibiotics pending results
Blood culture positive:
Streptococcus pneumoniae when patient is afebrile (without antipyretics) and well-appearing:
Consider repeat blood culture
May consider LP if clinical suspicion present
Complete 10 d of antibiotics
Follow up in 24–48 hr
Urine culture positive:
All organisms:
Admit if febrile or ill appearing
Outpatient antibiotics if afebrile and well
Blood culture positive:
Streptococcus pneumoniae with persistent fever OR all other pathogens
Admit for sepsis evaluation (including LP) and parenteral antibiotics pending results

15.13 Emergency Drugs in Pediatrics

adenosine	**SVT**: 0.01-0.02 mg/kg rapid IV push followed by saline flush; repeat at 2-min intervals and increase dose by 0.05 mg/kg each time until SVT resolves or max dose of 0.25 mg/kg reached; Children: First dose 0.1 mg/kg rapid bolus. Second dose 0.2 mg/kg rapid bolus **contraindication:** 2nd-/ 3rd-degree AV-block, sick sinus syndrome.
albuterol	PO: 0.3-0.6 mg/kg/d; MDI(> 4 yr): 1-2 puffs q4-6h prn; Neb: 0.1-0.15 mg/kg/dose
atropine	**Cardiac resuscitation**: 0.02 mg/kg IV push, repeat once if needed; if by ETT 0.04-0.06 mg/kg. Max- child: 0.5 mg, max- adolescent: 1 mg
diazepam	**Agitation, convulsions**: 0.2-0.5 mg/kg/dose IV q15-30min; max: < 5 yr: 5mg, > 5 yr: 10mg
dobutamine	2–20 µg/kg/min IV, titrate to effect; max: 40 µg/kg/min
epinephrine IV: use1:10,000 1ml = 0.1mg ET/SC: use 1:1,000 1ml = 1mg	**Cardiac arrest, bradycardia**: 0.01 mg/kg (0.1 ml/kg) IV or 0.1 mg/kg ET. Repeat the same dose q3-5 min until sinus rhythm or VT occurs. Higher repeat doses have been shown to be ineffective, and may in fact be detrimental. **Bronchodilation**: 0.01 ml/kg/dose SC q15min x3-4 doses or q4h PRN (max. 0.5 ml/dose). Alt: Nebulizer: 0.5 ml/kg 1:1000 diluted in 3ml NS (max: 2.5 ml (<4yro), 5 ml (>4yo)); Inhaler: 1-2 puffs q4hr PRN; **Anaphylaxis:** 0.01 mg/kg/dose IM/SC (max: 0.5mg)
etomidate	0.2–0.3 mg/kg IV
ipratropium bromide	Nebulizer: 0.25-0.5 mg/dose q20min x3; MDI: 4-8 puffs q2-4 hr
pancuronium	0.05–0.1 mg/kg/dose IV or 0.25–0.75 µg/kg/min continuous infusion ($t_{1/2}$: 45-90min)
prednisolone	**Acute asthma attack**: 2-4 mg/kg IV
propofol (1%, 2%)	Initial: 2–4 mg/kg/dose IV; Cont infusion: 5–10 mg/kg/h IV
sodium bicarb.	1 mmol/kg IV, use bicarb deficit formula, titrate to effect
s-ketamine	Initial: 0.2-1 mg/kg IV or 2-10 mg/kg IM Maintenance: 5-20 µg/kg/min IV infusion
succinylcholine	1–2 mg/kg IV

Source: Pediatrics Advanced Life Support (PALS) 2010 guidelines
http://circ.ahajournals.org/content/122/18_suppl_3/S876.full.pdf

15.14 Pediatric Intubation and Defibrillation Values

Age	NB	3 mo	6 mo	1 yr	2 yr	3 yr	5 yr	7 yr	10 yr	12 yr	15 yr
ETT diameter (mm)	3–3.5*	3–3.5*	3.5*	4.0*	4.5*	4.5–5*	5–5.5*	5.5–6*	6.5	7	7.5
	* uncuffed								cuffed		
Laryngoscope[1]	0 Mi	0-1 Mi	1 Mi	1 Mi	2 Mi	2 Mi /Mac	2 Mi /Mac	2 Mi /Mac	2-3 Mi / Mac	3 Mi /Mac	3 Mi /Mac
Defib. ini (2 J/kg) (J) max (4J/kg) (J)	7 14	12 24	15 30	20 40	24 48	28 56	36 72	44 88	65 130	80 160	100 200

Mi = Miller blade; Mac = Mac blade; [1] Rule of thumb: size = age/4 + 4

Source: Pediatrics Advanced Life Support (PALS) 2010 guidelines
http://circ.ahajournals.org/content/122/18_suppl_3/S876.full.pdf

15.15 Asthma Management

15.15.1 Stepwise approach to managing asthma (patients >5 years)

Step 1: Mild intermittent	Symptoms <2 times/week; night symptoms <2 times/month Asymptomatic and normal peak flow between exacerbations Exacerbations are brief (hours-days); Intensity may vary FEV1 or peak flow >80% of predicted
Step 2: Mild persistent	Symptoms >2 times/week but <1 time/day Exacerbations may affect activity Night symptoms >2 times/month FEV1 or peak flow >80% of predicted
Step 3: Moderate persistent	Daily symptoms Daily use of inhaled short-acting beta-2 agonist Exacerbations affect activity (Exacerbation > x2/wk – may last for days) Night symptoms > 1 time/week FEV1 or peak flow >60 but <80% of predicted
Step 4: Severe persistent	Continual symptoms; night symptoms are frequent Limited physical activity Frequent exacerbations FEV1 or peak flow <60% of predicted

Note: Presence of any one feature is sufficient to place a patient in that category. Patients are assigned to the most severe step. Patients may change categories over time.

15.15.2 Asthma treatment ladder

Severe persistent: Short acting inhaled beta-2 agonists as needed for symptoms. Daily medications: high-dose inhaled corticosteroids AND long acting inhaled β_2-agonists AND, if needed, corticosteroids. Systemic steroids are recommended for severe exacerbations
Moderate persistent: Short acting inhaled beta-2 agonists as needed for symptoms Daily Medications: Low-medium dose inhaled corticosteroids and long-acting inhaled β_2-agonists If needed, increase inhaled steroids to medium dose and add leukotriene inhibitor or theophylline Systemic steroids are recommended for severe exacerbations
Mild persistent: Short acting inhaled beta-2 agonists as needed for symptoms. Add low-dose inhaled corticosteroids. Alternative treatments include: Cromolyn, leukotriene modifier, nedocromil or theophylline. Systemic steroids are recommended for severe exacerbations
Mild intermittent: No daily medication needed. Severe exacerbations may occur separated by long periods of normal lung function. Quick relief: short acting inhaled beta-2 agonists as needed for symptoms. Systemic steroids are recommended for severe exacerbations
Source: 2007 Guidelines for Diagnosis and Management of Asthma, pages 329 and 331 http://www.nhlbi.nih.gov/guidelines/asthma/asthgdln.pdf

Step up - If patient is not controlled aggressively step up treatment to the next level
Step down - Review treatment every 1-6 months to evaluate for a possible step down in treatment in a stable patient.

15.15.3 Asthma action plan

Name____ Date _____ Based on your predicted peak flow and your personal best peak flow, for you 100% is ______

Green Zone is _____-_____ 80%–100% of your personal best
Use albuterol inhalers on an as-needed basis

Yellow Zone is -_____-_____ 50%–80% of your personal best
Take ___ puffs of Albuterol inhaler every _______ hours
Use nebulized albuterol every ______ hours
Take ___ puffs of ________ inhaled steroid ______ times per day on a daily basis
Begin oral steroids: Take ____ mg of ____________ every _____am, _____pm
Inform you doctor of a change in your symptoms (phone number _________)

Red Zone is <50% - Danger!
Take ___ puffs of albuterol, repeat ______ times
Call your doctor (phone number __________) or report to the nearest ER
Phone number for transportation: ______________

15.15.4 Management of status asthmaticus

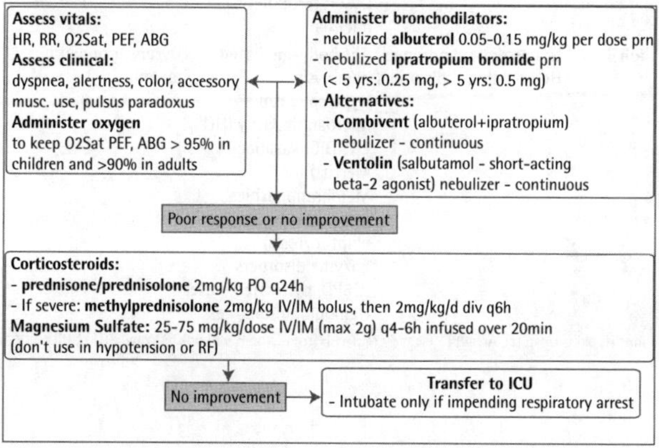
Assess vitals:
HR, RR, O2Sat, PEF, ABG
Assess clinical:
dyspnea, alertness, color, accessory musc. use, pulsus paradoxus
Administer oxygen
to keep O2Sat PEF, ABG > 95% in children and >90% in adults
Administer bronchodilators:
- nebulized albuterol 0.05-0.15 mg/kg per dose prn
- nebulized ipratropium bromide prn
(< 5 yrs: 0.25 mg, > 5 yrs: 0.5 mg)
- Alternatives:
- Combivent (albuterol+ipratropium) nebulizer - continuous
- Ventolin (salbutamol - short-acting beta-2 agonist) nebulizer - continuous
Poor response or no improvement
Corticosteroids:
- prednisone/prednisolone 2mg/kg PO q24h
- If severe: methylprednisolone 2mg/kg IV/IM bolus, then 2mg/kg/d div q6h
Magnesium Sulfate: 25-75 mg/kg/dose IV/IM (max 2g) q4-6h infused over 20min
(don't use in hypotension or RF)
No improvement
Transfer to ICU
- Intubate only if impending respiratory arrest

15.16 Pediatric Anemia

15.16.1 Classification of pediatric anemia

Retic count	Microcytic anemia	Normocytic anemia	Macrocytic anemia
Low	Iron deficiency Lead poisoning Chronic inflammation Aluminum toxicity Copper deficiency Protein malnutrition	Chronic inflammation RBC aplasia (TEC, infection, drug-induced) Malignancy Juvenile rheumatoid arthritis Endocrinopathies Renal failure	Folate deficiency Vitamin B12 deficiency Aplastic anemia Congenital bone marrow dysfunction (Diamond-Blackfan or Fanconi syndromes) Drug-induced Trisomy 21 Hypothyroidism
Normal	Thalassemia trait Sideroblastic anemia	Acute bleeding Hypersplenism Dyserythropoietic anemia	--
High	Thalassemia syndromes Hemoglobin C disorders	Antibody-mediated hemolysis Hypersplenism Microangiopathy (HUS, TTP, DIC, Kasabach-Merritt) Membranopathies (spherocytosis, elliptocytosis) Enzyme disorders (G6PD, pyruvate kinase) Hemoglobinopathies	Dyserythropoietic anemia Active hemolysis

Johns Hopkins Hospital, Arcara K, Tschudy M ,The Harriet Lane Handbook. Mosby 2011. 19th edition.

15.16.2 Common causes of microcytic anemia in children

	Iron deficiency	Beta thalassemia trait	Chronic inflammation
Reticulocyte count	Low	Normal to ↑	Normal
RDW	↑	↓	Normal
Ferritin	↓	Normal to ↑	Normal to ↑
Iron	↓	Normal	↓
TIBC	↑	Normal	↓
Electrophoresis	Normal	↑ HbA2	Normal
ESR	Normal	Normal	↑
Peripheral smear	Hypochromic microcytic	Normochromic, coarse basophilic stippling	Variable
Johns Hopkins Hospital, Arcara K, Tschudy M ,The Harriet Lane Handbook. Mosby 2011. 19th edition.			

15.16.3 Age-specific MCV

Age	MCV mean (fL)	Age	MCV mean (fL)
26-30 wks gestation	118.2	6 months - 2 years	78
28 weeks	120	2 years - 6 years	81
32 weeks	118	6 years - 12 years	86
1-3 days	108	12 - 18 years male	88
2 weeks	105	12 -18 years female	90
1 month	101	**Adult male**	90
2 months	95	**Adult female**	90
6 months	76		
Modified from: From: Johns Hopkins Hospital, Arcara K, Tschudy M ,The Harriet Lane Handbook. Mosby 2011. 19th edition.			

15.16.4 Iron deficiency anemia treatment

Preparations	
Ferrous sulfate	20% elemental Fe
Ferrous gluconate	12% elemental Fe
Polysaccharide-iron complex	(in mg of elemental Fe)
Goals	
Premature infants	Elemental iron 2-4 mg/kg/d PO divided 1-2 x/d
Children	Elemental iron 3-6 mg/kg/d PO divided 1-3 x/d
Adults	Elemental iron 60 mg/kg/d PO divided 2-4 x/d
Notes	
• Less GI irritation when given with or after meals • Vitamin C may enhance absorption • Liquid preparations may stain teeth (use dropper or straw for administration) • Constipation/nausea/abdominal pain and dark stools are common side effects	
Modified from Johns Hopkins Hospital, Arcara K, Tschudy M ,The Harriet Lane Handbook. Mosby 2011. 19th edition.	

15.17 Growth Charts

15.17.1 Boys: WHO height- and weight-for-age, 0 to 24 Mo

Birth to 24 months: Boys
Length-for-age and Weight-for-age percentiles

NAME ____________

RECORD # ____________

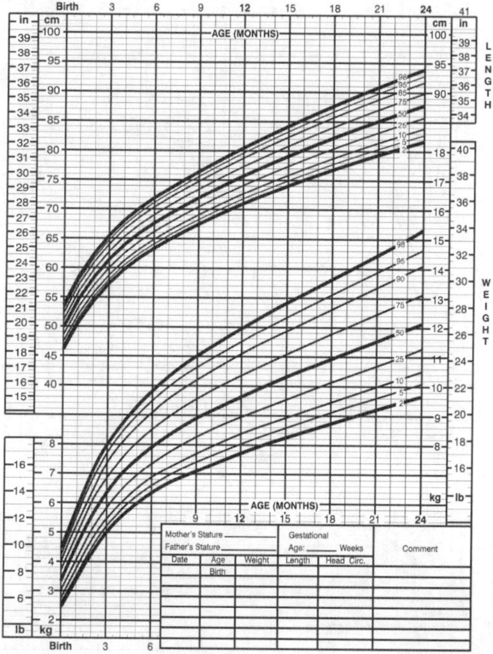

Published by the Centers for Disease Control and Prevention, November 1, 2009
SOURCE: WHO Child Growth Standards (http://www.who.int/childgrowth/en)

15.17.2 Boys: WHO weight-for-length and head circ., 0-24 Mo

Birth to 24 months: Boys
Head circumference-for-age and
Weight-for-length percentiles

NAME _____

RECORD # _____

Date	Age	Weight	Length	Head Circ.	Comment

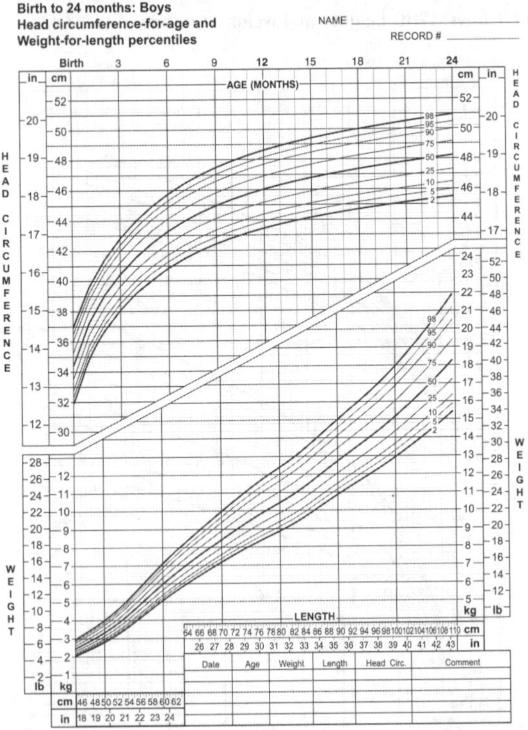

Published by the Centers for Disease Control and Prevention, November 1, 2009
SOURCE: WHO Child Growth Standards (http://www.who.int/childgrowth/en)

15.17.3Boys: CDC stature- and weight-for-age, 2–20 Yr

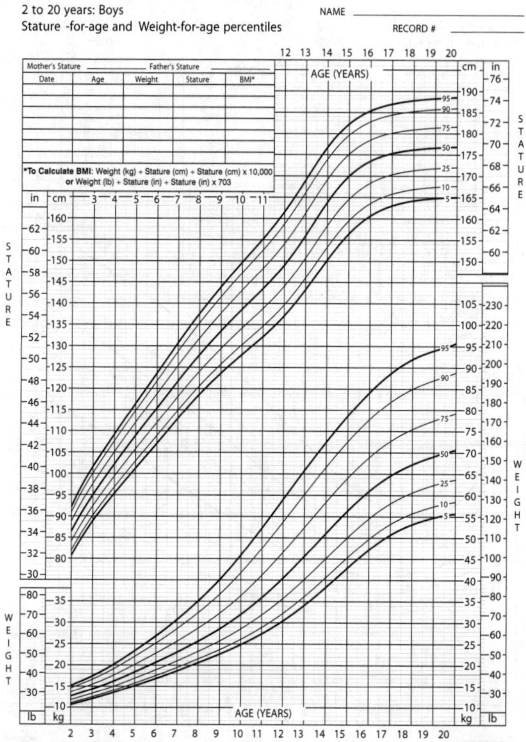

Published May 30, 2000 (modified 11/21/00).
SOURCE: Developed by the National Center for Health Statistics in collaboration with the National Center for Chronic Disease Prevention and Health Promotion (2000).
http://www.cdc.gov/growthcharts

CDC
SAFER · HEALTHIER · PEOPLE™

15.17.4Boys: CDC BMI-for-age, 2–20 Yr

2 to 20 years: Boys
Body mass index-for-age percentiles

NAME ______________

RECORD # ________

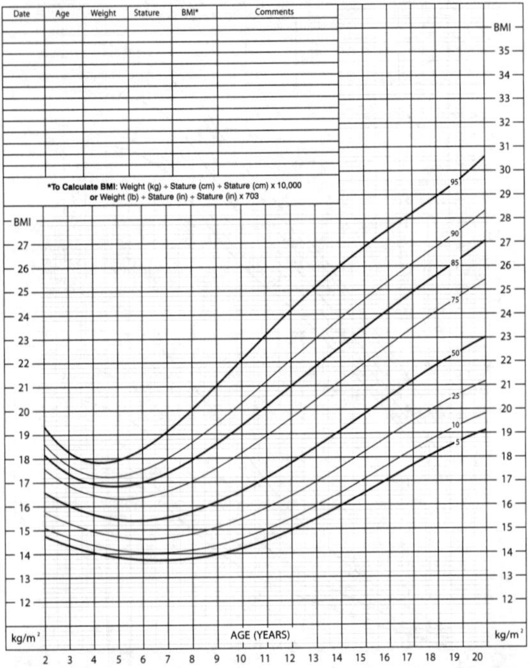

Published May 30, 2000 (modified 10/16/00).
SOURCE: Developed by the National Center for Health Statistics in collaboration with the National Center for Chronic Disease Prevention and Health Promotion (2000).
http://www.cdc.gov/growthcharts

CDC
SAFER · HEALTHIER · PEOPLE™

15.17.5Girls: WHO height- and weight-for-age, 0 to 24 Mo

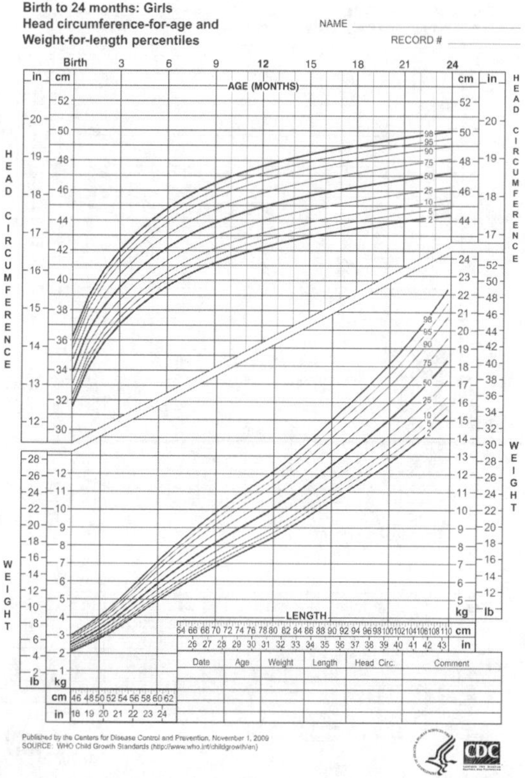
Birth to 24 months: Girls
Head circumference-for-age and
Weight-for-length percentiles
NAME
RECORD #
AGE (MONTHS)
Birth 3 6 9 12 15 18 21 24
HEAD CIRCUMFERENCE
WEIGHT
LENGTH
in
cm
kg
lb
98 95 90 75 50 25 10 5 2
64 66 68 70 72 74 76 78 80 82 84 86 88 90 92 94 96 98 100 102 104 106 108 110 cm
26 27 28 29 30 31 32 33 34 35 36 37 38 39 40 41 42 43 in
46 48 50 52 54 56 58 60 62
18 19 20 21 22 23 24
Date
Age
Weight
Length
Head Circ.
Comment
Published by the Centers for Disease Control and Prevention, November 1, 2009
SOURCE: WHO Child Growth Standards (http://www.who.int/childgrowth/en)
CDC

15.17.6Girls: WHO weight-for-length and head circ., 0–24 Mo

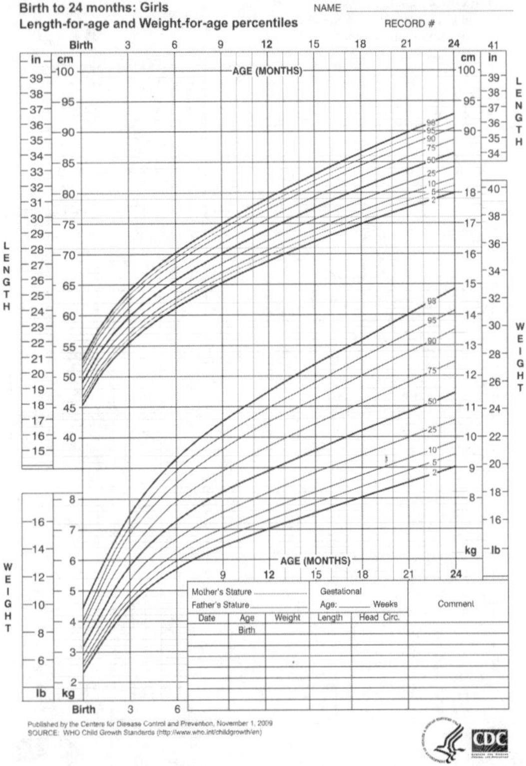

15.17.7Girls: CDC stature- and weight-for-age, 2–20 Yr

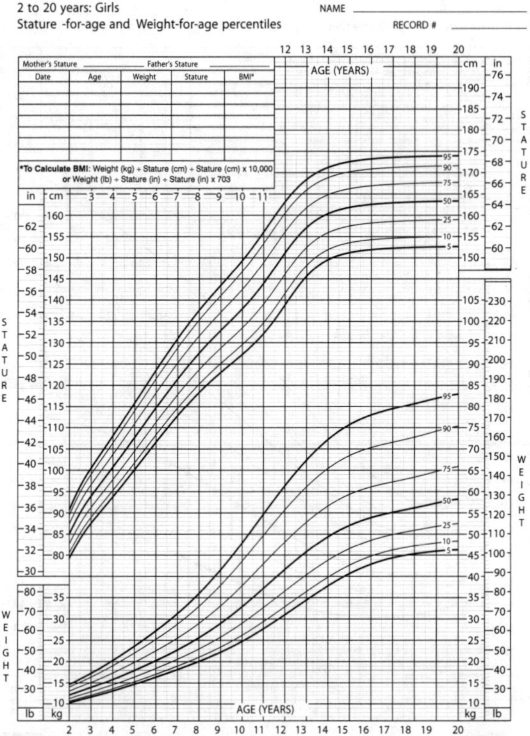

Published May 30, 2000 (modified 11/21/00).
SOURCE: Developed by the National Center for Health Statistics in collaboration with the National Center for Chronic Disease Prevention and Health Promotion (2000).
http://www.cdc.gov/growthcharts

CDC
SAFER · HEALTHIER · PEOPLE™

15.17.8Girls: CDC BMI-for age, 2–20 Yr

2 to 20 years: Girls
Body mass index-for-age percentiles

NAME ____________________

RECORD # __________

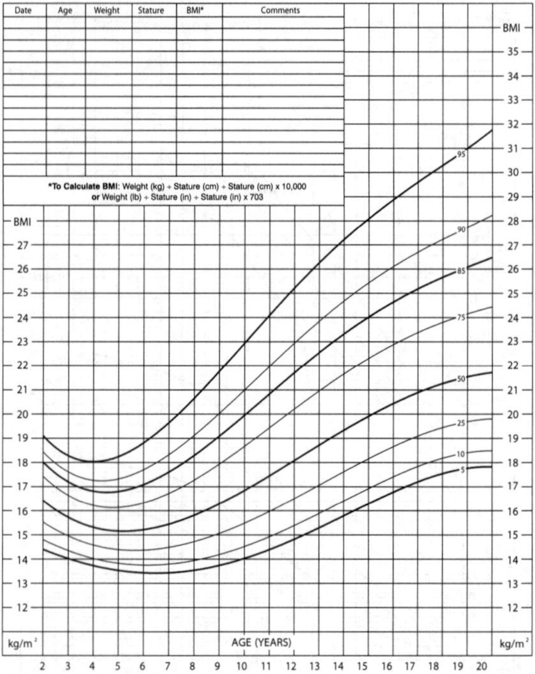

Published May 30, 2000 (modified 10/16/00).
SOURCE: Developed b y the National Center for Health Statistics in collaboration with
the National Center for Chronic Disease Prevention and Health Promotion (2000).
http://www.cdc.gov/growthcharts

CDC
SAFER · HEALTHIER · PEOPLE™

16 Psychiatry

Many of the definitions found in this chapter reference the Diagnostic and Statistical Manual of Mental Disorders, 4th Edition, Text Revision (DSM IV-TR).

16.1 Psychiatric Assessment (Mod. per AMDP)

Psychiatric History	
CC	Reason why patient has come for help, in patient's own words
HPI	- Demographic information: Age, race, gender, living situation, employment status (eg, "The patient is a 45-year old Caucasian man who lives with his mother, is divorced, and currently unemployed. He presents with ...") - Presenting symptoms: Onset, duration, progression - Stressors including relationship, work/school, financial/legal, other - Affective symptoms (→ 349) - Psychotic disorder (→ 351) - Cognitive symptoms (use mini-mental status exam) (→ 453) - Suicidal and homicidal symptoms - Substance use - Recent relevant treatment: compliance with medications, current medications and doses
Past psychiatric history	- Inpatient hospitalizations: # of hospitalizations, listing presenting symptoms, treatment and discharge plan for each - History of suicide attempts - History of violence - Past physical or sexual abuse - Outpatient treatment: Physician/clinic, therapy, case manager, day programs - Medication trials and side effects experienced
PMH	Medical illness, surgery, allergies, current medications
Substance abuse	For each drug: Age when drug was first started, route, frequency, quantity, longest period of abstinence, history of detox/rehab treatment, outpatient substance abuse treatment, physiological dependence (withdrawal tremors, seizures, DTs) and/or medical complications (hepatitis, pancreatitis, GI bleeds)

Family and marital history	Marital status, children, relationship with the patient, other family members with psychiatric/medical problems
Social history	Living situation, education, occupation, income, encounters with the law
Mental Status Exam	
Appearance	Age, grooming, appearance, race, gender, attitude (eg, "Pt is a 42-year-old fairly groomed, casually dressed, overweight Caucasian female, irritable but cooperative with interviewer")
Motor activity	Eg, decreased, normal, increased
Eye contact	Eg, poor, good, fair
Mood	Eg, Depressed, anxious, irritable, angry, elevated, euphoric
Affect	Blunted, constricted, mildly constricted, full range, labile; Specify whether affect is congruent/incongruent with mood, or whether it is odd or inappropriate
Speech	Describe rate, quantity, volume, quality (eg, "Increased rate and quantity, high volume with pressured quality")
Thought process	Disorganized, flight of ideas, loosening of associations, tangential, circumstantial, blocking, concrete, ruminations, perseverations, coherent, goal directed
Thought content	Hallucinations: Auditory, visual, tactile, olfactory; Delusions: Paranoia, ideas of reference, thought broadcasting; Suicidal or homicidal ideation
Insight	Eg, poor, good, fair
Judgment	Eg, poor, good, fair (in a patient with good command of the English language, this may be assessed by asking the patient what he or she would do in various situations, for example: "What would you do if you saw a letter on the ground next to a mailbox?")
Mini-Mental Status Exam (MMSE) - See Appendix (→ 453)	

16.2 Affective Symptoms - Differential

Depressive	**SIG E CAPS:** Sleep (increased/decreased), Interest, Guilt, Energy, Concentration, Appetite (increased/decreased), Psychomotor (agitation/retardation), Suicide (ideation, plan, intent, recent attempt, past attempt)
Manic	**DIG FAAST:** Distractibility, Insomnia, Grandiosity, Flight of ideas, increased goal directed Activities, Agitation, pressured Speech, Thoughtlessness
Anxiety	Screening question: Do you worry excessively? If answer is yes, use followup questions (see anxiety section)

16.3 Mood Disorders

The mood disorders listed do not include those caused by substance abuse, medications, or illness

Disorder	Definition and treatment
Major depressive disorder (MDD)	**Definition:** - Presence of at least one major depressive episode: Five or more depressive symptoms present for at least two weeks, leading to a change in functioning, and without any history of mania or hypomania - May have single episode, recurrent (> 1 episode), or chronic - Specify severity and presence/absence of psychosis **Treatment:** - First-line treatment: SSRIs +/- cognitive behavioral or interpersonal psychotherapy - Other options: Atypical antidepressants (venlafaxine, bupropion, mirtazapine, desyrel); TCAs; MAOIs; electro-convulsive therapy (ECT)

Disorder	Definition and treatment
Dysthymic disorder	**Definition:** - Depressed mood for most of the day, on most days, for at least 2 years. Must have **2 or more** depressive symptoms (SIG E CAPS) - The patient has not been without symptoms for more than 2 months at a time - If symptoms are severe enough to meet criteria for MDD, consider diagnosis of chronic MDD **Treatment:** - First-line treatment: SSRIs +/- cognitive behavioral or interpersonal psychotherapy - Other options: Atypical antidepressants: venlafaxine, bupropion, mirtazapine, desyrel, TCAs, MAOIs
Bipolar I	**Definition:** - Presence of **at least one** Manic Episode: A distinct period of elevated or irritable mood for **at least 1 week** and associated with **at least 3** manic symptoms - OR one mixed episode: Meet criteria for a major depressive episode and a manic episode for >1 week - Specify severity and presence/absence of psychosis **Treatment:** - First-line treatment: Discontinue or taper off antidepressant, if sole treatment, and begin mood stabilizer (lithium, valproic acid or carbamazepine) - Other options: Atypical antipsychotics
Bipolar II	**Definition:** Presence of **one or more** major depressive episodes AND **at least one** hypomanic episode: Meets criteria for a manic episode, but lasts **at least 4 days** and causes less impairment than mania, does not lead to hospitalization, and is not associated with psychosis. **Treatment:** Avoid antidepressant use without mood stabilizer present; Consider lamotrigine or atypical antipsychotic

Disorder	Definition and treatment
Cyclothymia	**Definition:** Numerous periods of hypomanic symptoms and depressive symptoms for > **2 years** The patient has not been without symptoms for more than 2 months at a time **Treatment:** Mood stabilizer; consider lamotrigine or atypical antipsychotic

16.4 Psychotic Disorders

16.4.1 Psychotic symptoms

The mood disorders listed do not include those caused by substance abuse, medications, or illness.

Positive symptoms	- Delusions and/or hallucinations - Disorganized speech, thought process, or behavior - Catatonia: Motor immobility, extreme negativism including mutism or resistance to all instructions - Bizarre voluntary movements including inappropriate postures, stereotyped movements, grimacing - Echolalia or echopraxia, excessive purposeless motor activity
Negative symptoms	- Affective flattening, alogia, avolition

16.4.2 Psychotic disorders

Disorder	Definition and treatment
Schizophrenia	- **Two or more** psychotic symptoms present for **at least one month** - Symptoms must be accompanied by decreased ability to function in one or more areas including school, work, self-care, relationships - Duration of **at least six months** (with at least one month of psychotic symptoms) **Treatment:** - First-line treatment: Atypical antipsychotics - Second-line treatment: Typical antipsychotics
Schizophreniform disorder	Presence of **two or more** psychotic symptoms for **between one and six months** **Treatment:** Same as for schizophrenia
Shizoaffective disorder	- Criteria met for schizophrenia plus either a manic, depressive, or mixed episode - To distinguish from bipolar pt must have **2 weeks** of psychotic symptoms after the mood symptoms have resolved **Treatment:** Atypical antipsychotic with mood stabilizer, +/- antidepressant medication
Delusional disorder	Non-bizarre delusions (i.e. situations that could occur in real life, like being stalked) that last for at least one month. Unlike schizophrenia, functioning is not impaired
Brief psychotic disorder	Presence of one or more psychotic symptoms **for less than one month** **Treatment:** First-line: Atypical antipsychotics Second-line: Typical antipsychotics
Shared psychotic disorder	A delusion develops in an individual in the context of a close relationship with another person who has an already established delusion (eg, husband and wife share a delusion that their daughter is poisoning them)

16.5 Anxiety Disorders

Disorder	Definition and treatment
Panic attack	- Discrete period of intense fear or discomfort with abrupt onset that must include **at least four** of the following symptoms: Palpitations or tachycardia, sweating, trembling, shortness of breath, sensation of choking, chest pain, nausea, dizziness, depersonalization, fear of losing control, fear of dying, numbness or tingling, chill/hot flushes - Indicate whether onset is spontaneous or situational (eg, triggered by crowds, enclosed spaces, etc.) - Indicate presence/absence of agoraphobia (fear of the inability to escape from a location or situation) **Treatment:** - Short-term: Benzodiazepines - Long-term: see panic disorder entry
Panic disorder	Must have **both of the following**: - Recurrent unexpected panic attacks - At least one of the attacks has been followed by one month or more of **at least one** of the following symptoms: Persistent concern about having additional attacks, worry about the implications or consequences of the attack, significant change in behavior related to the attacks - Specify whether panic attacks occur with or without agoraphobia (fear of the inability to escape from a location or situation) **Treatment:** - Short term: Benzodiazepines - Long term: SSRIs - Other options: TCAs, MAO inhibitors, cognitive behavioral therapy, relaxation training

Disorder	Definition and treatment
Specific phobia	A marked and persistent fear that is excessive and unreasonable which occurs with the presence or anticipation of a specific object or situation. Exposure to the object or situation evokes an immediate anxious response, possibly a panic attack. The individual recognizes the fear to be excessive, and tries to avoid the phobic situation. The individual's avoidance leads to significant impairment - Specify type of phobia: Animal (dogs, etc.), natural environment (heights, bridges, etc), blood/injection/injury (needles, etc.), situational (flying in planes, etc.) **Treatment:** Systemic desensitization (relaxation training + gradual exposure to phobic stimulus); can add benzodiazepine for short- term relief
Social phobia	A marked and persistent fear of a social or performance situation. The individual fears that they will act in a way or show symptoms that are embarrassing. The person recognizes that the fear is excessive and avoids the triggering situation - Identify specific triggers, for example, social settings, public speaking, performing - Identify fears, for example, criticism, confrontation, scrutiny **Treatment:** SSRIs, benzodiazepines, MAO inhibitors, beta blockers (only for performance-related anxiety), cognitive behavioral therapy

Disorder	Definition and treatment
Obsessive-compulsive disorder	Recurrent and intrusive obsessions and/or compulsions. The individual recognizes that the obsessions or compulsions are excessive and unreasonable, and experiences significant distress or functional impairment due to the symptoms. - **Obsessions:** Recurrent or persistent thoughts that are intrusive, inappropriate, and cause anxiety. Examples include contamination, harm to loved ones, symmetry. - **Compulsions:** Repetitive behaviors that the person feels driven to perform in response to an obsession or according to rules that must be applied rigidly. The compulsions are an unrealistic or exaggerated impulse aimed at preventing some dreaded event or situation. Examples include excessive hand washing, checking, counting, repeating, or praying. **Treatment:** First-line treatment: Higher dosed SSRIs; may need to add adjunctive therapy with options including buspirone, benzodiazepines, cognitive behavioral therapy
Post-traumatic stress disorder	Exposure to a traumatic event which involved actual or threatened serious injury to the exposed individual or others. The response to the traumatic event involved intense fear, helplessness, or horror. The event is persistently re-experienced by the exposed individual through nightmares, flashbacks or intrusive thoughts of the event. The individual displays persistent avoidance of any stimulus that is a reminder of the event. The individual experiences **at least two** persistent symptoms of increased arousal which were not present prior to the trauma. - Example symptoms: Exaggerated startle response, hypervigilance, insomnia, irritability, decreased concentration **Treatment:** - First-line: SSRIs - Other options: TCAs, MAO inhibitors, beta blockers, mood stabilizers, benzodiazepines, cognitive behavioral therapy, group therapy

Disorder	Definition and treatment
Generalized anxiety	Excessive anxieties and worries occurring **most days** over a period of **six months.** The individual finds it difficult to control the worry. The anxiety is associated with at least three of the following symptoms: Restlessness, fatigue, decreased concentration, irritability, muscle tension, insomnia. The anxiety or common symptoms cause significant distress and impairment in functioning. **Treatment:** - First-line treatment: SSRIs or venlafaxine - Other options: Benzodiazepines, TCAs, MAO inhibitors, cognitive behavioral therapy

16.6 Somatoform Disorders

These conditions should only be considered AFTER medical illness is ruled out. The key concept with this group of disorders is that the symptoms are **unintentionally produced** or feigned.

Disorder	Definition and treatment
Pain disorder	Pain in one or more anatomical sites which is the focus of the clinical presentation and is of sufficient severity to warrant medical attention. The onset of pain is preceded by psychological stress. The pain is not intentionally feigned, and causes significant distress or impairment in functioning. - Specify if acute (duration < 6 months), or chronic (duration > 6 months) **Treatment:** Multimodal physical, family, group and cognitive behavioral therapy; emphasize adjusting to living with some pain (not the complete removal of pain); avoid unnecessary medical workups and prevent iatrogenesis.

Disorder	Definition and treatment
Somatization disorder	A history of multiple physical complaints beginning before the age of 30 and occurring over a period of several years, resulting in the individual seeking treatment and leading to significant impairment in functioning. Over the course of the illness, the individual must display pain symptoms related to at **least four** different sites or functions, **at least two** gastrointestinal symptoms, **at least one** sexual symptom, and **at least one** pseudoneurological symptom: - **Pain symptoms:** Head, abdomen, back, joints, extremities, chest, rectum, pain during menstruation, sexual intercourse, or urination - **Gastrointestinal symptoms:** Nausea, bloating, vomiting, diarrhea, intolerance to several different foods - **Sexual symptoms:** Sexual indifference, erectile or ejaculatory dysfunction, irregular menses, excessive menstrual bleeding, vomiting throughout pregnancy - **Pseudoneurological symptoms:** Impaired coordination, paralysis or weakness, dysphagia, aphonia, urinary retention, hallucinations, loss of sensation, diplopia, blindness, deafness, seizures **Treatment:** Consistent, regularly scheduled appointments with empathic PMD; avoid unnecessary medical workups and prevent iatrogenesis; individual or group therapy; stress reduction education

Disorder	Definition and treatment
Conversion disorder	One or more symptoms or deficits affecting voluntary motor or sensory function that suggest a neurological or medical condition. The onset of symptoms is preceded by psychological stress. The symptom is not intentionally produced, and causes significant distress or impairment in functioning. Specify type of symptom or deficit: - **Motor:** Impaired coordination or balance, paralysis or localized weakness, dysphagia, aphonia, urinary retention, seizures - **Sensory:** Loss of touch or pain sensation, diplopia, blindness, deafness, hallucinations - Patient can have mixed symptoms **Treatment:** Non-confrontational individual therapy that addresses stressors +/- family therapy if family source of stress.
Hypochondriasis	Intense preoccupation with fears of having a serious disease based on the misinterpretation of bodily symptoms. The preoccupation persists despite appropriate medical evaluation and reassurance for at least six months. The preoccupation causes significant distress or impairment in functioning. **Treatment:** Consistent, regularly scheduled appointments with empathic PMD with palliation, not cure, as the goal; avoid unnecessary medical workups and prevent iatrogenesis; cognitive educational groups
Body dysmorphic disorder	Preoccupation with an imagined defect in appearance. If a slight physical anomaly is present, the individual's concern is markedly excessive. The preoccupation causes significant distress or impairment in functioning, and may lead to excessive efforts to correct the perceived defect, for example, multiple cosmetic surgeries. **Treatment:** Avoid unnecessary surgeries and medical workups; consider SSRIs; if preoccupation with defect is delusional, treat with antipsychotics.

16.7 Factitious Disorders

The individual must initially undergo full medical evaluation to rule out a medical etiology. The key concept with this group of disorders is that the symptoms are **intentionally produced**, and motivated by the desire to assume the sick role.

Disorder	Definition and treatment
Factitious disorder (Munchausen syndrome)	Intentional production or feigning of physical or psychological symptoms with the sole motivation of assuming the sick role. External incentives for the behavior (such as financial gain, avoiding work, avoiding legal responsibility), as in malingering, are absent. - Specify if symptoms are predominantly physical, psychological, or both. - Rule out malingering by establishing if external incentives are present. **Treatment:** No known specific psychiatric treatment; helpful to identify the disorder early to avoid unnecessary medical workups and prevent iatrogenesis; focus on management of symptoms rather than cure.
Factitious disorder by proxy (Munchausen by proxy)	Intentional production or feigning of physical or psychological symptoms in another person who is under the individual's care for the purpose of indirectly assuming the sick role. Example: A mother may induce symptoms in her child and seek medical attention for the child. **Treatment:** No known specific psychiatric treatment; helpful to identify early and involve child or adult protective services if case involves child or elderly person.

16.8 Dissociative Disorders

Before considering these diagnoses, one must initially rule out etiology due to substance use, medications, or medical conditions.

Disorder	Definition and treatment
Dissociative amnesia	One or more episodes of inability to recall important personal information, usually of a stressful or traumatic nature, that is too extensive to be explained by ordinary forgetfulness. The symptoms cause significant distress or functional impairment. **Treatment:** Individual psychotherapy aimed at restoring memories; consider hypnosis or Amytal interview.
Dissociative fugue	Sudden, unexpected travel away from home or usual work environment, with inability to recall one's past. Confusion about personal identity or assumption of new identity. The symptoms cause significant distress or functional impairment. **Treatment:** Individual psychotherapy aimed at restoring memories; consider hypnosis or Amytal interview.
Dissociative identity disorder	The presence of two or more distinct identities, each with its own enduring pattern of perceiving, relating to, and thinking about self and environment. **At least two** of these identities recurrently take control of the individual's behavior. Inability to recall important personal information. **Treatment:** Extensive individual psychotherapy
Depersonalization disorder	Persistent or recurrent experiences of feeling detached from one's mental processes or body, as if an outside observer of oneself. Reality testing remains intact, i.e. the individual is not psychotic. The episodes cause significant distress or functional impairment. **Treatment:** Extensive individual psychotherapy

16.9 Eating Disorders

Disorder	Definition and treatment
Anorexia nervosa	Refusal to maintain body weight at or above a minimally normal weight for age and height. Weight loss leading to maintenance of **body weight less than 85% of expected.** Intense fear of gaining weight or becoming fat. Disturbed perception of body weight with disproportionately high emphasis on body weight on self-evaluation. In postmenarcheal females, amenorrhea (the absence of at least three consecutive menstrual cycles). Specify type: - **Restricting:** Current episode does not include binge eating or purging behavior. - **Binge eating/purging:** Current episode includes binge eating or purging behavior. **Treatment:** Medically restore weight and electrolyte balance, treat malnutrition; nutritional education; individual, family and group therapy; no approved medication regimen.
Bulimia nervosa	Recurrent episodes of binge eating which includes larger than normal amount of food within a two hour period and a sense of lack of control during binge. Recurrent inappropriate compensatory behavior to prevent weight gain, such as induced emesis, laxative abuse, diuretics, enemas, or other medications, fasting, or excessive exercise. Symptoms occur at least twice per week for at least three months. Disproportionately high emphasis of body weight on self-evaluation. Specify type: - **Purging:** Current episode includes self-induced emesis, laxative, diuretic or enema abuse. - **Nonpurging:** Current episode includes other compensatory behaviors. **Treatment:** Medically restore electrolyte balance, and treat malnutrition; nutritional education; cognitive behavioral therapy, or combination of therapy modalities; group therapy; SSRIs are first-line medication option.

16.10 Substance Abuse and Dependence

16.10.1 Alcohol screening test (CAGE)

CAGE questionnaire		Score
C	**Cut down:** Have you ever felt you ought to cut down on your drinking (drug use)?	1
A	**Annoyed:** Have people annoyed you by criticizing your drinking (drug use)?	1
G	**Guilty:** Have you ever felt bad about your drinking (drug use)?	1
E	**Eye-opener:** Have you ever had a drink (used drugs) to steady your nerves in the morning?	1
Needs a specialist referral if total points ≥2.		

16.10.2 Substance abuse vs. dependence

Substance abuse	Substance dependence*
Maladaptive pattern of substance use leading to clinically significant impairment or distress, shown by **at least one** of the following **over a 12-month period**:	Maladaptive pattern of substance use leading to clinically significant impairment or distress, shown by **at least 3** of the following **over a 12-month period**:
- Failure to fulfill obligations at work, school or home - Recurrent use in situations that are physically hazardous (example: driving) - Recurrent substance-related legal problems - Continued use despite persistent social or interpersonal problems	- Tolerance - Withdrawal - Substance taken in larger quantity or over longer period than intended - Persistent desire to cut down or control use - Great deal of time is spent obtaining, using, or recovering from substance - Social, occupational, or recreational tasks are sacrificed to use substance - Use continues despite physical and psychological problems
*Specify with or without physiological dependence (evidence of tolerance or withdrawal indicates physiological dependence)	

16.10.3 Drug intoxication and withdrawal

Keep in mind that **3 drugs can be lethal in withdrawal: Alcohol, barbiturates, and benzodiazepines.**

Intoxication symptoms	Withdrawal symptoms	Treatment
Alcohol		
Disinhibition, lability, slurred speech, ataxia, incoordination, nystagmus, coma	Tremulousness, tachycardia, hypertension, nausea, seizures, agitation, hallucinations, delirium tremens (DT)	**Short-term:** Long acting benzodiazepines tapered over several days; treat symptoms with antiemetics, antipsychotics **Long-term:** AA (self help) group therapy; consider therapeutic environment; consider acamprosate, naltrexone, or disulfiram
Opioids		
Euphoria, CNS depression, N/V, constipation, pupillary constriction via excitation of the Edinger-Westphal nucleus of the oculomotor nerve leading to enhanced parasympathetic stimulation to the eye, seizures, respiratory depression	Anxiety, insomnia, anorexia, sweating, fever, rhinorrhea, piloerection, nausea, vomiting, diarrhea	**Short-term:** In cases of overdose leading to respiratory depression: IV naloxone For less severe withdrawal: methadone substitution, clonidine +/- naltrexone, or buprenorphine; treat symptoms with antiemetics, antidiarrheal medications **Long-term:** NA group therapy, individual, groups and family therapy; consider therapeutic environment; methadone maintenance, L-alpha acetylmethadol, buprenorphine, or naltrexone

Intoxication symptoms	Withdrawal symptoms	Treatment
MDMA (Ecstasy)		
Euphoria, enhanced sensation, intense feelings of empathy, emotional warmth, impulsivity, paranoia, tremors, decreased appetite, tachycardia, hypertension, pupillary dilation, hyperthermia, seizures, cardiac arrhythmias	Lethargy, fatigue, depressed mood, long-term use can lead to persistent psychosis	**Short-term:** Treat symptoms, could include antipsychotics, antidepressants **Long-term:** Self help group therapy; consider therapeutic environment
Amphetamines		
Anxiety, euphoria, insomnia, decreased appetite, delusions, hallucinations; N/V, diarrhea, pupillary dilation, tremor, hypertension, tachycardia, diaphoresis, cardiac arrhythmias, sudden cardiac death	Lethargy, fatigue, headache, depressed mood, irritability, hypersomnolence, hunger	**Short-term:** Treat symptoms **Long-term:** Self-help group therapy; consider therapeutic environment
Cocaine/Crack		
Anxiety, agitation, euphoria, insomnia, decreased appetite, paranoia, grandiosity, hallucinations; pupillary dilation, hypertension, tachycardia, diaphoresis, N/V, vasoconstriction, seizures, cardiac arrhythmias, sudden cardiac death	Lethargy, fatigue, depressed mood, irritability, intense craving, increased appetite, hypersomnolence, suicidality	**Short-term:** Treat symptoms **Long-term:** CA group therapy; cognitive behavioral therapy; consider therapeutic environment

Intoxication symptoms	Withdrawal symptoms	Treatment
Phencyclidine (PCP, "Angel dust")		
Agitation, hostility, delusions, impulsivity, homicidality, fever, hallucinations, tachycardia, ataxia, vertical and horizontal nystagmus; dissociative anesthesia (insensitivity to pain without loss of consciousness); coma	Sudden onset of violence, recurrence of symptoms due to reabsorption from lipid stores; CNS effects may persist for a week; can be detected in urine up to eight days after ingestion	**Short-term:** Treat symptoms **Long-term:** Self help group therapy; consider therapeutic environment
Lysergic acid diethylamide (LSD, "Acid")		
Anxiety or depression, delusions, hallucinations, flashbacks; pupillary dilation, increased blood pressure, piloerection, increased body temperature, hyperreflexia	Long-term use can lead to persistent psychosis	**Short-term:** Treat symptoms **Long-term:** Self-help group therapy; consider therapeutic environment
Marijuana		
Euphoria, drowsiness, impaired short-term memory, temporal slowing, amotivation, social withdrawal, increased appetite, dry mouth, conjunctival injection, paranoia, hallucinations	Anxiety, irritability, tremor, diaphoresis, muscle aches	**Short-term:** Treat symptoms **Long-term:** Self-help group therapy

Intoxication symptoms	Withdrawal symptoms	Treatment
Barbiturates		
Sedation, hypnosis, nausea, dizziness, anesthesia (loss of sensation), respiratory depression, cardiovascular depression, coma (low safety margin)	Anxiety, agitation, tremulousness, N/V, tachycardia, weakness, insomnia, seizures, delirium, **cardiac arrest**	**Short-term:** Determine tolerance level by admin pentobarbital, then use phenobarbital; if hemodynamically unstable consider shorter-acting benzodiazepine **Long-term:** Self-help group therapy; consider therapeutic environment
Benzodiazapines		
Euphoria, disinhibition, anterograde amnesia, sedation, lability, ataxia, slurred speech, nystagmus, respiratory depression, coma	Anxiety, agitation, tremulousness, insomnia, hallucinations, N/V, tachycardia, hypertension, seizures	**Short-term:** Long-acting benzodiazepines tapered over several days; treat symptoms with antiemetics, antipsychotics **Long-term:** Self-help group therapy; consider therapeutic environment

16.11 Personality Disorders

These disorders include the following characteristics and are coded on **Axis II**:

1) An enduring pattern of thoughts and behavior that deviates from the norm within the individual's culture, displayed in **at least two** of the following areas:
   - **Cognition** (ways of perceiving and interpreting self and others).
   - **Affective** symptoms (range, intensity, and appropriateness)
   - **Interpersonal** functioning
   - Impulse control
2) This enduring pattern is pervasive across multiple areas in the individual's life: occupational, social, relationships.
3) The pattern leads to significant distress and impairment in functioning.
4) The pattern is chronic and usually begins in late adolescence or early adulthood.
5) Personality disorders cannot be diagnosed until individual is at least eighteen years old, but individuals can display characteristics of a personality disorder starting in childhood.

Cluster A Personality Disorders	
Paranoid personality disorder	Pervasive distrust of others, including at **least four** of the following: 1) suspects that others are exploiting, harming or deceiving him/her. 2) preoccupied with doubts about trustworthiness of others. 3) reluctant to confide in others because of suspiciousness. 4) reads hidden threatening meaning into benign comments. 5) persistently bears grudges. 6) perceives attacks on his/her character or reputation and at times reacts angrily. 7) suspects without justification the infidelity of sexual partner. **Treatment:** Individual supportive psychotherapy
Schizoid personality disorder	Pervasive detachment from others and restricted range of emotions, including **at least four** of the following: 1) does not desire or enjoy close relationships. 2) chooses solitary activities. 3) has little interest in sexual relationships. 4) lacks pleasure in activities. 5) lacks close friends other than family. 6) appears indifferent to the praise or criticism of others. 7) seems cold and detached to others. **Treatment:** Individual supportive psychotherapy
Schizotypal personality disorder	Pervasive pattern of discomfort within close relationships, as well as cognitive or perceptual disturbances and eccentric behavior, including **at least five** of the following: 1) ideas of reference (excluding delusions). 2) odd beliefs or magical thinking. 3) unusual perceptual experiences, including bodily illusions. 4) odd thinking and speech. 5) suspiciousness or paranoia. 6) odd or constricted affect. 7) odd behavior or appearance. 8) lack of close friends other than family. 9) excessive social anxiety associated with suspiciousness towards others. **Treatment:** Individual supportive psychotherapy; social skills training

Cluster B Personality Disorders	
Antisocial personality disorder	Pervasive disregard for and violation of the rights of others, including **at least three** of the following: 1) repeatedly engaging in criminal behavior. 2) repeatedly lying or conning others for personal profit. 3) impulsivity. 4) irritability and aggressiveness, with frequent fighting. 5) disregard for safety of others. 6) consistent irresponsibility. 7) lack of remorse **Treatment:** No known effective psychiatric treatment
Borderline personality disorder	Pervasive pattern of instability of relationships, self-image and affect, along with marked impulsivity, including **at least five** of the following: 1) desperate efforts to avoid abandonment by others. 2) unstable and intense relationships which alternate between intense idealization and devaluation. 3) unstable self-image. 4) impulsivity in at least two areas that are self-destructive. 5) recurrent suicidal behavior, gestures, threats, or self-mutilating behavior. 6) highly reactive and rapidly shifting mood. 7) chronic feelings of emptiness. 8) difficulty containing affect, including displays of temper. 9) transient stress-related paranoia or dissociative symptoms. **Treatment:** Individual and group psychotherapy; Dialectical behavioral therapy; Medications as indicated to target symptoms of impulsivity, mood instability, and transient psychosis.

Histrionic personality disorder	Pervasive pattern of excessive emotionality and attention seeking, including **at least five** of the following: 1) discomfort in situations where he/she is not the center of attention. 2) inappropriate seductive or provocative behavior. 3) rapidly shifting and shallow expression of affect. 4) draws attention to self with physical appearance. 5) excessively dramatic speech lacking detail. 6) exaggerated expression of emotion. 7) easily influenced by others. 8) feels relationships are more intimate than they are in reality. **Treatment:** Individual psychodynamic psychotherapy; medications as indicated for episodes of psychosis.
Narcissistic personality disorder	Pervasive pattern of grandiosity, need for admiration, and lack of empathy, including **at least five** of the following: 1) grandiose sense of self. 2) preoccupied with fantasies of success, power, beauty or ideal love. 3) believes he or she is unique and only associates with others of higher status. 4) requires excessive admiration. 5) has a sense of entitlement. 6) exploits others to achieve goals. 7) lacks empathy. 8) envies others or believes others are envious of him/her. 9) displays arrogance. **Treatment:** Individual psychodynamic psychotherapy.

Cluster C Personality Disorders	
Avoidant personality disorder	Pervasive pattern of social inhibition, feelings of inadequacy, and hypersensitivity to negative evaluation, including **at least four** of the following: 1) avoids interpersonal contact due to fear of criticism or rejection. 2) is unwilling to form relationships unless certain of being liked. 3) is hesitant in intimate relationships due to fear of being ridiculed. 4) preoccupied with being criticized or rejected in social situations. 5) feels inadequate compared to others. 6) views self as inferior to others. 7) hesitates to take risks due to fear of embarrassment. **Treatment:** Individual and group therapy with cognitive behavioral focus; consider anxiolytics to manage situational anxiety.
Dependent personality disorder	Pervasive and excessive need to be cared for that leads to submissive and clingy behavior and fears of separation, including **at least five** of the following: 1) needs excessive advice and reassurance from others to make minor decisions. 2) needs others to assume responsibility for major areas of life. 3) reluctant to disagree with others due to fear of disapproval. 4) lacks self-confidence to initiate projects. 5) excessively seeks nurturance and support from others, to the point of volunteering to do unpleasant things to gain approval. 6) discomfort from being alone due to fears of being unable to care for self. 7) desperately seeks new relationship when old relationship ends due to fear of being alone. 8) preoccupied with fears of being left alone to care for self. **Treatment:** Individual and group therapy with cognitive behavioral focus; assertiveness and social skills training.

Obsessive-compulsive personality disorder	Pervasive pattern of preoccupation with orderliness, perfectionism, and self-control, at the expense of flexibility, openness and efficiency, including **at least 4** of the following: 1) preoccupied with details, rules, order, to the extent that the major point of the activity is lost. 2) unable to complete tasks due to high level of perfectionism. 3) excessively devoted to work to the exclusion of friendships and leisure. 4) displays inflexibility about moral or ethical issues. 5) is unable to discard worthless objects even when they have no sentimental value. 6) hesitates to delegate tasks due to fear that task will not be carried out as he/she would do. 7) hoards money for future possible disasters. 8) behaves rigidly and stubbornly. **Treatment:** Individual and group therapy

16.12 DSM-IV Multiaxial Diagnosis

Axis	Psychiatric diagnosis	Examples
Axis I	Mood disorders, psychotic disorders, anxiety disorders, somatoform disorders, factitious disorders, dissociative disorders, eating disorders, substance abuse, developmental disorders, learning disabilities	Depression, generalized anxiety disorder, bipolar disorder, schizophrenia, somatization disorder, factitious disorder, dissociative identity disorder, bulimia nervosa, alcohol dependence, autism, reading disorder
Axis II	Personality disorders, mental retardation	Antisocial personality disorder, mild mental retardation
Axis III	General medical condition	Diabetes mellitus, hypertension, asthma
Axis IV	Psychosocial, relationship, occupational, educational, social, environmental problems	Fired from job last week, wife died last month, failed semester in school, divorce or separation
Axis V	Global Assessment of Functioning (see below)	Judgment of the overall level of functioning

GAF - Global Assessment of Functioning (Mod. per DSM-IV)	
Score	**Criteria (rate LOWEST possible score)**
100-91	No symptoms. Superior functioning in a wide range of activities.
90-81	Minimal or absent symptoms. Good functioning in all areas, satisfied with life.
80-71	Mild symptoms, but expectable reactions to psychosocial stressors. Slight impairment in social, work, or school functioning.
70-61	Some mild symptoms (depressed mood). Some difficulty in social, work, or school functioning.
60-51	Moderate symptoms (panic attacks). Any moderate difficulty in social, work, school functioning.
50-41	Serious symptoms. Any serious impairment in social, work, or school functioning, no friends/job.
40-31	Major impairment in several areas, eg, work, school, relationships, judgment, thinking or mood. Other symptoms (hallucinations, delusions, severe obsessive rituals). Passive suicidal ideation.
30-21	Behavior influenced by hallucinations or delusions. Serious impairment in judgment or communication. Inability to function in all areas. Suicidal ideation.
20-11	Suicide attempts, some severe violence. Severe manic excitement, or agitation. Occasionally fails to maintain minimal personal hygiene. In physical danger due to medical problems.
10-1	Serious suicidal act, frequent severe violence. Extreme manic excitement, or extreme agitation. Persistently fails to maintain minimal personal hygiene. In acute, severe danger (medical problems).
0	Not enough information available to provide GAF.

16.13 Psychotropic Medications

16.13.1 Antipsychotics - typical/conventional

Generic name	Brand name	Therapeutic range	Potency
haloperidol*	Haldol	0.5 - 5 mg bid	High
droperidol	Inapsine	2.5 -15 mg qd	High
fluphenazine*	Prolixin	0.5 - 10 mg qd	High
thiothixene	Navane	2 - 5 mg bid	High
trifluoperazine	Stelazine	2 - 5 mg bid	Medium
perphenazine	Trilafon	8 -16 mg bid	Medium
thioridazine	Mellaril	100 - 400 mg bid	Low
chlorpromazine	Thorazine	100 - 400 mg bid	Low

MA: Typical antipsychotics decrease positive psychotic symptoms by D2 receptor antagonism
* Medication is available in decanoate form

16.13.2 Side effects of typical antipsychotics

Side effect	Manifestations
Cognitive/Affective	Increased negative symptoms and cognitive deficits.
Extrapyramidal (EPS)	Acute dystonia (abnormal muscle tone), akathisia (motor restlessness), parkinsonism (tremor, rigidity, bradykinesia), and **tardive dyskinesia** (TD) (involuntary stereotypic orofacial movements). TD is a long-term irreversible side effect!
Endocrine	Increased prolactin secretion can lead to galactorrhea, amenorrhea, gynecomastia (see endocrine chapter (→ 107))
Anticholinergic	Dry mouth, urinary retention, constipation, blurred vision, sedation.
Antihistaminergic	Sedation, weight gain.
alpha-1 adrenergic	Orthostatic hypotension, dizziness, sedation.

Side effect	Manifestations
Neuroleptic malignant syndrome (NMS)	Rare but potentially LETHAL!! Characterized by fever, rigidity, autonomic instability, increased creatine phosphokinase (CPK) levels, and mental status changes. The patient should be managed in the MICU and the treatment is to immediately discontinue the antipsychotic medication and lower patient's body temperature, administer IV fluids, **dantrolene** (direct muscle relaxant) and/or **bromocriptine** (dopamine agonist).
Note: In general, lower-potency medications have increased anticholinergic side effects, higher-potency medications have increased extrapyramidal side effects	

16.13.3 Antipsychotics - atypicals

Generic name	Brand name	Therapeutic range
clozapine	Clozaril	100 - 300 mg bid
olanzapine	Zyprexa	5 - 20 mg daily
quetiapine	Seroquel	50 - 400 mg bid
risperidone*	Risperdal	1 - 6 mg daily
ziprasidone	Geodon	20 - 80 mg bid
aripiprazole	Abilify	10 - 30 mg qd
Iloperidone	Fanapt	6-12 mg bid
paliperidone	Invega	3-12 mg daily
MA: Atypical antipsychotics also decrease positive psychotic symptoms by D2 receptor antagonism *Medication is available in decanoate form Ref: American Psychiatric Association practice guidelines		

16.13.4 Atypical antipsychotic side effects

Side effect	Manifestations
General	Due to serotonin antagonism atypicals have decreased incidence of extrapyramidal symptoms and TD, decreased negative symptoms, and less incidence of increased prolactin levels. In general, they also have less anticholinergic, antihistaminergic and alpha-adrenergic side effects. Atypicals have largely replaced typicals as the first-line treatment for schizophrenia and acute psychosis for these reasons.
Weight gain, dyslipidemia, DM	All atypical anti-psychotics can potentially cause weight gain, dyslipidemia, and development of diabetes mellitus. The current recommendations for monitoring patients while on atypical antipsychotics are as follows: - Prior to or upon beginning atypical antipsychotic: 1) Review personal and family history of DM, obesity, dyslipidemia, hypertension, and cardiovascular disease 2) Check BMI [body weight(kg) / height $(m)^2$], waist circumference (at level of umbilicus), blood pressure, fasting glucose and fasting lipid panel - Following initiation of treatment, check the following at the indicated intervals: - After 4 weeks: Check BMI - After 8 weeks: Check BMI - After 12 weeks: Check BMI, blood pressure, fasting glucose and lipid panel - Every 3 months thereafter: Check BMI - Annually: Check personal and family history, waist circumference, blood pressure, fasting glucose - Every 5 years: Check fasting lipid panel
Clozapine toxicity	Clozapine is associated with a 1-2% incidence of **agranulocytosis,** requiring careful monitoring of WBCs and absolute neutrophil count (ANC) according to the following schedule: - First 6 months: Weekly - Next 6 months: Biweekly - After first year: Monthly Discontinue if WBC is below 3000 or ANC is below 1500.

16.13.5 Antidepressants - serotonin-specific reuptake inhibitors (SSRIs)

Characteristics	
Mechanism of action	Block serotonin presynaptic reuptake pumps. Over time, long-lasting blockade of the reuptake pumps leads to downregulation of the postsynaptic neurotransmitter receptors, which correlates with the onset of anti-depressant action.
Clinical uses	First-line treatment for depression due to increased safety and tolerability, decreased toxicity vs. TCAs and MAO inhibitors. Most side effects short-term, with tolerance developing over time. Can observe decreased efficacy over time.
Toxicity: serotonin syndrome	- Rare; associated with concomitant MAOI use - **Mental status changes** including disorientation, agitation - **Autonomic symptoms** including hyperthermia, diaphoresis, tachycardia, hypertension, flushing, vomiting, diarrhea, cardiac arrhythmias - **Neuromuscular hyperactivity** including muscle rigidity, tremor, myoclonus, hyperreflexia, bilateral Babinski signs. Treatment is discontinuation of serotonergic agents, IVFs, monitoring of vital signs, benzodiazepines, and possibly **cyproheptadine** (serotonin antagonist).

Generic name	Brand name	Therapeutic range
fluoxetine	Prozac	20 - 60 mg qd
sertraline	Zoloft	20 - 200 mg qd
paroxetine	Paxil	10 - 50 mg qd
fluvoxamine	Luvox	50 - 150 mg bid
citalopram	Celexa	20 - 60 mg qd
escitalopram	Lexapro	10 - 20 mg qd

16.13.6 Tricyclic antidepressants (TCAs)

Characteristics	
Mechanism of action	Block serotonin and norepinephrine presynaptic reuptake pumps, leading to accumulation of serotonin and norepinephrine within the synapse. Over time, long-lasting blockade of the reuptake pumps leads to downregulation of the postsynaptic neurotransmitter receptors, which correlates with the onset of antidepressant action.
Clinical uses	Second- or third-line treatment for refractory depression, pts with severe pain or fibromyalgia, severe insomnia or weight loss. Avoid in suicidal pts at risk for overdosing, overweight pts, pts with cardiac illness or on multiple medications, pts with dementia
Side effects	- **Antihistaminergic:** Sedation, weight gain - **Anticholinergic:** Constipation, urinary retention, dry mouth, blurry vision, sedation - **alpha-1 adrenergic:** Dizziness, orthostatic hypotension, sedation
Toxicity	- **"Three C's":** **C**onvulsions (seizures), **C**oma, **C**ardiotoxicity (arrhythmias) - Presenting signs: Arrhythmias, hypotension, and **anticholinergic toxicity**, including hyperthermia, dry skin, flushing, dilated pupils, intestinal ileus, urinary retention, and sinus tachycardia. Treatment includes IVFs, cardiac monitoring, **physostigmine**, and sodium bicarbonate.

Generic name	Brand name	Therapeutic range
clomipramine	Anafranil	150 - 250 mg qd
imipramine	Tofranil	150 - 300 mg qd
desipramine	Norpramin	100 - 200 mg qd
trimipramine	Surmontil	75 - 150 mg qd
amitriptyline	Elavil	50 - 150 mg qd
nortriptyline	Pamelor	50 - 150 mg qd
protriptyline	Vivactil	5 - 10 mg qd
maprotiline	-	75 - 150 mg qd
amoxapine	-	200 - 300 mg qd
doxepin	Sinequan	150 - 300 mg qd

16.13.7 Antidepressants - monoamine oxidase inhibitors (MAOIs) (non-selective)

Characteristics	
Mechanism of action	Bind irreversibly to MAO to inhibit the enzyme from destroying norepinephrine, serotonin and dopamine, leading to accumulation of these neurotransmitters within the synapse. Over time, long-lasting blockade of MAO by an MAO inhibitor leads to downregulation of the postsynaptic neurotransmitter receptors, which correlates with the onset of antidepressant action.
Clinical uses	Second- or third-line treatment for refractory depression, atypical depression (hyperphagia, hypersomnia)
Side effects	Insomnia, orthostatic hypotension, sexual dysfunction, dietary restrictions, multiple drug interactions/restrictions
Toxicity	These are particularly dangerous medications as tyramines are present within food (fermented cheeses, smoked or aged meats, Chianti, champagne, and avocados) and can lead to increased endogenous NE levels. With the presence of an irreversible MAO inhibitor, large levels of NE accumulate within the synapse, leading to **hypertensive crisis**. A special diet and close blood pressure monitoring are required to take these medications, and they are contraindicated with SSRIs and beta agonists. Toxicity treatment involves the use of a **nonselective beta blocker** such as **labetalol**, or **carvedilol** (Coreg) which have beta-1, beta-2, and alpha-1 activity. It is contraindicated to use a cardioselective beta-1 blocker alone, such as metoprolol (Lopressor) or atenolol (Tenormin), because unopposed alpha-adrenergic activity leads to vasoconstriction and a further rise in BP.

Generic name	Brand name	Therapeutic range
phenelzine	Nardil	15 - 30 mg tid
tranylcypromine	Parnate	10 - 20 mg tid
isocarboxazid	Marplan	10 - 20 mg tid

16.13.8 Antidepressants - heterocyclics

Generic name	Brand name	Therapeutic range	Indications
trazodone	Desyrel	50-400 mg qd	Depressed pts with insomnia
mirtazapine	Remeron	7.5-40 mg qd	Pts who have experienced intolerable side effects with SSRIs, and/or depressed pts with insomnia, anxiety
bupropion	Wellbutrin	150-450 mg qd	Pts with decreased concentration, distractability, psychomotor slowing, pts not responsive to or with significant side effects to SSRIs (no sexual side effects), pts who are also interested in smoking cessation
venlafaxine	Effexor	75-300 mg qd	Pts with atypical depression, refractory depression, psychomotor slowing
duloxetine	Cymbalta	40-60 mg qd	Pts with atypical depression, refractory depression, psychomotor slowing, diabetic neuropathy

16.14 Key Points

When to admit to psychiatric unit:
When the patient poses a danger to him/herself and/or to others, including but not limited to psychosis, suicidal or homicidal thoughts, dementia, or any condition that seriously impairs judgment.

Capacity:
The patient must understand and be able to verbalize the procedure and medical illness involved, verbalize the benefits and risks of undergoing the procedure in question, and the potential risks of refusing the procedure. The patient has the right to refuse any procedure even without capacity, unless it is immediately life-threatening.

16.15 5 Board-Style Questions

1) A 57-year-old female patient with a history of recurrent treatment for refractory depression and no chronic medical issues has been experiencing worsening depressive symptoms following the end of a four-year relationship with her boyfriend. The patient has been maintained on tranylcypromine over the past few years, and during most recent visit to her primary medical doctor, sertraline was added to her medication regimen. The patient now presents to the emergency room with complaints of colorful visual hallucinations, flushing, diarrhea, hypertension, confusion, hyperreflexia and myoclonus. The likely diagnosis is:
   a) Cholinergic crisis
   b) Hypertensive crisis
   c) Serotonin syndrome
   d) Alcohol withdrawal

2) A 35-year-old male patient is brought to the emergency room by a friend. The patient is hypoventilating and has blue lips, pinpoint pupils, severe constipation and is disoriented to place and time. Which of the following drugs is most likely to be responsible for the symptoms:
   a) Alcohol
   b) Codeine
   c) LSD
   d) Cocaine
   e) Diazepam

3) Which of the following metabolic abnormalities is commonly found in patients with bulimia nervosa, purging type?
   a) Decreased serum bicarbonate
   b) Decreased serum potassium
   c) Increased serum chloride
   d) Increased serum calcium

4) A 26-year.old male patient with history of chronic paranoid schizophrenia presents to the emergency room with disorientation to place and time, agitation, stiffness of his arms and legs, temperature of 102.9^0 F, hypertension and tachycardia. The patient has been taking haloperidol and sertraline as prescribed by his psychiatrist. What is the first step in treating this patient?
   a) Discontinue haloperidol, administer IV fluids and bromocriptine
   b) Administer atypical antipsychotic to control agitation
   c) Discontinue sertraline, administer IV fluids and benzodiazepine
   d) Send blood cultures, chest x-ray and urinalysis with microanalysis to determine cause of fever

5) A 60-year-old male patient with history of recurrent refractory depression was recently discharged from the psychiatric hospital where he received a course of electroconvulsive therapy to treat his depression, and was restarted on his previous dose of amitriptyline. He presents to the emergency room with confusion, dilated pupils, flushing, dry skin, decreased bowel sounds, and sinus tachycardia. Which of the following is the best current treatment option?
   a) bromocriptine
   b) labetalol
   c) diphenhydramine
   d) lorazepam
   e) physostigmine

17 Pulmonary and Critical Care

17.1 Physical Exam Findings

	Percussion	Breath sounds
Pneumothorax	Hyperresonant	Decreased
Pneumonia	Dull	Bronchial
Pleural effusion	Dull	Decreased
COPD	Hyperresonant	variable

17.2 Chest X-Ray Interpretation

1) Identify name of patient and date of film
2) Assess film quality:
   Body position - Check for rotation based on symmetrical alignment of clavicles in relation to vertebral column.
   Penetration - Should see pulmonary vessels through the heart, but not the vessels at the periphery. Intervertebral spaces should be clear in the upper lung fields but obscured near the diaphragm.
   Inspiration - Good inspiratory effort exposes the **6th rib anteriorly** or the **10th rib posteriorly**
3) Assess bones/soft tissues/lines/endotracheal tubes
4) Assess heart borders and mediastinum
5) Assess hila
6) Assess lungs: diaphragms, pleura, bronchi, vessels, parenchyma

17.3 Exposure-Related Lung Findings

Disease	Findings
Asbestosis	Fibrosis at bases that spares the costophrenic angles, associated with mesothelioma, calcified plaques in the pleura or diaphragm
Silicosis	Hilar eggshell calcifications, upper lung nodules, hilar lymphadenopathy, increased incidence of TB
Coal worker's pneumoconiosis	Upper lung nodules
Berylliosis	Hilar lymphadenopathy, upper lung nodules, non-caseating granulomas

17.4 Key Differentials

Findings	Diseases
Upper lung fibrocalcifications	TB, coal worker's pneumoconiosis, berylliosis, silicosis
Reticular nodular infiltrates	*Nocardia, Actinomyces, H. Influenzae, Klebsiella, Histoplasmosis, Cryptococcus*, adenovirus, Varicella, CMV, measles, sarcoidosis, BOOP (cryptogenic organizing pneumonitis)
Bronchiectasis	Infection, cystic fibrosis, alpha-1 antitrypsin deficiency, Kartagener's syndrome, hypogammaglobulinemia
Honeycombing	IPF, sarcoidosis, asbestosis, berylliosis, collagen vascular disease
Cystic lung disease	Cystic fibrosis, LAM, tuberous sclerosis, eosinophilic granuloma
Caseating granulomas	Fungal, silicosis, berylliosis, tularemia, TB, sarcoidosis, rheumatoid arthritis
Bilateral hilar adenopathy	Sarcoidosis, lymphoma, histoplamosis, toxoplasmosis, TB

17.5 Management of Hypoxemia

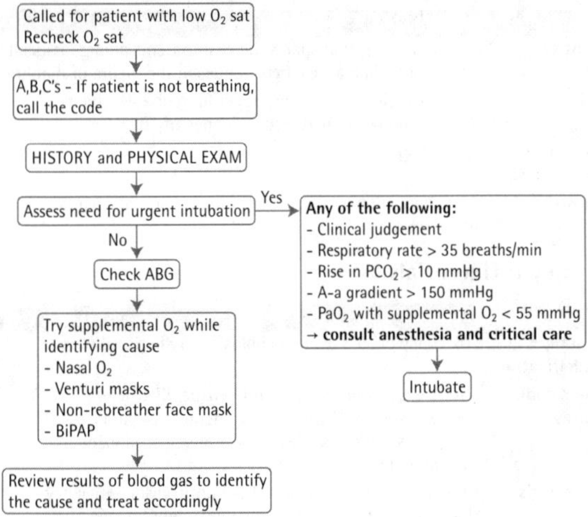
Called for patient with low O_2 sat
Recheck O_2 sat
A,B,C's - If patient is not breathing, call the code
HISTORY and PHYSICAL EXAM
Assess need for urgent intubation
Yes
Any of the following:
- Clinical judgement
- Respiratory rate > 35 breaths/min
- Rise in PCO_2 > 10 mmHg
- A-a gradient > 150 mmHg
- PaO_2 with supplemental O_2 < 55 mmHg
→ consult anesthesia and critical care
Intubate
No
Check ABG
Try supplemental O_2 while identifying cause
- Nasal O_2
- Venturi masks
- Non-rebreather face mask
- BiPAP
Review results of blood gas to identify the cause and treat accordingly

17.6 Pleural Effusions

17.6.1 Thoracentesis tubes

Chemistry - Red or yellow top	LDH, total protein, amylase, glucose, triglycerides
Hematology - Purple top	Cell count, differential
Microbiology - 10ml per culture bottle	Gram stain, culture (culture bottles), TB culture and smear (fungal collection tubes)
Pathology	Cytology
"Didya" tube - Extra tube	"Did you send the fluid for...PCR for TB and adenosine deaminase activity?"

17.6.2 Pleural effusion visual inspection

Finding	Causes
Bloody fluid	Malignancy, PE, trauma
Pale yellow (straw)	Normal, transudate, or exudate
White	Chylothorax
Yellow-green	Rheumatoid pleurisy
Dark brown-black	Long-standing bloody effusion, rupture of amebic liver abscess, aspergillus
Pus	Empyema
Anchovy paste	Amebic liver abscess

17.6.3 Pleural fluid analysis

Pleural fluid sample	Exudate	Transudate
Protein/serum protein ratio	> 0.5	< 0.5
LDH/serum LDH ratio	> 0.6	< 0.6
LDH in relation to upper limits of normal serum LDH	> 2/3	< 2/3
Protein	> 2.9 g/dL	< 2.9 g/dL
Cholesterol	> 45 mg/dL	< 45 mg/dL
Most common etiologies	Infection, malignancy, PE, connective tissue disease, sub-phrenic disorders (pancreatitis), hemithorax, chylothorax	CHF, nephrotic syndrome, constrictive pericarditis, cirrhosis, PE, myxedema hypoalbuminemia

* The first 3 criteria comprise **Light's criteria**

Remember: only one out of 3 criteria is needed to diagnose an exudative effusion

17.6.4 Specific pleural fluid findings

Pleural fluid findings	Differential diagnosis
Glucose < 60mg/dL **or** pH < 7.30	Rheumatoid pleurisy, empyema, malignant effusions, tuberculosis, lupus pleuritis, esophageal rupture
Amylase > Serum amylase	Acute pancreatitis, chronic pancreatic pleural effusion, esophageal rupture, malignancy
Lymphocytes > 85%	Tuberculous effusion, lymphoma, sarcoidosis, chronic rheumatoid pleurisy, yellow nail syndrome, chylothorax
Eosinophils > 10%	Pneumothorax, hemothorax, pulmonary infarction, asbestos pleural effusion, parasitic disease, fungal infection, drugs, malignancy
Mesothelial cells Finding > 5% (normally present in small numbers)	Excludes tuberculosis
Triglycerides > 115 (chylous effusion)	Trauma, mediastinal lymphoma, lymphangioleiomyomatosis
Triglycerides < 115 (pseudochylous effusion)	TB, rheumatoid arthritis

17.7 Spirometry

17.7.1 Lung volumes and capacities

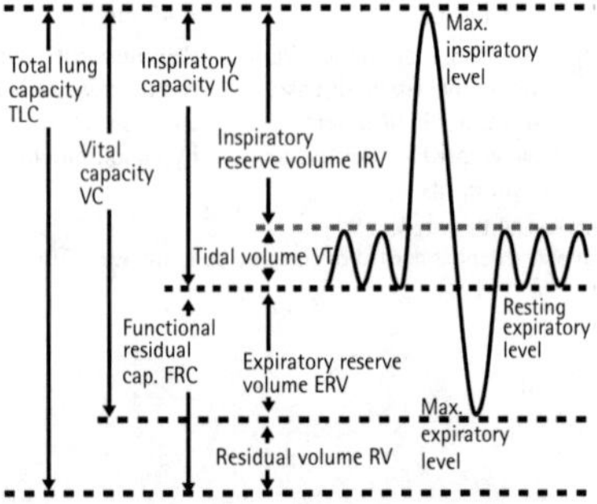

17.7.2 Normal flow volume curve

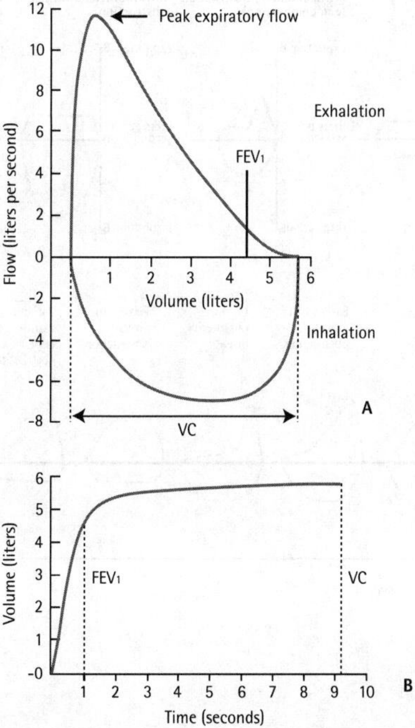

17.7.3 Flow volume loop examples

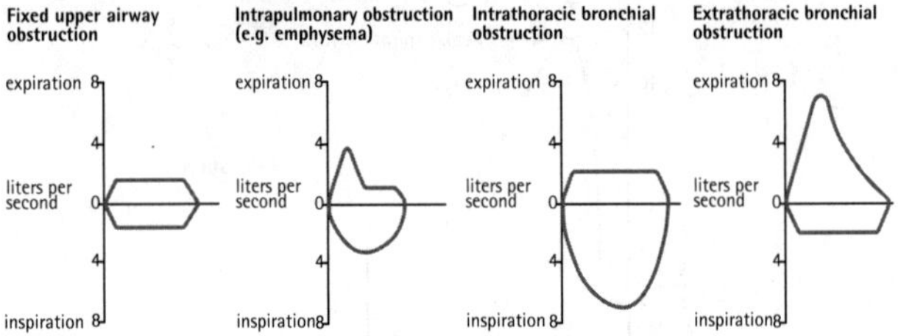

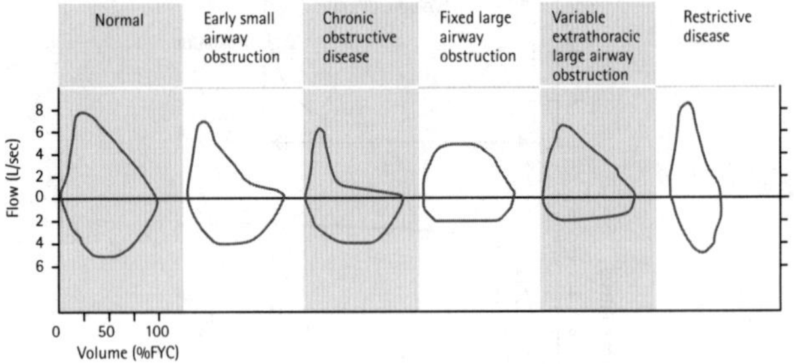

17.7.4 Diagnosis on pulmonary function testing

PFT finding	Likely causes
Fixed extrathoracic obstruction	Tumors, thyroid, tracheal stenosis
Dynamic extrathoracic obstruction	Epiglottitis, vocal cord dysfunction
Dynamic intrathoracic obstruction	Intrathoracic tracheomalacia

17.7.5 PFT interpretation

	FEV1	FEV1/FVC	TLC	DLCO
COPD	⇓	⇓	⇑	⇓
Asthma	⇓	⇓	Nl/⇑	Nl
Interstitial lung disease	⇓	Nl	⇓	⇓
Chest wall stiffness	⇓	Nl	⇓	Nl

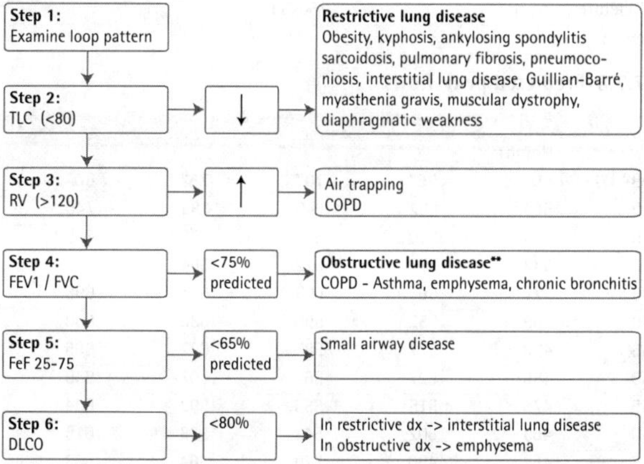

** Check for reversibility. If the FEV1 improves by 12% or 200cc post nebulizer treatment, the patient has a positive bronchodilator response.

17.7.6 Criteria for staging COPD

Degree	FEV1 (% of predicted)
Mild	> 80
Moderate	50-80
Severe	30-49
Very severe	<30 or <50 + chronic respiratory failure
Adapted from Executive Summary: Global Strategy for Diagnosis, Management, and Prevention of COPD, Dec 2009	

17.7.7 Criteria for assessing restrictive disease

Degree	TLC (% of predicted)
Mild	70-lower limit of normal
Moderate	60-69
Moderately severe	50-59
Severe	< 50

17.7.8 Predicted peak flows

Normal Males (Flow Values are in L/min)					
	Height				
Age (years)	60"	65"	70"	75"	80"
20	554	602	649	693	740
25	543	590	636	679	725
30	532	577	622	664	710
35	521	565	609	651	695
40	509	552	596	636	680
45	498	527	583	622	665
50	486	527	569	607	649
55	475	515	556	593	634
60	463	502	542	578	618
65	452	490	529	564	603
70	440	477	515	550	587

Normal Females (Flow Values are in L/min)

Age (years)	Height				
	55"	60"	65"	70"	75"
20	390	423	460	496	529
25	385	418	454	490	523
30	380	413	448	483	516
35	375	408	442	476	509
40	370	402	436	470	502
45	365	397	430	464	495
50	360	391	424	457	488
55	355	386	418	451	482
60	350	380	412	445	475
65	345	375	406	439	468
70	340	369	400	432	461

From Leiner GC, Abramowitz S, Small MJ, et al. American Review of Respiratory Disease, 1963. Nov;88:644-51.

17.8 Asthma

17.8.1 Stepwise approach to managing asthma in patients > 5 years

Step 1: Intermittent	Symptoms < 1 time/week Exacerbations are brief (hours-days), intensity may vary Nocturnal symptoms ≤ 2 times/month FEV1 or peak flow ≥ 80% of predicted
Step 2: Mild persistent	Symptoms > once a week but < 1 time/day Exacerbations may affect activity Nocturnal symptoms > 2 times/month FEV1 ore peak flow ≥ 80% of predicted
Step 3: Moderate persistent	Daily symptoms Daily use of inhaled short-acting beta-2 agonist Exacerbations affect activity Nocturnal symptoms > 1 time/week FEV1 or peak flow >60 but <80% of predicted
Step 4: Severe persistent	Daily symptoms Limitation of physical activity Frequent exacerbations Frequent nocturnal symptoms FEV1 or peak flow ≤60% of predicted

Note: Presence of any one feature is sufficient to place a patient in that category. Patients are assigned to the most severe step. Patients may change categories over time.
Adapted from Global Strategy for Asthma Management and Prevention, Global Initiative for Asthma (GINA) 2008

17.8.2 Asthma treatment steps

Step 1	Step 2	Step 3	Step 4	Step 5
Rapid-acting β2 agonists as needed				
Controller options	Select one	Select one	Select one or more	Add one or both
	Low-dose ICS	Low-dose ICS + LABA	Medium/high dose ICS + LABA	Oral steroids (lowest dose)
	Leukotriene modifier	Medium/high dose ICS Low-dose ICS + leukotriene modifier	Leukotriene modifier Theophylline	Anti-IgE treatment
		Low-dose ICS + Theophylline		

ICS= Inhaled corticosteroids LABA= long acting beta agonists
Preferred options in shaded boxes. Adapted from GINA 2009 (Global Initiative for Asthma) pg 59

Asthma action plan

Name____ Date _____
Based on your predicted peak flow and your personal best peak flow, for you 100% is ______

Green Zone is _____-_____ 80–100% of your personal best
Take controller medicine(s) and avoid asthma triggers
Use albuterol inhalers on an as-needed basis

Yellow Zone is -____-_____ 50–80% of your personal best
Take ___ puffs of Albuterol inhaler every _______ hours
Use nebulized albuterol every ______ hours
Take ___ puffs of ________ inhaled steroid ______ times per day on a daily basis
Begin oral steroids: Take ____ mg of ____________ every _____am, _____pm
Inform you doctor of a change in your symptoms (phone number _________)

Red Zone is <50% - Danger!
Take ___ puffs of Albuterol- repeat ______ times
Call your doctor (phone number ___________) or report to the nearest ER
Important phone number for transportation is ______________

17.8.3 Management of status asthmaticus

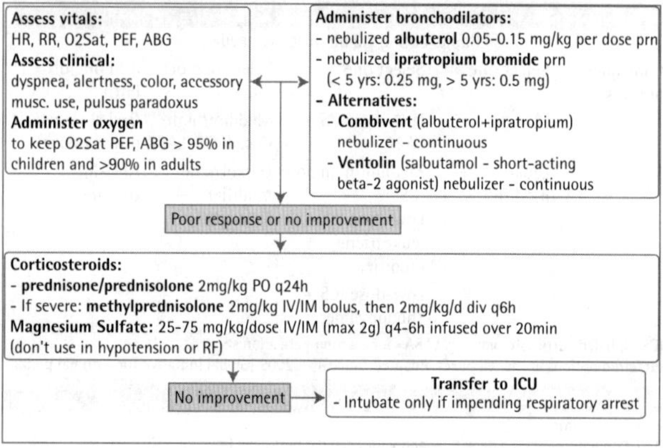
Assess vitals:
HR, RR, O2Sat, PEF, ABG
Assess clinical:
dyspnea, alertness, color, accessory musc. use, pulsus paradoxus
Administer oxygen
to keep O2Sat PEF, ABG > 95% in children and >90% in adults
Administer bronchodilators:
- nebulized albuterol 0.05-0.15 mg/kg per dose prn
- nebulized ipratropium bromide prn (< 5 yrs: 0.25 mg, > 5 yrs: 0.5 mg)
- Alternatives:
- Combivent (albuterol+ipratropium) nebulizer - continuous
- Ventolin (salbutamol - short-acting beta-2 agonist) nebulizer - continuous
Poor response or no improvement
Corticosteroids:
- prednisone/prednisolone 2mg/kg PO q24h
- If severe: methylprednisolone 2mg/kg IV/IM bolus, then 2mg/kg/d div q6h
Magnesium Sulfate: 25-75 mg/kg/dose IV/IM (max 2g) q4-6h infused over 20min
(don't use in hypotension or RF)
No improvement
Transfer to ICU
- Intubate only if impending respiratory arrest

17.9 COPD

17.9.1 Admission criteria for COPD

- High-risk comorbidities including pneumonia, cardiac arrhythmia, congestive heart failure, diabetes mellitus, renal failure, or liver failure
- Inadequate response of symptoms to outpatient management
- Marked increase in dyspnea
- Inability to eat or sleep due to symptoms
- Worsening hypoxemia
- Worsening hypercapnia
- Changes in mental status
- Inability to care for oneself (i.e. lack of home support)
- Uncertain diagnosis

17.9.2 COPD exacerbation therapy

Inhaled beta-2 agonists	albuterol MDI 180 µg (2 puffs) or 2.5mg nebulized every 1-2 hours
Anti-cholinergic bronchodilators	ipratropium bromide MDI 36 µg (2 puffs) every 4 hours or 500 µg nebulized every 2-3 hours
Corticosteroids	**methylprednisolone** (Solumedrol) 125 mg IV every 6 hours for 3 days then: Hospitalized: methylprednisolone 60 mg IV qd x 4 days, 40 mg IV qd x 4 days, 20 mg IV qd x 4 days Outpatient : **prednisone** 60 mg PO qd with 20 mg taper q 3-4 days (NEJM 1999: 340: 1941)
Antibiotics	Hospitalized: ampicillin-sulbactam, levofloxacin, moxifloxacin, piperacillin-tazobactam Hospitalized with risk for pseudomonas: ciprofloxacin, high dose levofloxacin, beta lactam with anti pseudomonal activity Outpatient: amoxicillin, doxycycline or trimethoprim-sulfamethoxazole, macrolide
Supplemental O_2	Target O_2 sat is ~90%-92% and PaO_2 of 60-65% Venturi masks are more precise than nasal cannula BiPAP may prevent the need for intubation
MDI = metered dose inhaler; BiPAP = bilevel positive airway pressure	

17.9.3 Indications for O_2 therapy

- PaO_2 < 55 mmHg or O_2 saturation < 88%
- PaO_2 between 56-59% or saturation <89% along with any of the following:
  - Pulmonary hypertension
  - Cor pulmonale
  - Erythrocytosis with hematocrit >55%

17.10 Pulmonary Embolus (PE)

17.10.1 Algorithm for assessing probability of PE - 3 steps

Step 1: Calculate the Clinical Probability of PE	
Variable	**Points**
Clinical signs and symptoms of DVT (leg swelling, pain)	3
Alternative diagnosis less likely than PE	3
Heart rate >100 beats/min	1.5
Immobilization >3 days or surgery in the previous 4 weeks	1.5
Previous PE or DVT	1.5
Hemoptysis	1
Malignancy: Receiving treatment, treated in the last 6 months or palliative	1
Christopher Study Investigators, JAMA 2006;295:172-179	
Unlikely ≤ 4 points (go to step 2)	
Likely > 4 points (go to step 3)	

Step 2: PE Unlikely

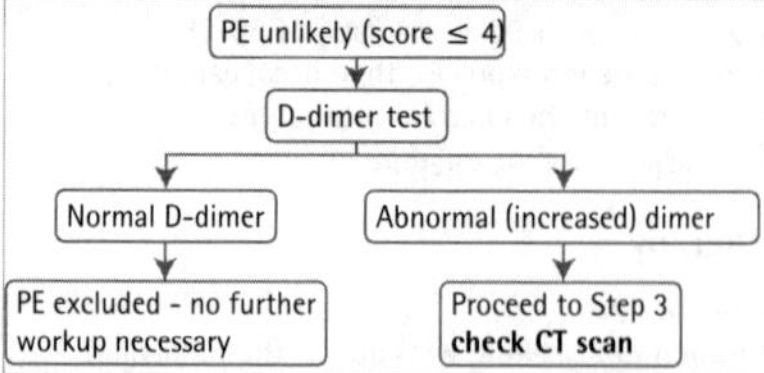

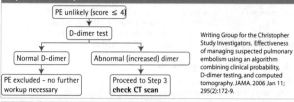

Writing Group for the Christopher Study Investigators. Effectiveness of managing suspected pulmonary embolism using an algorithm combining clinical probability, D-dimer testing, and computed tomography. JAMA. 2006 Jan 11; 295(2):172-9.

Step 3: PE Likely

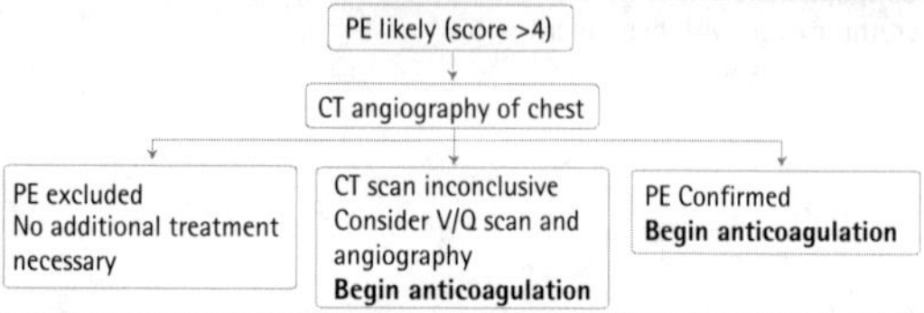

17.10.2 Treatment of PE

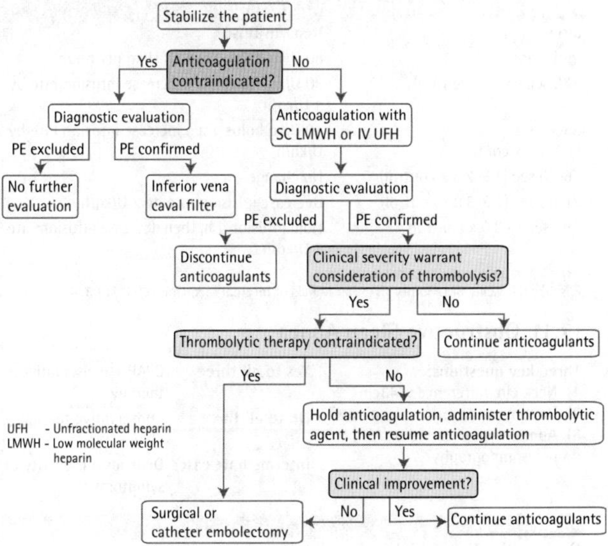

Reproduced with permission from: Tapson VF. Treatment of acute pulmonary embolism. In: UpToDate, Rose, BD (Ed), UpToDate, Waltham, MA, 2007. ©2007 UpToDate
For more information visit www.uptodate.com

17.10.3 Heparin dosing

Weight-based Nomogram for IV Heparin Infusion	
aPTT	**Heparin Dose**
Initial dose	80 U/kg bolus, then 18 U/kg per hour
<35 sec (<1.2 x control)	80 U/kg bolus, then increase infusion rate by 4 U/kg/h
35-45 sec (1.2-1.5 x control)	40 U/kg bolus, then increase infusion rate by 2 U/kg/h
46-70 sec (1.5-2.3 x control)	No change
71-90 sec (2.3-3.0 x control)	Decrease infusion rate by 2 U/kg/h
>90 sec (> 3.0 x control)	Hold infusion 1 h, then decrease infusion rate by 3 U/kg/h
aPTT: activated partial thromboplastin time. Raschke RA, Reilly BM, Guidry JR, et al. Annals of Internal Medicine 1993; 119:874.	

17.11 Obstructive Sleep Apnea

Three key questions: 1) Neck circumference > 43cm? 2) Daytime symptoms - sleepiness? 3) Apnea-hypopnea index (AHI) > 5 on polysomnography?	**Yes to all three**	CPAP + conservative therapy
	No to all three	Conservative therapy only
	Intermediate cases	Depends on severity of symptoms

Treatment for Sleep Apnea	
Conservative therapy (all patients)	Weight reduction Avoiding alcohol or sedating medications Lateral sleeping position
Continuous positive airway pressure (CPAP)	Shown to decrease somnolence, BP and to improve the quality of life, mood, and alertness
Flemons, New England Journal of Medicine 2002. 347:489-504.	

17.12 Management of Spontaneous Pneumothorax

Stable patients with small pneumothorax	Supplemental oxygen and observation for 3-6 hours and discharged home if repeat x-ray excludes progression. Give a followup appointment in 1-2 days with repeat chest x-ray. The patient should be admitted if followup is unreliable.
Stable patients with large pneumothorax	Supplemental oxygen and hospital admission for re-expansion of the lung using a small-bore catheter or chest tube placement.
Clinically unstable patients with large pneumotharaces	Supplemental oxygen and hospitalization for small-bore catheter or chest tube placement
Prevention of recurrence	Offered after a second pneumothorax (except in pilots or scuba divers). Preferred intervention is thoracoscopy (95-100% success rates) rather than chemical pleurodesis (78-91% success rates).

American College of Chest Physicians Delphi Consensus Statement. Chest 2001; 119:590-602

17.13 ARDS

17.13.1 Definition

- Bilateral radiographic infiltrates
- Ratio: $PaO_2/FiO_2 \leq 200$. Acute lung injury if $PaO_2 / FiO_2 \leq 300$
- No clinical evidence for elevated left atrial pressure. If measured, the pulmonary capillary wedge pressure is <18mmHg

17.13.2 Ventilator settings in ARDS

Mode	Assist control
Tidal volume goal	6 ml/kg of predicted body weight
Plateau pressure goal	$\leq$ 30 cm of H_2O
Ventilator rate and pH goals	Initial rate <35 breaths per minute to achieve arterial pH of >7.30 if possible
Inspiration: expiration time	1:1 - 1:3
Oxygenation goal - PaO_2	55 - 80 mmHg
Oxygenation goal - O_2 sat	85 - 95%
Weaning	Can be attempted by means of pressure support when level of PaO_2 is acceptable with PEEP <8 cm of H_2O and FiO_2 <0.40

Allowable combinations of PEEP and FIO_2	FiO_2	0.3	0.4	0.4	0.5	0.5	0.6	0.7	0.7	0.7	0.8	0.9	0.9	0.9	1.0
	PEEP	5	5	8	8	10	10	10	12	14	14	14	16	18	18-24

Source: The National Heart, Lung, and Blood Institute ARDS Clinical Trials Network. New England Journal of Medicine 2004;351:327-36.

17.14 Critical Care

17.14.1 Shock

Hemodynamic Monitoring in Shock				
	PCW	CO	SVR	Pressors of choice
Cardiogenic (acute MI, tamponade)	↑	↓	↑	Dobutamine, dopamine
Hypovolemic (hemorrhage, dehydration)	↓	↓	↑	Fluids/blood, NE
Distributive (sepsis, anaphylaxis)	↓/nl	↑	↓	NE, high-dose dopamine
Obstructive (massive PE)	nl	↓	↑/nl	NE, dopamine

Vassopressor Use in the Treatment of Shock				
	Receptor/Action	Inotropic	HR	SVR
dopamine low-dose 1-2 µg/kg/min	D1	↔	↔	↔/↓
dopamine high-dose >10 µg/kg/min	beta-1 → alpha-1	↑↑	↑	↑↑
norepinephrine	alpha-1, alpha-2, beta-1	↑↑	↔/↓	↑↑↑
dobutamine	beta-1, beta-2 > alpha-2	↑↑	↔/↓	↓↓
phenylephrine	alpha-1	↔	↔	↑↑↑
vasopressin	ADH analog	↑(weak)	↔	↑
amrinone/milrinone	PDE inhibitors	↑	↔/↑	↓

Treatment for Anaphylaxis	
epinephrine	0.5 mg (1:1000 solution) SubQ/IM q5-15min PRN; then 1-4 µg/min IV in severe anaphylactic shock
diphenhydramine	50 mg IV
methylprednisolone	125 mg IV or hydrocortisone 500 mg IV
albuterol	0.5 mg in 2.5 ml NS for resistant bronchospasm
Patients with moderate to severe reactions should be admitted to the hospital for close observation to watch for recurrence of symptoms. Consider Epi-pen at time of discharge.	

17.14.2 Swan-Ganz catherization pressures

Chamber	Normal Pressure	Causes of increase
RA	0-7 mmHg	- Right ventricular infarction - Pulmonary hypertension - Pulmonic stenosis - Left-to-right shunts - Tricuspid valvular disease - Volume overload - Impaired right ventricular contractile function
RV	RV systolic pressure: 5-25 mmHg RV end-diastolic pressure: 3-12 mmHg	- Pulmonary hypertension - Pulmonic stenosis - Acute pulmonary embolism
PA	PA systolic pressure: 15-25 mmHg PA diastolic pressure: 8-15 mmHg	- Volume overload Elevated pulmonary vascular resistance: - Left heart failure of any cause - All forms of primary lung disease - Mitral valvular disease - Pulmonary embolism - Hypoxemia with pulmonary vasoconstriction - Idiopathic pulmonary arterial hypertension - Left-to-right shunts
PCW	< 12 mmHg	- Mitral stenosis - Left ventricular systolic dysfunction - Primary left ventricular diastolic dysfunction - Left ventricular volume overload - Myocardial ischemia or infarction with decreased left ventricular compliance

17.14.3 Common modes of mechanical ventilation

Mode	Characteristics	Benefits	Problems	Example Vent Settings	Caveats
A/C (Assist Control)	Ventilator automatically delivers set tidal vol at the set rate. In addition, a full tidal volume is delivered if pt's insp. effort is suff. to trigger vent. (i.e. effort exceeds set point)	Common initial vent mode, as it decreases the work of breathing to help "rest" ventilatory muscles	Poor synchrony between pt-triggered breaths and the vent may cause auto-PEEP (breath stacking)	AC: RR 12/min Tidal vol: 10ml/kg FIO2: 100% I:E: 1:3 PEEP: 5 mmHg	In ARDS the tidal vol should be ↓ to 6mg/kg, and RR may be ↑ to 20. Goal is to decrease FIO_2 to <60% to prevent O_2 toxicity!
SIMV (Synchronized Intermittent Mandatory Ventilation)	Ventilator automatically delivers a set tidal vol at the set rate **only if there are no pt-initiated breaths.** Pt-initiated breaths are augmented by a specified amount of pressure support	Prevents auto-PEEP, helps maintain respiratory muscle function; facilitates weaning	Respiratory muscle fatigue	SIMV: RR 10/min Tidal vol: 10ml/kg FIO2: 50% I:E: 1: 3 PEEP: 5 mmHg Press Support: 10 mmHg	Pts who are not triggering their own breaths probably do not benefit from SIMV
CPAP (Continuous Positive Airway Pressure)	Ventilator provides pressure support only when the pt breathes	Comfortable for the pt who has adequate respiratory function. Used during weaning trials	Close monitoring is required because all breaths must be triggered by the pt.	CPAP: 10/5 (PS 10 and PEEP 5 mmHg)	Pts with accessory muscle use on CPAP should be switched back to SIMV or A/C

17.14.4 Sepsis

Sepsis Definitions	
SIRS (Systemic Inflammatory Response Syndrome)	2 or more of the following: - Temperature > 38°C or < 36°C - Heart rate > 90 beats/min - Respiratory rate > 20 breaths/min or $PaCO_2$ < 32 mmHg - WBC > 12,000 cells/mm^3, < 4000 cell/mm^3 or with > 10% immature forms (bands).
Sepsis	SIRS + suspected infection
Severe sepsis	Sepsis + organ dysfunction, hypoperfusion Organ dysfunction includes: Areas of mottled skin; capillary refilling of ≥ 3 s; urinary output of < 0.5 mL/kg for at least 1 h or renal replacement therapy; lactate >2 mmol/L; abrupt change in mental status or abnormal EEG findings; platelet count of <100,000 cells/mL or disseminated intravascular coagulation; acute lung injury/ARDS; and cardiac dysfunction (echocardiography)
Septic shock	Severe sepsis with systemic mean BP of <60 mm Hg (< 80 mm Hg if previous hypertension) despite adequate fluid resuscitation(40 to 60 mL/kg saline solution)
Refractory septic shock	Need for dopamine at >15 mcg/kg/min, or norepinephrine or epinephrine at >0.25 mcg/kg/min to maintain mean BP at >60 mm Hg (80 mm Hg if previous hypertension)
Annane, D et al. Septic shock. Lancet 2005; 365:63	

Goals of Therapy in Septic Shock**- Early Goal Directed Therapy	
Central venous pressure measured through central venous line	8 - 12 mmHg
Mean arterial pressure	≥ 65 mmHg
Urine output	≥ 0.5 ml/kg/hr
Central venous oxygen saturation	≥ 70%
**Rivers E; Nguyen B; Havstad S et al. Early goal-directed therapy in the treatment of severe sepsis and septic shock. New England Journal of Medicine 2001 Nov 8;345(19):1368-77.	

Early Considerations for the Septic Patient		
Issue	**Monitor**	
Sufficient fluids?	**Physical exam:** - Dry mucous membranes - Poor skin turgor - Axillary sweat **Vitals:** - Blood pressure - Mean arterial pressure - Heart rate	**Labs:** - BUN/CR ratio - Urine Na concentration - Fractional excretion of sodium (FeNA) - Urine osmolarity **Tissue perfusion:** - Urine output - Mental status (if not sedated)
Need for intubation?	Clinical decision based on patient's respiratory status	
Adequate IV access?	Critical patients require 2 large bore IV's at the very least	
Vasopressors	After adequate fluid resuscitation, vasopressors should be used to maintain the mean arterial blood pressure	
Special considerations		
Insulin	Administer insulin to maintain blood glucose at target <180 mg/dL	
Steroids	For patients with severe septic shock (systolic blood pressure <90 mmHg for more than one hour despite both adequate fluid resuscitation and vasopressor administration), may consider initiation of intravenous corticosteroid therapy within eight hours after the onset of shock. Response to ACTH testing should not be used to select patients for corticosteroid therapy.**	

** N Engl J Med. 2008;358(2):111-24

Early Goal Directed Therapy Algorithm

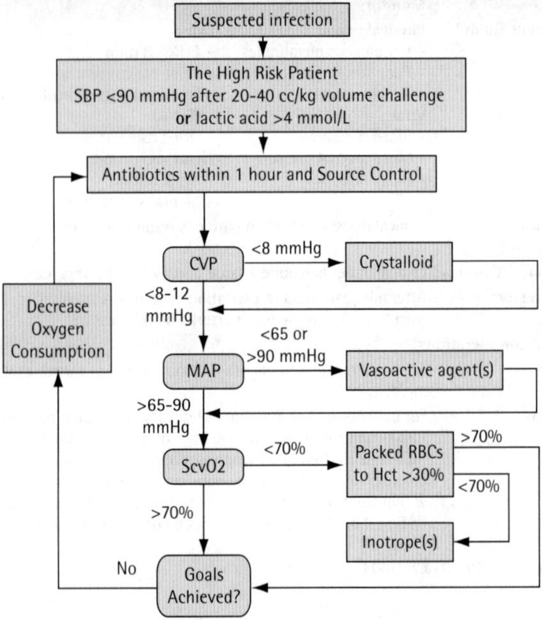

Otero RM, Nguyen HB, Huang DT, et al. Early Goal-Directed Therapy in Severe Sepsis and Septic Shock Revisited: Concepts, Controversies, and Contemporary Findings. Chest 2006;130:1579

17.14.5 Hypoxia

Five Causes of Hypoxia in the ICU			
Cause	**Explanation**	**Etiology**	**Treatment**
Shunt	Deoxygenated blood bypasses functioning portions of the lungs. Increased A-a gradient	Cardiogenic: - Acute MI - Left ventricular failure - Mitral valve disease - Diastolic dysfunction Noncardiogenic: - ARDS - Aspiration - Sepsis - Pancreatitis - Pneumonia - Drug reactions (ASA, narcotics) - Mixed (eg, MI with sepsis)	Treat underlying cause Does not correct with supplemental O_2
Ventilation-perfusion mismatch	Imbalance between blood flow and aeration of the lungs. Normal A-a gradient.	- COPD - Pulmonary vascular disease (PE, pneumonia) - Parenchymal disease (sarcoidosis)	Supplemental O_2
Low inspired O2	Decreased oxygen tension at the level of the alveoli. Low $FIO_2 \rightarrow PAO_2 \downarrow$	High altitude	Supplemental O_2 or descend from high altitude
Hypo-ventilation	Decreased respiratory rate or effort leads to decreased PaO_2 and increased PCO_2 PaO_2 will fall 1.25 mmHg for each 1 mmHg increase in PCO_2	- CNS depression - Neural conduction abnormality - Disease of the chest wall	Decrease sedation and/or identify cause
Diffusion impairment	Reduced efficiency of gas exchange with stress or exercise, but may be normal at rest	Interstitial lung disease	Supplemental O_2
Oxygen content (ml/dl) = 1.36 x Hgb (g/dl) x O_2 Sat + 0.003 x PaO_2 (mm/Hg)			

17.14.6 Hypercapnia in the ICU

Cause	Explanation	Etiology	Treatment
↑ CO_2 production	Respiratory acidosis	Fever Sepsis Seizures ↑ Carbohydrate load	Intubate early for rising PCO_2
↑ dead space	Areas of the lung are ventilated but not perfused. ↑ A-a gradient.	COPD Asthma Cystic fibrosis Pulmonary fibrosis	May tolerate higher PCO_2 to maintain respiratory drive
↓ minute ventilation	Normal A-a gradient	**Central lesions:** - Spinal cord lesion - CVA - Herniation **Peripheral lesions:** - Guillain-Barré syndrome - Myasthenia gravis - ALS - Botulinum toxin **Muscle disorders:** - Polymyositis - Muscular dystrophy **Drug overdose:** Metabolic abnormality - Hypothyroidism - Hypokalemia	Intubate early for rising PCO2 Identify reversible causes early (eg, consider nalaxone)

17.14.7 Intubation techniques

Verification of endotracheal tube placement	
Visualization	Watch the tube pass between the cords, or use fiber optic scope.
Auscultation	Hear bilateral breath sounds that are equal with each bagged breath. Also, no increased stomach sounds or gastric distension.
End tidal CO2	Easy Cap or end tidal CO2 monitor demonstrates that exhaled air is different from inhaled air.
Radiographic	Chest x-ray confirms end of the ET tube 3-5 cm above the carina.

17.15 5 Board-Style Questions

1) What is the best challenge test to diagnose exercise-induced asthma (exercise-induced bronchospasm)?

2) A 55-year-old woman returns to her pulmonologist's office complaining that her pneumonia has not improved even after a course of oral antibiotics. Initial chest X-ray revealed a LLL alveolar infiltrate. Now, two weeks later, the infiltrate has migrated to the RML. Current symptoms include malaise, fatigue, and cough for 4 weeks. The diagnosis of COP (cryptogenic organizing pneumonitis) is considered. What is the recommended treatment for COP?

3) A 42-year-old man with HIV/AIDS and a CD4 count of 23 presents with progressive SOB. The patient is comfortable at rest, but when he ambulates more than a few steps his SaO_2 drops to from 98% to 88% and he becomes short of breath. CXR reveals bilateral interstitial infiltrates. LDH is elevated, and ABG reveals a PaO_2 of 68% on room air. The patient is admitted for presumed PCP (pneumocystis jiroveci pneumonia). How should this patient be treated?

4) A 62-year-old woman is evaluated in the emergency department for fever, non-productive cough, and two-day history of myalgia, headache, and diarrhea. The patient has a 50-pack/year smoking history. On physical examination the patient is slightly disoriented. Temperature is 38.9°C (102°F), pulse of 89/min, respiratory rate of 20. Chest x-ray is poor quality and will need to be repeated. Laboratory results are only significant for a WBC count of 10.9 with 85% neutrophils, thrombocytopenia, and hyponatremia. A Gram stain of respiratory secretions shows many neutrophils, but no microorganisms. Which of the following is the single most important laboratory test for this patient?
   a) Serologic testing for Legionella
   b) Direct fluorescent antibody testing for Legionella
   c) Rapid urinary antigen test of Legionella antigen
   d) A rapid (2-to-3 hour) real-time PCR assay for Legionella
   e) Respiratory culture for Legionella on specific culture media

5) A 70-year-old man with respiratory failure, receiving mechanical ventilation, becomes restless. He is found to have a drop in his blood pressure, becomes acutely tachycardic and triggers the high pressure alarm. Peak pressure is found to be 60 with a plateau pressure of 52. The patient is noted to have decreased breath sounds on the right side and deviation of the trachea to the left. What should be done for this patient?

18 Rheumatology

18.1 Approach to Arthralgia Limited to 1 or Several Joints

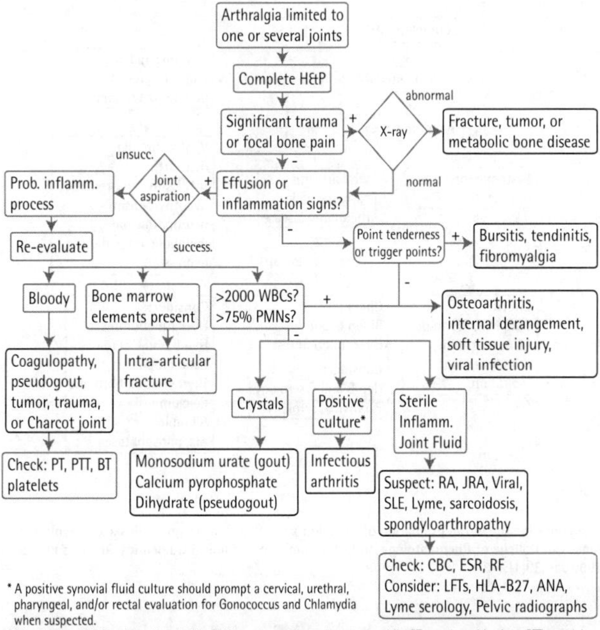

* A positive synovial fluid culture should prompt a cervical, urethral, pharyngeal, and/or rectal evaluation for Gonococcus and Chlamydia when suspected.

Abbreviations: WBCs=white blood cells; PMNs=polymorphonuclear neutrophils; PT=prothrombin time; PTT=partial thromboplastin time; RA=rheumatoid arthritis; JRA=juvenile rheumatoid arthritis; SLE=systemic lupus erythematosus; CBC=complete blood cell count; ESR=erythrocyte sedimentation rate; RF=rheumatoid factor; LFTs=liver function tests; ANA=antinuclear antibodies

Guidelines for the initial evaluation of the adult patient with acute musculoskeletal symptoms. American College of Rheumatology Ad Hoc Committee on Clinical Guidelines. Arthritis Rheum. 1996 Jan;39(1):1-8.

18.2 Approach to Arthralgia in Multiple Joints

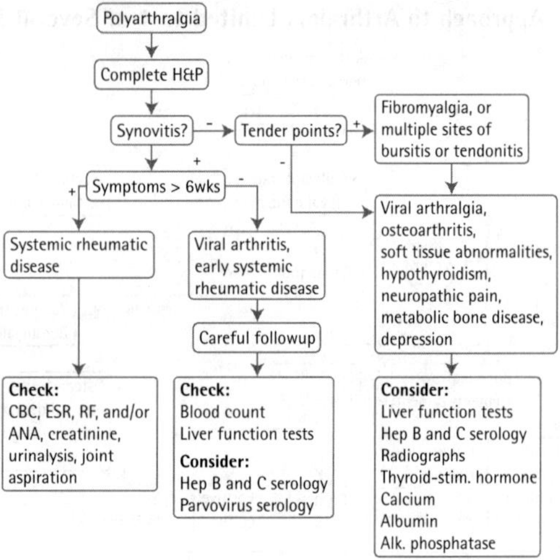

Guidelines for the initial evaluation of the adult patient with acute musculoskeletal symptoms. American College of Rheumatology Ad Hoc Committee on Clinical Guidelines. Arthritis Rheum. 1996 Jan;39(1):1-8.

18.3 Synovial Fluid Analysis

Joint Aspiration Tubes		
Chemistry	Red or yellow top	LDH, total protein, glucose
Hematology	Purple top	Cell count, differential
Microbiology	Clear sterile tube +/- fungal isolator	Gram stain, culture

Differential Diagnosis

	Normal	Non-inflammatory	Inflammatory	Septic arthritis	Hemorrhagic hemarthrosis
Examples	Normal	Osteoarthritis, trauma	RA, gout, SLE, pseudogout, psoriatic arthritis, reactive arthritis	Bacteria, mycobacteria, fungus	Trauma, hemophilia, hemangioma
Clarity	Transparent	Transparent	Transparent-opaque	Opaque	Bloody
Color	Clear	Yellow	Yellow-opalescent	Yellow-green	Red
Viscosity	High	High	Low	Variable	Variable
WBC (count/mm^3)	<200	200-2,000	2,000-100,000	>100,000	200-2,000
PMN %	<25	<25	≥50	≥75	50 - 75
Culture	Negative	Negative	Negative	Often positive	Negative
Tot. protein (g/dL)	1 - 2	1 - 3	3 - 5	3 - 5	4 - 6
LDH	Low	Low	> serum LDH	Variable	~ serum LDH
Glucose	~ serum LDH	~ serum LDH	Low (>25 g/dL)	Very low (<25 g/dL)	~ serum LDH
Next step	None	Pain meds	Microscopic crystal analysis Clinical clues to diagnosis	IV Abx +/- emergent arthroscopic lavage and drainage	Stop anti-coagulation, check x-ray

* Ratios represent synovial fluid to serum ratios

18.4 Common Crystal Diseases

Disease	Type of crystal	Microscopy	Treatment
Gout	Monosodium urate	Needle-like intracellular and extracellular; negative birefringent on polarized light	See gouty arthritis management section
Pseudogout	Calcium pyrophosphate dihydrate (CPPD)	Positively birefringent on polarized light	Intra-articular glucocorticoids, NSAIDS and colchicine

18.5 Gouty Arthritis Management

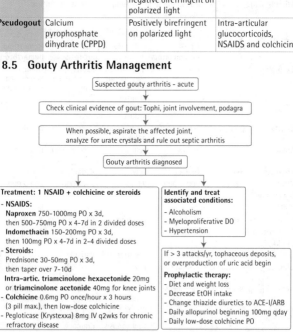

Suspected gouty arthritis - acute

↓

Check clinical evidence of gout: Tophi, joint involvement, podagra

↓

When possible, aspirate the affected joint, analyze for urate crystals and rule out septic arthritis

↓

Gouty arthritis diagnosed

↓

Treatment: 1 NSAID + colchicine or steroids

- **NSAIDS:**
  Naproxen 750-1000mg PO x 3d, then 500-750mg PO x 4-7d in 2 divided doses
  Indomethacin 150-200mg PO x 3d, then 100mg PO x 4-7d in 2-4 divided doses
- **Steroids:**
  Prednisone 30-50mg PO x 3d, then taper over 7-10d
  Intra-artic. triamcinolone hexacetonide 20mg or **triamcinolone acetonide** 40mg for knee joints
- **Colchicine** 0.6mg PO once/hour x 3 hours (3 pill max.), then low-dose colchicine
- Pegloticase (Krystexxa) 8mg IV q2wks for chronic refractory disease

↓

Identify and treat associated conditions:

- Alcoholism
- Myeloproliferative DO
- Hypertension

↓

If > 3 attacks/yr, tophaceous deposits, or overproduction of uric acid begin

Prophylactic therapy:

- Diet and weight loss
- Decrease EtOH intake
- Change thiazide diuretics to ACE-I/ARB
- Daily allopurinol beginning 100mg qday
- Daily low-dose colchicine PO

Terkeltaub RA. Clinical practice. Gout. N Engl J Med. 2003 Oct 23;349(17):1647-55.

18.6 Fibromyalgia

Criteria for diagnosis

Both of these criteria must be satisfied:

1. Widespread pain; ie, all areas of the body
2. Pain in 11 of 18 tender points (9 on each side) on digital exam ("tender" is not considered to be "painful"). See diagram:

Fibromyalgia Tender Point Sites

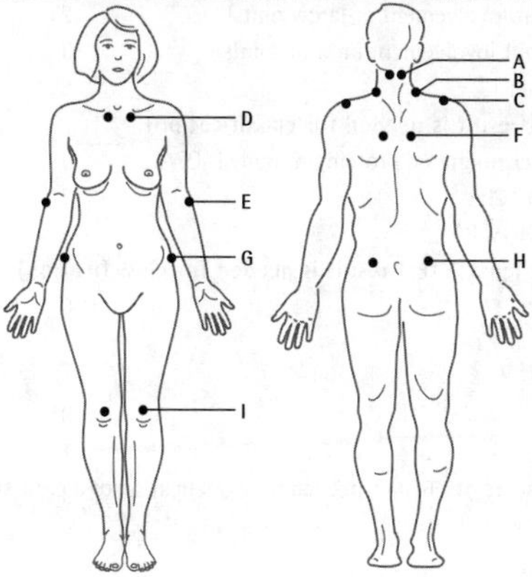

- A Suboccipital at hairline (insertion point of trapezius, splenius capitis mm.)
- B Lgg. transversaria C5–C7
- C Superiolateral border of Trapezius m. near clavicular insertion
- D 2nd costochondral joint
- E Approx. 2cm distal to lateral epicondyle of the humerus
- F Levator scapulae m. at superior angle of the scapula
- G Greater trochanter, posterior to the trochanteric prominence
- H Gluteus medius m.
- I Knee, medial to the Pes anserinus

Treatment for Fibromyalgia	
Step 1	Explain the disease to the patient
Step 2	Tricyclic antidepressant: **amitriptyline** 25-50 mg PO qhs
Step 3	Low-impact aerobic activities (walking, swimming, cycling) and referral for cognitive and behavioral therapy
Step 4	Referral to specialist (pain clinic, rheumatologist, psychiatrist) for consideration of additional medications **(pregabalin, SSRI, duloxetine, milanacipran)**

18.7 Rheumatoid Arthritis

18.7.1 Classification criteria for RA

Criteria	Score
A. Joint involvement	
1 large joint	0
2-10 large joints	1
1-3 small joints (with or without involvement of large joints)	2
4-10 small joints (with or without involvement of large joints)	3
>10 joints (at least one small joint)	5
B. Serology (at least one test result is needed for classification)	
Negative RF and negative anti-citrullinated protein antibody (ACPA)	0
Low positive RF or low-positive ACPA	2
High positive RF or high-positive ACPA	3
C. Acute-phase reactants (at least 1 test result is needed for classification)	
Normal CRP and normal ESR	0
Abnormal CRP or normal ESR	1
D. Duration of symptoms	
<6 weeks	0
≥6 weeks	1
Add score of categories A-D; a score of ≥6/10 is needed for classification of a patient as having definite RA	

18.7.2 Management of rheumatoid arthritis

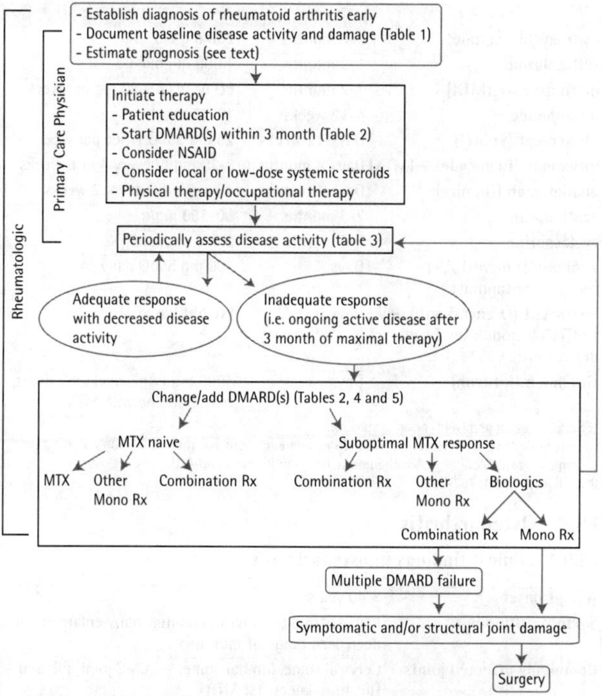

American College of Rheumatology Subcommittee on Rheumatoid Arthritis Guidelines. Guidelines for the management of rheumatoid arthritis: 2002 Update. Arthritis Rheum. 2002 Feb;46(2):328-46.

18.8 DMARD (Disease-Modifying Antirheumatic Drugs)

Drug	Time to benefit	Usual maintenance dose
hydroxychloroquine*	2-6 months	200 mg bid
sulfasalazine	1-3 months	1,000 mg bid-tid
methotrexate (MTX)	1-2 months	PO or IV: 7.5-20 mg per week
leflunomide	4-12 weeks	10-20 mg/d
etanercept (Enbrel)	Days-12 weeks	25 mg SubQ twice per week
infliximab (Remicade) + (MTX)	Days-4 months	3-10 mg IV every 4 or 8 weeks
adalimumab (Humira)	Days-4 months	40 mg SubQ every 2 weeks
azathioprine	2-3 months	50-150 mg/d
cyclosporine	2-4 months	2.5-4 mg/kg/d
anakinra (Kineret) IL-1 receptor antagonist	Days	100 mg SubQ daily
abatacept (Orencia) antibody to CTLA4 modulates T-cell activation	Days	Weight based
rituximab (Rituxan)	Days	1000 mg IV q2 weeks x 2 doses, may combine with MTX

*Check eye exam and G6PD prior to starting.
American College of Rheumatology 2008 Recommendations For the Use of Nonbiologic and Biologic Disease-Modifying Antirheumatic Drugs in Rheumatoid Arthritis. Arthritis & Rheumatism 59(6): 762-784 .

18.9 Osteoarthritis

18.9.1 Clinical findings in osteoarthritis

Age at onset	> 40 years
Symptoms/findings	Pain, stiffness, synovitis, crepitus, bony enlargement, decreased range of motion
Commonly affected joints	Cervical spine, lumbar spine, 1st CMC joint, PIP and DIP, hips, knees, 1st MTP
Uncommon joints	Shoulder, wrist, elbow, MCP joints
Synovial fluid	Clear, WBC <2000/mm3, normal viscosity

Radiographic findings	Joint space narrowing, subchondral sclerosis, osteophytes
Presentation	Young adult: monoarticular Middle age: pauciarticular, large joints
Natural history	Slowly progressive, variable

18.9.2 Management of osteoarthritis

Non-Pharmacologic Therapy

- Education and counseling regarding weight reduction, joint protection, and energy conservation
- Range-of-motion, aerobic, and muscle strengthening exercises
- Physical therapy and occupational therapy for patients with functional limitations
- Assistive devices for ambulation and activities of daily living
- Appropriate footwear, orthotics (eg, wedged insoles)
- Self-management resources (eg, American Arthritis Foundation self-help course and book)
- Complementary alternative medicine (eg, glucosamine)

Pharmacologic Therapy	
Non-NSAID analgesics	Initial drug of choice: **acetaminophen** 4 g/day Note patients with hepatic toxicity risk factors, especially those on aspirin. Reassess and taper as tolerated.
Other agents	Nonacetylated salicylate, tramadol, opioids, intra-articular glucocorticoids or hyaluronate, topical capsaicin or methyl salicylate
NSAID analgesics	Patients who are **not at cardiovascular risk** and are not using aspirin Patients at **no or low NSAID GI risk**: - Use a traditional NSAID - If GI symptoms develop, add an antacid, H2 blocker, or proton pump inhibitor (PPI) Patients who are **at cardiovascular risk** (consider aspirin) Patients at **no or low NSAID GI risk**: - Use traditional NSAID plus PPI if GI risk warrants gastroprotection - Consider non-NSAID therapy Patients at **NSAID GI risk**: - A gastroprotective agent must be added if a traditional NSAID is prescribed. - Consider non-NSAID therapy.
Modified from: Michigan Quality Improvement Consortium. Medical management of adults with osteoarthritis. Southfield (MI): Michigan Quality Improvement Consortium; 2005 Aug. 1	

18.10 Back Pain

Alarm Symptoms in Back Pain

- Age >50 years
- History of known cancer
- Unexplained weight loss
- Failure to improve in one month
- No relief with conservative therapy

Approach to the Patient with Back Pain

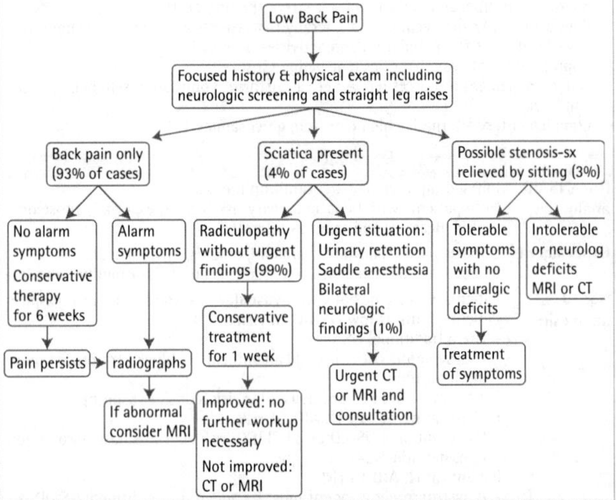

Jarvik JG, Deyo RA. Diagnostic evaluation of low back pain with emphasis on imaging. Ann Intern Med. 2002 Oct 1;137(7):586-97.

18.11 Autoantibodies in Connective Tissue Diseases

	ANA% and pattern	RF %	RNP %	Other
SLE	95, diffuse, speckled, rim	20	30-50	ds DNA 50-70%, Smith 30%
Drug induced SLE	95, diffuse	20	20	Antihistone Antibodies
Scleroderma	90, speckled, nucleolar	30	30	Scl-70, anticentromere, U3-RNP antibodies
CREST	90, speckled, nucleolar	30	30	Anticentromere
Mixed connective tissue disease	95, diffuse, speckled	50	100	
Dermatomyositis and polymyositis	80	33	0	Jo-120% Anti-SRP, Anti Mi-2
Sjogren's syndrome	90, diffuse, speckled	75	15	Ro/SSA 55%, La/SSB 40%

ANA = antinuclear antibody; RF = rheumatoid factor; RNP = ribonucleoprotein

18.12 Lupus

Diagnosis	
SOAP BRAIN MD* (presence of >4 of the following)	
Serositis	Pleurisy, pericarditis
Oral ulcers	Oral or nasopharyngeal, usually painless; palate is most specific
Arthritis	Nonerosive Jaccoud type
Photosensitivity	Unusual skin reaction to light exposure
Blood disorders	Leukopenia, lymphopenia, thrombocytopenia, Coombs-positive anemia
Renal involvement	Proteinuria (>0.5 g/d or positive on dipstick testing; cellular casts)
Antinuclear Abs (ANAs)	Higher titers generally more specific (>1:160)
Immunologic phenomena	Lupus erythematosus (LE) cells; anti-double-stranded DNA (dsDNA); anti-Smith (Sm) antibodies; antiphospholipid antibodies (anticardiolipin immunoglobulin G [IgG] or immunoglobulin M [IgM] or lupus anticoagulant); biologic false-positive serologic test results for syphilis
Neurologic DO	Seizures or psychosis
Malar rash	Fixed erythema over the cheeks and nasal bridge
Discoid rash	Raised rimmed lesions with keratotic scaling + follicular plugging

* "SOAP BRAIN MD" acronym presents all 11 criteria used by American College of Rheumatologists The presence of 4 of the 11 criteria has a sensitivity of 85% and a specificity of 95%.

18.12.1 Management of lupus

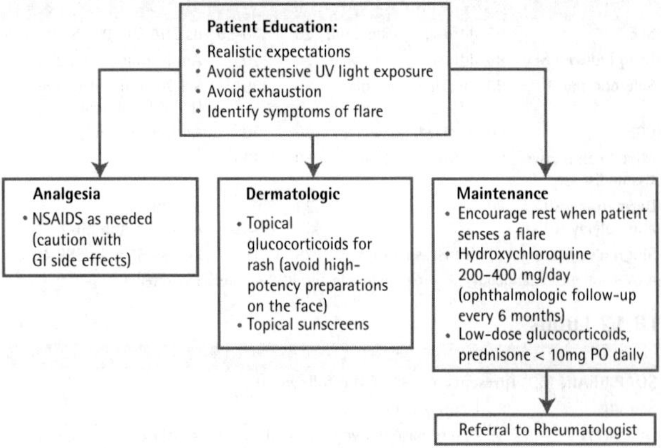

Modified from: Guidelines for referral and management of systemic lupus erythematosus in adults. American College of Rheumatology Ad Hoc Committee on Systemic Lupus Erythematosus Guidelines. Arthritis Rheum. 1999 Sep;42(9):1785-96.

18.12.2 Agents used in lupus nephrits

Agent	Mechanism of action
Steroids	Decrease inflammation; suppresses the immune system by reducing activity and volume of the lymphatic system
Mycophenolate mofetil	Cytostatic effect on T and B lymphocytes; inhibits inosine monophosphate dehydrogenase
Cyclophosphamide	Alkylating agent; prevents cell division by cross-linking DNA strands and decreasing DNA synthesis; has potent immunosuppressive activity
Azathioprine	Antagonizes purine metabolism and may inhibit synthesis of DNA, RNA, and proteins; The 6-thioguanine nucleotides mediate the majority of azathioprine's immunosuppressive and toxic effects.
Rituxan	Monoclonal antibody directed against the CD20 antigen on B-lymphocytes
Calcineurin inhibitors (Cyclosporin and Tacrolimus)	Inhibits transcription of interleukin-2 and several other cytokines, mainly in T-helper lymphocytes.
Hydroxychloroquine	Inhibits locomotion of neutrophils and chemotaxis of eosinophils; impairs complement-dependent antigen-antibody reactions

18.13 Seronegative Spondyloarthropathies

Common Features
- Negative RF and ANA - Sacroiliitis and spondylitis - Peripheral asymmetric arthritis - Enthesopathy - HLA-B-27 associated - >1 organ system involvement (joints, eyes, urethritis, mucocutaneous lesions)

Specific disorder	Common Features	Treatment
Ankylosing spondylitis	Inflammation and ossification of the joints and ligaments of the spine and sacroiliac joints	Physical therapy and exercise Naproxen 500mg PO BID TNF-α antagonists (etanercept, infliximab, adalimumab)
Psoriatic arthritis	7% of patients with psoriasis Nail findings: pitting is common, sausage digits may be present	NSAIDS, methotrexate 7.5-20 mg/week, other DMARDs
Inflammatory bowel disease	Asymmetric oligoarthritis, urethritis, conjunctivitis and characteristic skin and mucous membrane lesions. More common in young men, especially those with HIV. Associated with Chlamydia infection in some patients. Also, arthritis after dysentery caused by Shigella, Salmonella, Yersinia, or Clostridium	Acute inflammation: NSAIDS Infection: antibiotics (only for documented infection) Chronic disease: Sulfasalazine or methotrexate, intra-articular injection, DMARDs
Reactive arthritis	10-20% of patient with Crohn's disease or ulcerative colitis. Commonly affect knee and ankle	Antibiotics are not effective NSAIDS, DMARDs, physical therapy, and local injection of glucocorticoids

18.14 Vasculitis

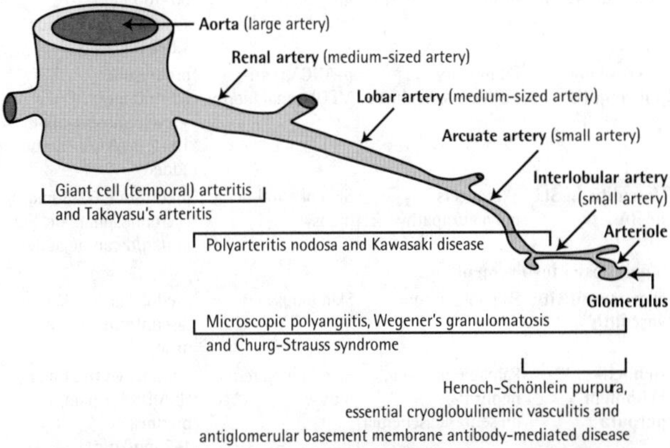

Clinical Features and Diagnostic and Treatment Approaches to Vasculitis			
Type of vasculitis	**Clinical features**	**Diagnostic tests**	**Treatment**
Large Vessel Involvement			
Temporal arteritis	Headache, jaw claudication, vision changes	Temporal artery biopsy	prednisone 40-60 mg/d
Takayasu's arteritis	Finger ischemia, arm claudication	Aortic arch arteriogram	prednisone 45-60 mg/d
Medium Vessel Involvement			
Polyarteritis nodosa	Skin ulcers, nephritis, mononeuritis multiplex, mesenteric ischemia	Skin biopsy, renal biopsy, sural nerve biopsy, mesenteric angiogram, Hep B/C testing	prednisone 60-100 mg/d +/- cyclophosphamide 1.5-2 mg/kg/d

Wegener's granulomatosis	Sinusitis, pulmonary infiltrates, nephritis	c-ANCA (anti-PR3), lung biopsy	prednisone 60-100 mg/d + cyclophosphamide 1.5-2 mg/kg/d
Microscopic polyangiitis	Pulmonary infiltrates, nephritis	p-ANCA (anti-MPO), renal biopsy	prednisone 60-100 mg/d + cyclophosphamide 1.5-2 mg/kg/d can be added
Vasculitis in SLE or RA	Skin ulcers, polyneuropathy	Skin or sural nerve biopsy	prednisone 60-80mg/d, cyclophosphamide 1-2 mg/kg/d can be added
Small Vessel Involvement			
Hypersensitivity vasculitis	Palpable purpura	Skin biopsy	prednisone 20-60 mg/d, discontinue inciting drug
Henoch-Schönlein purpura	Palpable purpura, nephritis, mesenteric ischemia	Skin biopsy, renal biopsy	Supportive treatment, NSAIDS for pain, prednisone 1-2 mg/kg/d*
* Not based on randomized controlled trials			

18.15 5 Board-Style Questions

1) A 24-year-old woman is admitted to the hospital for chest pain. She is found to have pericarditis, and also found to have synovitis in her hands, most prominently in the MCP and PIP joints. Both ANA and rheumatoid factor are positive. The patient is found to have 1.5 grams of protein in her urine. What is the most likely diagnosis in this patient?

2) A 43-year-old man who smokes 1 pack of cigarettes per day presents to his primary care provider with a new rash on his foot. He is found to have an ischemic ulcer on the distal portion of the right great toe. Biopsy of the lesion confirms the presence of inflammatory thrombi. What is the diagnosis, and what should be recommended for this patient?

3) A 68-year-old man with a long history of osteoarthritis presents to his primary care provider for pain, swelling and tenderness of his right leg. He reports a long history of knee swelling that he has attributed to arthritis. On exam he has edema exclusively below the knee, and a small hematoma over the medial malleolus. What is the most likely diagnosis, and what test should be performed?

4) A 52-year-old woman with carpal tunnel syndrome, diagnosed on nerve conduction velocity studies, reports feeling more tired than normal, and has gained 8 pounds in the past 2 months. What diagnosis should be considered?

5) A 50-year-old woman with rheumatoid arthritis for more than ten years is admitted to the hospital with pneumonia. She is found to be leukopenic, and the absolute neutrophil count is 900/mm^3. Physical exam reveals marked splenomegaly and rheumatoid nodules. Rheumatoid factor is positive. There is no malar rash, anti-ds DNA is negative. What is the most likely diagnosis?

19 Statistics

19.1 The 2x2 Bayesian Table

To understand the 2x2 table, imagine 1000 fans attending a U2 concert. They enter the stadium at the side entrance labeled TEST.

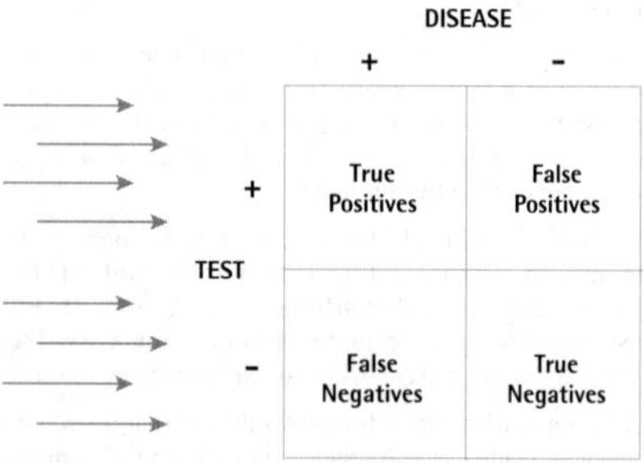

The fans wearing U2 t-shirts are told to follow the upper corridor. Those with other t-shirts follow the bottom corridor. The guards are pretty good, but occasionally a fan who is not wearing a U2 t-shirt sneaks past to the upper corridor. These are the false positives. Likewise, those, who are actually wearing a U2 shirt, but are not recognized and sent to the lower corridor, are the false negatives.

19.2 Sensitivity and Specificity

Sensitivity:

Sensitivity is the rate of true positives
Sensitivity = TP / (TP + FN)
Screening tests have a high sensitivity

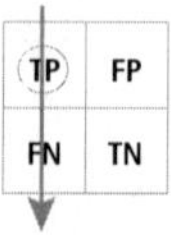

SnOut – Sensitivity rules out:
When a test has a high sensitivity, a negative result rules OUT the diagnosis. That is, if the number of false negatives is low (high sensitivity), the negative predictive value (NPV) will tend to be high. Thus, a negative test result in a test that has a high sensitivity tends to rule out the diagnosis.

Specificity:
Specificity is the rate of true negatives
Specificity = TN / (TN + FP)
Confirmatory tests have a high specificity

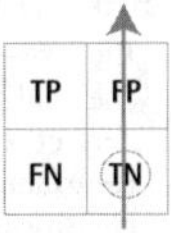

SpIn – Specificity rules in:
When a test has a high specificity, a positive result rules IN the diagnosis. That is, when the number of false positives is low (high specificity) the positive predictive value (PPV) will be high. Thus, a positive test result with a test that has high specificity tends to rule in the diagnosis.

19.3 Positive and Negative Predictive Values

Positive Predictive Value (PPV or PV+):
PPV is the fraction of patients with a positive test result who actually have the disease.
PPV = TP / (TP+FP); also called the post-test probability

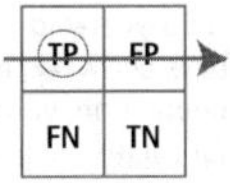

Negative Predictive Value (NPV or PV-):
NPV is the fraction of patients with a negative test result who in fact do not have the disease.
NPV = TN / (TN+FN)

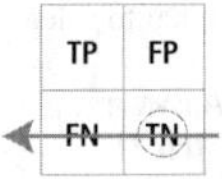

19.4 Likelihood Ratios

Likelihood Ratio + :
Probability of a positive test result in patients who have the disease divided by the probability of a positive test result in patients without the disease.
True positive rate / false positive rate = (sensitivity) / (1-specificity)

Likelihood Ratio - :
Probability of a negative test result in patients with the disease divided by the probability of a negative test result in patients without the disease.
False negative rate / true negative rate = (1-sensitivity) / (specificity)

Likelihood ratio	Change from pre-test to post-test probability
> 10 or < 0.1	Large, often conclusive
5-10 or 0.1-0.2	Moderate
2-5 or 0.2-0.5	Small, sometimes important
0.5-2	Rarely important

19.5 The Gold Standard

- The procedure that is used to define the true state of the patient.
- The gold standard must be reasonable and sensible, but does not have to be a perfect test.
- For example, coronary angiography is considered the gold standard for the identification of coronary artery disease.
- While an Autopsy would be the gold standard in most diseases, it would not be reasonable in a living patient (statistics humor).

19.6 Examples

19.6.1 Example 1

A 55-year-old man comes to your office. He has no cardiac risk factors, exercises 6 days per week, and eats a healthy diet. Based on the prevalence of CAD in his population, you estimate his pre-test probability of CAD to be approximately 1%. Calculate the positive and negative predictive values if he were to undergo an exercise stress test. How many false negatives would there be (use a population of 1,000 to calculate)? Exercise stress ECG: sensitivity 33%, specificity 99%.

Answer:

Step 1)

Use the pre-test probability to determine the number of patients with and without disease in a population of 1,000:

1% of 1000 = 10 have disease

1000 - 10 = 990 don't have disease

		DISEASE +	DISEASE -	
TEST	+	TP	FP	
TEST	-	FN	TN	
		10	990	=1,000

Step 2)

Use the given sensitivity and specificity of the stress test to calculate each cell in the 2 x 2 table:

10 x 33% = 3, 10 x 67% = 7

990 x 99% = 980, 990 x 1% = 10

		DISEASE +	DISEASE -	
TEST	+	3	10	
TEST	-	7	980	
		10	990	=1,000

Step 3)
Calculate the PPV and NPV using the filled-in 2x2 table:
PPV = TP / (TP+FP) = 3/(3+10) = 0.23
NPV = TN / (FN+TN) = 980/(7+980) = 0.99

Interpretation:
If the test is positive, the patient has a 23% chance of having CAD, given the pre-test probability of 1%. If the test is negative, the patient has a 99% chance of NOT having CAD. That is, if the test is negative, the patient has a 1% chance of having CAD.

This example illustrates that when the prevalence of a disease is low, a negative test is not very helpful. A positive test may not be convincing enough to prompt further testing. However, given the dire consequences of a missed diagnosis, a probability of 23% may be high enough to prompt a more definitive test.

19.6.2 Example 2

A 58-year-old man with intermittent, exertional chest pain is evaluated by his primary care provider. He has a 50-year/pack history of smoking and a first-degree relative who had an MI at age 50. He also has hypertension and hyperlipidemia. At this time he is requesting your permission to begin a strenuous cardiovascular exercise program at his gym.

You estimate his probability of coronary artery disease is approximately 90%. Calculate the positive and negative predictive values if he were to undergo an exercise stress test. How many false negatives would there be?
Exercise stress ECG: sensitivity 33%, specificity 99%.

Answer:
Step 1)
Use the pre-test probability of 90% to determine how many patients have and don't have disease. Assume a population of 1,000 and set up the 2 x 2 table just like in example 1, step 1.
1000 x 90% = 900 with CAD
1000 x 10% = 100 without CAD

Step 2)
Use the given sensitivity and specificity to calculate each cell in the 2 x 2 table:
900 x 33% = 297, 900 x 66% = 603
100 x 99% = 99, 100 x 1% = 1

		DISEASE +	DISEASE -	
TEST	+	297	1	
TEST	-	603	99	
		900	100	=1,000

Step 3)
Calculate the PPV and NPV from the filled in 2x2 table:
PPV = TP / (TP+FP) = 297/(297+1) = 0.99
NPV = TN / (FN+TN) = 99/(603+99) = 0.14

Interpretation:
If the test is positive, the patient has a 99%+ chance of having CAD (pretest probability was 0.9). If the test is negative, the patient has a 14% chance of NOT having CAD. That is, if the test is negative, the patient still has an 86% chance of having CAD.

This illustrates that when the prevalence of disease is high, a positive test is not very helpful. In this situation, even a negative stress test would likely prompt you to perform a more definitive test.

19.7 Screening Biases

19.7.1 Selection bias

Occurs because the people who elect to undergo screening are often different (more health-conscious, for example) from those who do not:

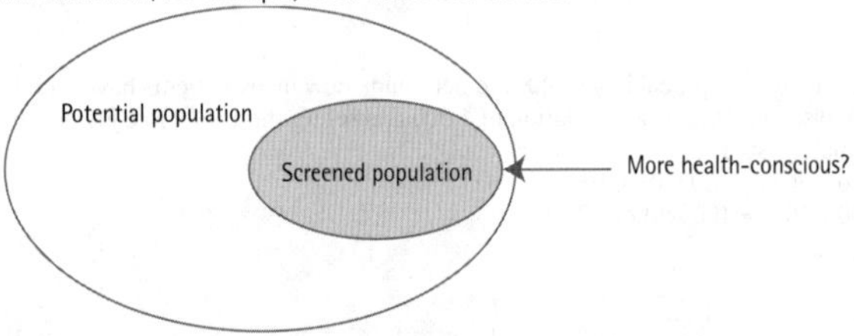

19.7.2 Lead time bias

Occurs because patients who are screened for a disease appear to live longer than an unscreened patient with the same disease. Actually, all patients with the disease may live for the same amount of time, but the screened patient will know about the disease longer.

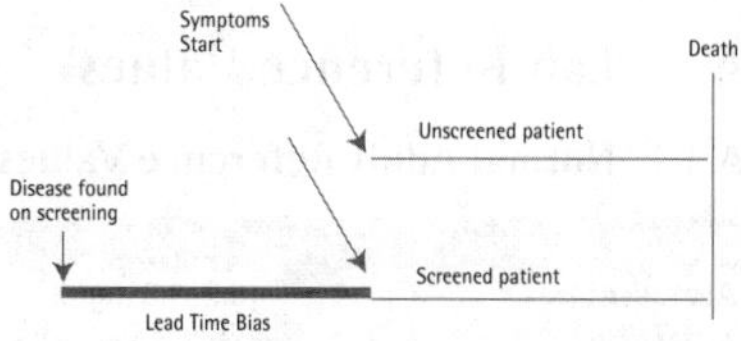

19.7.3 Length bias

Occurs because an asymptomatic disease (asymptomatic cancer), on average, is more indolent than a symptomatic disease (eg, cancer causing biliary or bowel obstruction). It is the asymptomatic diseases that are detected by screening.

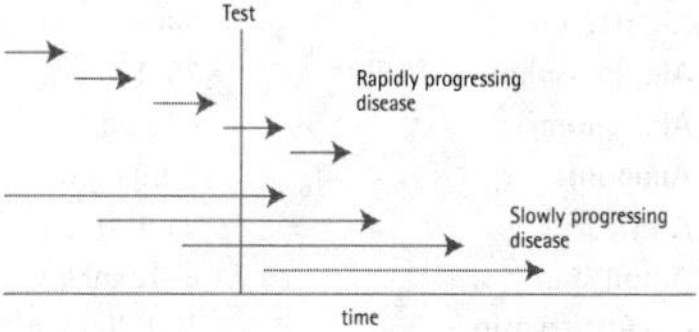

19.7.4 Overdiagnosis

Occurs when a disease is so indolent that the patient would likely die of other causes not related to the disease.

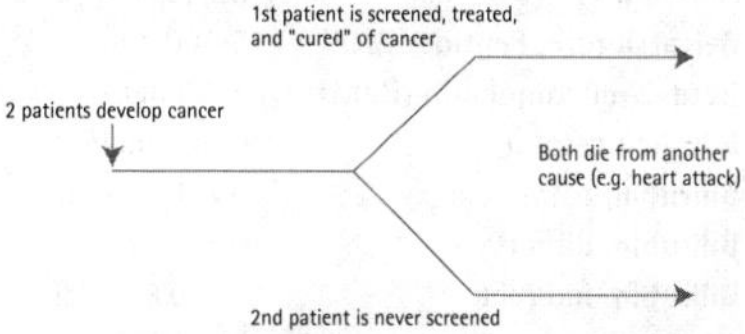

20 Appendix

A Lab Reference Values

A.1 Normal Adult Reference Values

Bloou d Chemistry	
Acetoacetate	0.2–1.0 mg/dl
ACTH	M: 7-69 pg/ml, F: 6-58 pg/ml
AFP	<20 ng/ml
Albumin	3.1–5.4 g/dL
Aldolase	0–8 U/L
Aldosterone	Supine: <16 ng/dl, Upright: 4-31 ng/dl
Alk. Phosphatase (AP)	30-120 U/L
Aluminum	<15 µg/L
Ammonia	0-50 µg/dl
Amylase	<170 U/L
Anion Gap	8–12 mEq/L
α_1-Antitrypsin	100-200 mg/dl
AST (SGOT)	15-45 U/L
ALT (SGPT)	**M:** 10-40 U/L, **F:** 7-35 U/L
B-Natriuretic Peptide (BNP)	5-100 pg/ml
Beta-2-microgobulin (B2M)	< 1.9 mg/L
Bile Acids, total	0-10 µmol/L
Bilirubin, total	0.2-1.0 mg/dl
Bilirubin, direct	0-0.3 mg/dl
Bilirubin, indirect	0.2–0.6 mg/dl
CA 15-3	<31 U/ml
CA 19-9	<37 U/ml
CA 27-29	<38-40 U/ml
CA 125	<30–35 U/ml
Calcitonin	**M:** <11.5 pg/ml, **F:** <4.6 pg/ml

Calcium, total	8.6–10.0 mg/dl (2.2-2.5 mmol/L)
Calcium, ionized	4.6-5.3 mg/dl (1.2-1.3 mmol/L)
Carcinoembryonic Antigen CEA	0–3.8 ng/ml
CEA, Smoker	0–5.5 ng/ml
Ceruloplasmin	16-66 mg/dl
Chloride	98–108 mEq/l
Cholesterol, total	<200 mg/dl (<5.2 mmol/L)
LDL Cholesterol	<150 mg/dl
HDL Cholesterol	**M**: >45 mg/dl, **F**: >55 mg/dl
Cholinesterase	3100 - 6300 U/L
Citrate	1.7–3.0 mg/dl
Complem. C3	88-201 mg/dl
Complem. C4	16-47 mg/dl
Copper, total	M: 70-140 µg/dl, F: 80-155 µg/dl
Cortisol, AM (7-9am) **Cortisol, PM (3-5pm)**	4.3-22.4 µg/dl 3.1-16.6 µg/dl
Creatinine	**M:** 0.7-1.3, **F:** 0.6–1.1 mg/dl
Creatinine Kinase-CK	**M**: 15-105 U/L, **F**: 10–80 U/L
CK-MB (Heart)	0–12 U/L (<5% of total)
C-Reactive Protein-CRP	<0.5 mg/dl
Ferritin	**M:** 20-250 ng/ml, **F:** 10–120 ng/ml
Fluoride	<0.05 mg/dl
Folate serum	3–20 ng/ml [7–45 nmol/L]
Folate RBC	140–628 ng/ml
γ-Glutamyl Transferase-GGT	**M:** 11-50 U/L, **F:** 7-32 U/L
Gastrin, fasting	<100 pg/ml
GH	**M:** <1 ng/ml, **F:** <10 ng/ml
Glucose	74-106 mg/dl [4.1-5.9 mmol/L]
Glutathione	24–37 mg/dl [0.77–1.2 mmol/L]
Hemoglobin A1C	4.8 - 6.0%
Haptoglobin	30-200 mg/dl
HBDH, alpha	140–350 U/l

Immunoglobulins IgA	85–385 mg/dl
IgD	0–8 mg/dl
IgE	<25 µg/dl
IgG	700-1600 mg/dl
IgM	40-230 mg/dl
Iron	**M**: 65-175 µg/dl [11.6–31.3 µmol/L]
	F: 50-170 µg/dl [9.0-30.4 µmol/L]
Ketones quantitative	0.5–3.0 mg/dl
Lactate	**Venous:** 5-20 mg/dl, **Arterial:** 5-14 mg/dL
LAP	**M:** 80–200 U/ml, **F:** 75–185 U/ml
LDH	100-190 U/L
Lead	<10 µg/dl
Lipase	10-220 U/dl
Magnesium	1.3-2.1 mEq/L
5'-Nucleotidase (5NT)	<15 U/L
Osmolality	275–295 mOsm/kg
Oxalate	1.0–2.4 µg/ml [11–27 µmol/L]
Pepsinogen	25–100 ng/ml
Phenylalanine	0.8-1.8 mg/dl
Phosphatase, alkaline	30–120 U/L
Phosphatase, acid	0-4.3 U/L
Phosphate	3–4.5mg/dl [0.97–1.45mmol/L]
Potassium	3.5–5.1 mEq/L
Prealbumin	10–40 mg/dl
Prolactin	**M:** 4-15.2 ng/ml; **F:**4.8-23.3 ng/ml
Protein, total **Albumin** **α-1 globulins** **α-2 globulins** **β globulins** **γ globulins**	6–8 g/dl 3.1-5.4 g/dl 0.1-0.4 g/dl 0.4-1.1 g/dl 0.5-1.2 g/dl 0.7-1.7 g/dl

PSA	<4 ng/ml
PTH	10-65 pg/ml
Pyruvate	0.3-0.9 mg/dl (0.03-0.10 mmol/L)
Rheumatoid Factor (RF)	<30 U/ml
Renin activity	0.9–3.3 ng/ml/h
Sodium	135–145 mEq/L
T_4, total	4.5–12 µg/dl [58–155 nmol/L]
$T_{4,\ free}$	0.8–2.4 ng/dl [10–31 pmol/L]
T_3, total	110–230 ng/dl [1.2-1.5 nmol/L]
T_3, free	0.93-1.70 ng/dl
T_3 uptake	24–34%
Testosterone total	**M**: 300–800 ng/dl, **F**: 20–82 ng/dl
Tot. Iron Bind. Capacity (TIBC)	250-425 µg/dl (44.8-76.1 µmol/L)
Transferrin	215–380 mg/dl
Triglycerides	<200 mg/dl
Troponin I	0-0.5 ng/ml
TSH	0.3-4.2 µU/ml
Urea Nitrogen (BUN)	6–20 mg/dl
Uric Acid	**M:** 3.5-7.2 mg/dl **F:** 2.4-6.4 mg/dl
Vit. A	26–72 µg/dl [0.9–2.5 µmol/L]
Vit. B_1-Thiamine	5.3-7.9 µg/dl [0.16-0.23 µmol/L]
Vit. B_2-Riboflavin	4-24 µg/dl [106-638 µmol/L]
Vit. B_6	3.6–18 ng/ml [15–73 nmol/L]
Vit. B_{12}	200–600 pg/ml [148–443 pmol/L]
Vit. C	0.4–1.5 mg/dl [23–85 µmol/L]
Vit. D_3, 1,25-dihydroxy	15–60 pg/ml [36–144 pmol/L]
Vit. D, 25-hydroxy	10–55 ng/ml [25–137 nmol/L]
Zinc	70-120 mg/dl[10.7-18.4 mmol/L]

Pleural, Pericardial, or Peritoneal Fluid	Transudate	Exudate
Amylase		> 500 U/ml
Erythrocytes (RBC)	< 10,000/µl	variable
Proteins total Pleural/Serum Ratio	< 3 g/dl < 0.5	> 3 g/dl > 0.5
Glucose	same as serum	less than serum
Leukocytes (WBC)	< 1000/µl	> 1000/µl
LDH Pleural/Serum LDH Ratio	< 200 U/L < 0.6	> 200 U/L > 0.6
pH	7.4-7.5	< 7.4
Specific Gravity	< 1.016	> 1.016

Gases	arterial	venous	Met. Acidosis	Resp. Acidosis	Met. Alkal.	Resp. Alkal.
pH	7.35–7.44	7.33–7.43	↓	↓	↑	↑
pCO_2	35–45 mmHg	36-48 mmHg	normal	↑*	normal	↓*
HCO_3^-	21-27 mEq/L	22–29 mEq/L	↓*	normal	↑*	normal
pO_2	70–100 mmHg	37–47 mmHg	*= Primary change			
O_2-Sat	>95%	60–85%				
Base excess	-2 to 3					

Hematology	
Hemoglobin	**M**: 13.5-17.5 g/dl **F**: 12–16 g/dl
Methemoglobin	<2 % of total Hb
Hematocrit	**M**: 41–53 % **F**: 36–47 %
Erythrocyte count (RBC)	**M**: 4.5–5.7 $\times 10^6$/µl **F**: 3.9–5.0 $\times 10^6$/µl
MCV	80–100 fl
MCH	26-34 pg/cell
MCHC	31-37 g/dl
Leukocytes (WBC), total	4.5-11 $\times 10^3$/µl
Neutrophils	1.8–7.7 $\times 10^3$/µl, 40-84%

Bands	< 8%
Eosinophils	0–0.45 x10^3/µl, < 6%
Basophils	0–0.2 x10^3/µl, < 2%
Monocytes	0.2–0.9 x10^3/µl), 2-8%
Lymphocytes, total	1.0–4.8 x10^3/µl, 20-50%
B-cell (CD19)	0.1-0.5 x10^9/L, 6-19%
T-cells total (CD3)	0.7-2.1 x10^9/L, 55-83%
T-Helper (CD4)	0.3-1.4 x10^9/L, 28-57%
T-Suppressor (CD8)	0.2-0.9 x10^9/L, 10–39%
CD4/CD8 ratio	1.0-3.6
Platelets	150–350 x10^3/µl
Reticulocytes	M: 0.5–2.5 % F: 0.8-4.1 %
Coag. Inhibitors - AT III	0.74-1.26 U/ml
Protein C	0.64-1.28 U/ml
Protein S	0.60-1.13 U/ml
Coag. Factors - Factor VIII	0.50-1.49 U/ml
vonWillebrand (vWF)	0.50-1.58 U/ml
Bleeding Time (BT)	1-7 min
Prothrombin time (PT)	11–14 sec
Part. Thrmbplst. time (aPTT)	27-40 sec
Thrombin time (TT)	15-18 sec
D-Dimer	< 0.50 µg/ml
Fibrinogen	150–400 mg/dl
Fibrin deg. prod. (FDP)	Normal titer: < 1:25 Borderline: 1:25 - 1:50 Positive: > 1:50
Sed rate (ESR)	M: <50yr: 0-15, 50-65yr: 0-20, >65yr: 0-38 mm/h F: <50yr: 0-20, 50-65yr: 0-30, >65yr: 0-53 mm/h

Cerebrospinal Fluid	
Opening pressure	< 20 cmH20 (200 mmH2O)
Albumin	13.4-23.7 mg/dl
Chloride	700–750 mg/dl
Protein, total	18-58 mg/dl
Glucose	approx. 2/3 of normal serum levels
Immunoglobulins - IgA IgG IgM IgG, Synthesis rate	0.1–0.3 mg/dl 0.4–5.2 mg/dl 0.01–1.30 mg/dl (–) 9.9 to (+) 3.3 mg/d
Lactate	10–25 mg/dl [1.1–2.6 mmol/L]
Lactic Acid Dehydrogenase	5-30 U/L (10% of serum value)
Leukocytes, total (WBC) Lymphocytes Monocytes Neutrophils Eosinophils	<5 /mm^3 60–70% 30–50% 1–3% rare
Pyruvate	0.078–0.081 mEq/L
RBC	0

Urine and Urinalysis	
Albumin	50–80 mg/24h (at rest)
Ammonia Nitrogen	30–50 mEq/d (30–50 mmol/d)
Amylase	0-15 U/h
Bilirubin	negative
Blood	negative
Calcium	100–300 mg/d
Casts, microscopic - Hyaline Casts - Other	< 5 /hpf 0
Chloride	50–250 mEq/d
Copper	15–60 µg/d
Coproporphyrin	100-300 µg/d [150-460nmol/d]
Cortisol, free	10–100 µg/d [27–276 nmol/d]

Creatinine	**M:** 1.0–2.0 g/d, **F:** 0.8–1.8 g/d
Cystine	10–100 mg/d [0.08–0.83 mmol/d]
δ-Aminolevulinic acid	1–7 mg/d [0.1–0.6 mg/dl]
Dopamine	60–580 μg/d
Epinephrine	<3-38 μg/d
Fat	negative
Fructose	30–65 mg/h
Glomerular filtration rate	125 ml/min (GFR) (varies with age, gender, race)
Glucose	<0.5 g/d [<2.78 mmol/d]
5-HIAA	2–6 mg/d [10.4-31.2 μmol/d]
Homovanillic acid (HVA)	0.7-7.8 mg/d
Hydroxyproline, total	15–45 mg/d
Ketones, total	negative
17-Ketos	**M:** 7–25 mg/d [24–88 μmol/d] **F:** 4–15 mg/d [14–52 μmol/d]
17-OCHS	**M:**4.5-10 mg/d, **F:** 2.5-10 mg/d
Leukocyte esterase	negative
Magnesium	1-24 mEq/d
Metanephrine	24–96 μg/d
Nitrite	negative
Norepinephrine	15–80 μg/d [88.5-472 nmol/d]
Osmolality **12h fluid rest**	50–1400 mOsmol/kg >850 mOsmol/kg/d
Oxalate	M: 7-44 mg/d [80-502 μmol/d] F: 4–31 mg/d [46–353 μmol/d]
Pentoses	2.0–5.0 mg/kg/24h
pH	4.5-8.0
Phosphorus	3.5-4.5 mg/dL
Porphobilinogen	0–2.0 mg/d [0–8.8 μmol/d]
Porphyrins	
Coproporphyrin	**M:** <97 μg/d, **F:** <61 μg/d
Uroporphyrin	**M:** <47 μg/d, **F:** <23 μg/d

Potassium	25–125 mEq/d
Protein, total	<150 mg/d
Protein, hourly	< 4 $mg/m^2/h$
RBC, microscopic	< 5 RBCs/hpf
Sodium	130-315 mEq/d
Specific Gravity	1.005–1.030
Urea-Nitrogen	6–17 g/d [0.21–0.60 mol/d]
Uric acid	250-750 mg/d
Urobilinogen	0.2-1.0 mg/dl
Vanillylmandelic a. (VMA)	2.0–7.0 mg/d
Volume	600–2500 ml/d
WBC, microscopic	< 5 WBCs/hpf

Stool	
Fat	<6 g/d (2.5–5.5 g/24h) (<30.4 % of dry weight)
Trypsin Activity	positive (2 + to 4 +)
Wet Weight	<197.5 g/d (74–155 g/d)
Dry Weight	<66.4 g/d (18–50 g/d)

A.2 Normal Cardiovascular Values

Hemodynamic Pressures	
CVP - RA RV	6 mmHg 25/0-6 mmHg
Pulmonary Artery (PA)	25/12 mmHg
Wedge Pressure	10-12 mmHg
LA Pressure	10-12 mmHg
LV Pressure	120/0-12 mmHg
SBP	120/80
Pulmonary Normal Values	
PaO_2 (Art. O_2 Part Press)	80-100 mmHg
SaO_2 (Art. O_2 Sat)	95-100%
CaO_2 (Art. O_2 Content)	17-20 ml O_2/dl blood
$PaCO_2$ (Art. CO_2 Part Press)	40 mmHg
$CaCO_2$ (Art. CO_2 Content)	23-27 mmol/L
PvO_2 (Ven. mixed O_2 part press)	35-45 mmHg
CvO2 (Ven. mixed O_2 content)	12-15 ml CO_2/dl blood
$PACO_2$ (Alv. CO_2 part press)	40 mmHg

A.3 Pediatric Reference Lab Values

A.3.1 Serum Values

	Newborn (term)	Child/Adult
Ammonia	90-150 mcg/dl	0-50 mcg/dl
Alkaline Phosphatase	150-420 U/l	30-120 U/l
ALT (SGPT)	< 45 U/l	< 40 U/l
AST (SGOT)	< 75 U/l	< 45 U/l
Bili total/direct	< 8.7/0.6 mg/dl	< 1.2/0.6 mg/dl
Bicarbonate ($HCO3^-$)	17-24 mEq/l	22-26 mEq/l
Calcium Ca^{2+} total	7.6–10.4 mg/dl	8.6–10.0 mg/dl
Chloride Cl^-	98–113 mEq/l	98–108 mEq/l
Cholesterol	53–192 mg/dl	<200 mg/dl
HDL-Cholest.	> 60 mg/dl	> 60 mg/dl
LDL-Cholest.	< 150 mg/dl	< 150 mg/dl
Creatinine	0.3–1.0 mg/dl	0.5–1.3 mg/dl
Creatinine Clearance	38–62 ml/min/1.73m^2	98–156 ml/min/1.73m^2
GGT	0 - 130 U/l	9-40 U/l
Glucose	40–60 mg/dl	74–106 mg/dl
Iron	100–250 µg/dl	50–175 µg/dl
LDH	290-775 U/l	100-190 U/l
Lead	< 10 µg/dl	< 10 µg/dl
Magnesium	1.3–2.0 mEq/l	1.3–2.0 mEq/l
Osmolality	275–295 mOsm/kg	275–295 mOsm/kg
Phosphorus	4.5–9.0 mg/dl	3.5–4.5 mg/dl
Potassium K^+	3.6–5.9 mEql/l	3.5–5.1 mEq/l
PTT	35–65 sec	27-40 sec
Sodium Na^+	133–146 mEq/l	133–146 mEq/l
Triglycerides	32 - 106 mg/dl	< 200 mg/dl
Urea (BUN)	4 - 12 mg/dl	6 - 20 mg/dl
Uric acid	2.4 - 6.4 mg/dl	2.4 – 7.2 mg/dl

A.3.2 Urine Lab Values

	Newborn	Child/Adult
Chloride Cl^-	40–220 mEq/d	40–220 mEq/d
Erythrocytes	< 5 RBC/hpf	< 5 RBC/hpf
Potassium K^+	25–125 mEq/d	25–125 mEq/d
Calcium Ca^{2+}	2.5–7.5 mEq/d	2.5–7.5 mEq/d
Leukocytes	< 5 WBC/hpf	< 5 WBC/hpf
Sodium Na^+	40–250 mEq/d	40–250 mEq/d
Phosphate	16–58 mEq/d	16–58 mEq/d

A.3.3 CSF Lab Values

	Newborn	Child/Adult
Opening pressure	8-11 cmH2O	< 20 cmH2O
Leukocytes	0-25 WBC/mm^3	0 - 5 WBC/mm^3
Protein	20 - 170 mg/dl	18-48 mg/dl
Erythrocytes	0	0
Glucose	34 - 119 mg/dl	40 - 80 mg/dl
Lactate	1.2–2.1 mEq/l	1.2–2.1 mEq/l
Glucose CSF/ Blood ratio	0.44 - 1.30	0.50

B Conversions & Formulas

B.1 Temperature

°C = 5/9 x (°F - 32)	°F = (°C x 9/5) + 32
95 °F = 35 °C	102.2 °F = 39 °C
96.8 °F = 36 °C	104 °F = 40 °C
98.6 °F = 37 °C	105.8 °F = 41 °C
100.4 °F = 38 °C	212 °F = 100 °C

B.2 Length

1 inch [in] = 2.54 cm	1 centimeter [cm] = 0.3937 in
1 foot [ft] = 0.3048 m	1 meter [m] = 3.28 ft
1 yard [yd] = 0.9144 m	1 meter [m] = 1.0936 yd
1 mile = 1.609347 km	1 kilometer [km] = 0.6214 mile

B.3 Mass (weight)

1 pound [lb] = 0.4535924 kg	1 kilogram [kg] = 2.20462 lb
1 ounce [oz] = 28.35 g	1 gram [g] = 0.0353 oz
1 grain = 0.0648 g	1 milligram [mg] = 0.01543 grain

B.4 Volume

1 gallon [gal] = 3.785 l	1 liter [l] = 0.26417 gal
1 fluid ounce [fl oz] = 29.57353 mL	1 milliliter [ml] = 0.034 fl oz

B.5 Medical Formulas

B.5.1 Electrolyte Physiology Formulas

Calculated Anion Gap = [Na+] - [HCO_3-] - [Cl-] *the AG will increase 2.5 points for every 1 point drop in the serum Albumin below 4	Normal range: 8-12 mEq/L
Calculated Osmolarity = 2[Na] + [Glucose]/18 + [BUN]/2.8	Nomal range: 275-295 mEq/L
Osmolar Gap = measured osmolality - calculated osmolarity	Normal range: < 10 mEq/L
Δ gap (delta-delta) = Δ Anion gap (measured - expected)/ Δ HCO_3 (expected - measured)	1 in uncomplicated metabolic acidosis
Corrected Serum Calcium (mg/dl) = SerCa + 0.8 x (normal serum albumin - measured serum albumin) = 0.8 x (4 - measured - measured serum albumin)	Normal albumin = 4.0 g/dl
Na Deficit (mEq) = TBW x (120 mEq/L* - measured Na) TBW = Total body water = 0.5 x weight (kg) in women = 0.6 x Weight (kg) in men In the elderly the TBW factor should be reduced to 0.45 in women, and 0.5 in men *Correct to Na = 120 mEq/L initially.	Normal Na: 140 mEq/L
Water deficit (L) = TBW x [(S_{Na}/140) - 1] TBW = Total body water = 0.5 * Weight (kg) in women = 0.6 * weight (kg) in men In the elderly the TBW factor should be reduced to 0.45 in women, and 0.5 in men S_{Na} = Serum sodium	Normal Na: 140 mEq/L

B.5.2 Nephrology Formulas

Formula	Interpretation
Fractional Excretion of Na^+ (FENa) $= (U_{Na}/S_{Na})/(U_{Cr}/S_{Cr}) \times 100$ Represents % of filtered Na that is excreted in the urine. U and S are serum and urine conc. of creatinine and sodium in (mg/dl) and (mEq/L) $U_{Na/Cr}$= Urine sodium/creatinine $S_{Na/Cr}$ = Serum sodium/creatinine	>2%: Diuretics, chronic renal failure, non-oliguric ATN <1%: Pre-renal azotemia, Cirrhosis or hepatorenal syndrome, CHF, non-oliguric ATN, Meds (NSAIDs, ACE-I)
Estimated Adult GFR - Cockcroft-Gault Formula $= [(140\text{-age(yrs)}) \times \text{Wt (kg)}] / [72 \times S_{Cr}\text{(mg/dl)}] \times$ (0.85 if female) S_{Cr} = Serum creatinine	Normal GFR rates: Men: 90–139 ml/min Women: 80–125 ml/min Renal impairment: < 60 ml/min
Estimated Adult GFR - MDRD Levey Formula $= 186 \times S_{Cr}^{-1.154} \times \text{Age (yrs)}^{-0.203} \times$ (0.742 if female) $\times$ (1.21 if African American) S_{Cr} = Serum creatinine	Men: 90–139 ml/min Women: 80–125 ml/min Renal impairment: < 60 ml/min
Estimated Pediatric GFR - Schwartz Formula = Height (cm) $\times K/S_{Cr}$ (mg/dl) K= 0.45 infants-1yr, 0.55 in children and adolescent girls, 0.65 in adolescent boys. S_{Cr} = Serum creatinine	Value given in ml/min/1.73m^2
24 Hour Urine Creatinine Clearance $= [U_{Cr}\text{(mg/dl)} \times \text{Vol (ml)}] / [S_{Cr}\text{(mg/dl)} \times \text{time(min)}]$ S_{Cr} = Serum creatinine	Men: 90–139 ml/min Women: 80–125 ml/min Renal impairment: < 60 ml/min

B.5.3 Cardiovascular Formulas

Body Surface Area (BSA) (m^2) = Sqrt[(height in cm)(weight in kg)/3600] Alternative: BSA = $(\text{weight in kg})^{0.425} \times (\text{height in cm})^{0.725} \times 71.84 / 10{,}000$	Standard BSA = 1.73 m^2
Cardiac output (CO) - Fick Equation = SV x HR = VO2 / [C(a-v)O2] SV = Stroke volume (ml); HR = Heart rate (bpm); VO2 = Oxygen uptake (l/min); C(a-v)O2 = Difference between arterial and mixed venous O2 content (ml O2/dl blood).	Normal = 5.4 L/min

Arterial O2 content (CaO2) (ml O2 /dl blood) = (Hb x 1.34) x SaO2 + (PaO2 x 0.0031) Hb = Serum hemoglobin (g/dl), SaO2 = arterial O2 saturation (fraction), PaO2 = arterial O2 partial pressure (mmHg)	Normal: 16–22 mls O^2/dl blood
Mixed venous O2 content (CvO2) (mlO2/dl blood) = (Hb x 1.34) x SvO2 + (PvO2 x 0.0031) Hb = Serum hemoglobin (g/dl), SaO2 = venous O2 saturation (fraction), PvO2 = venous O2 partial pressure (mmHg)	Normal: 14.5–15.5 mls O^2/dl blood
Arterial-mixed venous O2 content diff C(a-v) O2 (ml O2/dl blood) = (Hb x 1.34) x (SaO2 - SvO2)	Normal 3.5-5.5 ml O2/dl blood
Mean Arterial Pressure (MAP) (mmHg) = DBP + SBP/3	Normal: 80–95 mmHg
Systemic Vascular Resistance (SVR) (dynes-sec/cm^5) = (MAP - CVP) x 79.9/CO	Normal: 770–1500 dynes-sec/cm^5
Pulmonary Vascular Resistance (PVR) (dynes-sec/cm^5) PVR = (MPAP - PAOP) x 79.9/CO	Normal: 20–120 dynes-sec/cm^5
Stroke Volume (SV) (ml) = CO/HR SV Index (SVI)= SV/BSA (or CI/HR); BSA = Body surface area; CI = Cardiac Index = CO/BSA; HR = Heart Rate (bpm)	Normal: SV: 55–100 ml; SVI: 35–60 ml/beat/m^2
Absolute Reticulocyte Count (ARC) = (Reticulocyte % / 100) * RBC **Corrected ARC** = ARC / Reticulocyte Maturation Time (days) RBC = RBC count in million/µl	Normal Values: % Retic count: 0.5–1.5 % (2.5–6.5% in newborns)
Reticulocyte Maturation Times (RMT) Values: Hct (%) RMT (days) Hct (%) RMT (days) > 40 1.0 15-24 2.5 35-39 1.5 5-14 3.0 25-34 2.0	
Reticulocyte Index (RI) = % Retic count * Hct / 45	Normal Values: % Retic Count: 0.5 - 1.5%; RI: 1-3%

B.5.4 Pulmonology formulas

A-a gradient (AAG) (mmHg) AAG = PAO2 - PaO2 AAG = (150 - PaCO2/0.8) - PaO2	Normal = (age + 4)/4 +/- 2
Minute Volume (VE) (L/min) = VT x #breaths/min	Normal: 6 L/min
Alveolar Ventilation (VA) = (VCO2/PACO2) x K VCO2 = rate of CO2 production (ml) / min; PaCO2 = Alveolar CO2 part. press. (mmHg); K = constant of 863 mmHg	Normal: 4.2 l/min
Compliance (C) = Δ volume / Δ pressure	
Static Compliance (SC) = VT / (plateau pressure - PEEP) VT - Tidal volume (ml) Plateau press = Inspiratory phase plateau pressure value when pt is on ventilator (mmHg) PEEP = Peak end-expiratory pressure (mmHg).	Normal: 50–85 ml/cm H2O
Dynamic Compliance (DC) = VT / (peak inspiratory pressure - PEEP) VT = Tidal volume (ml); peak insp press = Pressure at the peak of the inspiratory effort (mmHg); PEEP = Peak end-expiratory pressure (mmHg)	Normal: 75–125 ml/cm H2O

C Writing Orders and Notes

C.1 History and Physical Exam

CC	"In the patient's own words"
HPI	Mr X is a 65 year old man with a history of Y who presents to the emergency room with Z. **CODIERS:** - **C**ourse - **O**nset - **D**uration - **I**ntensity (quality, radiation, location) - **E**xacerbation - **R**emission - **S**igns and Symptoms that may be associated
ROS	Review of Systems. (→ 454)
PMH	Disorder and date of diagnosis
PSH	Type of surgery and date
ALL	Allergies to any medications with type of reaction
SOC	Social history including smoking, EtOH, IVDA, profession, living situation
FH	Parents/siblings medical history (or age and cause of death) and diseases that run in the family
PE	
General	Apparent age and distinguishing characteristics
Vitals	Temp Tmax, HR, BP, RR, O2Sat, Height, Weight, I/Os
HEENT	Head: evidence of trauma, sinus tenderness (ex: NCAT) Eyes: pupils, sclera, movements (ex: PERRL, EOMI) Ears: tympanic membrane, canals (ex: Tms clear) Nose: mucosa, exudates, turbinates appearance (ex: nose clear, pink turbinates) Throat: oral mucosa, tonsils oral pharynx (ex: throat clear, MMM)
Neck	JVD, thyroid exam, lymph nodes (ex: neck supple, no cervical LAD)
Lungs	Auscultation, fremitus, percussion (ex: CTA-b/l)

CV	PMI, pulses, auscultation, carotids (ex: RRR, s1s2 wnl, no s3, s4 no murmur) **Pulses** 4+ bounding 2+ expected 0 not present **Murmurs** 1/6 very quiet (only heard by cardiologist) 2/6 quiet 3/6 easily audible, no thrill 4/6 loud + thrill present 5/6 audible with stethoscope half on chest 6/6 audible without stethoscope
Abdomen	Bowel sounds, distension, pain (ex: S/NT/ND +NBS no rebound/guarding)
Extremities	Edema, pulses, clubbing, microfilament (ex: no LE edema, +2 DP pulses b/l)
Rectal	Inspection, prostate, hemoccult (ex: no masses, prostate wnl, hemoccult +)
Neurologic	Refer to neuro exam section for more details → 269 Motor strength, reflexes (ex: motor: 5/5, reflexes +2 throughout) Mini Mental Status Exam → 453 **Power-Motor strength:** 0/5 no contraction 1/5 trace contraction 2/5 weak contraction, less than force of gravity 3/5 movement stronger than force of gravity 4/5 movement against some resistance 5/5 normal, movement against full resistance **Reflexes** 0 absent 1+ reduced (hypoactive) 2+ normal 3+ increased (hyperactive) 4+ clonus

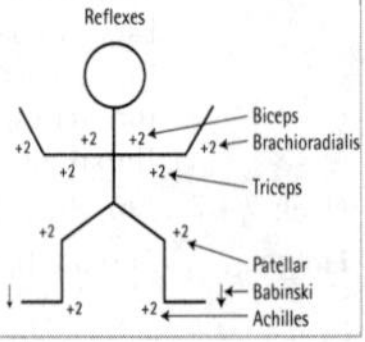

C.2 Mini Mental Status Exam

Date Orientation		**Repeating a Phrase**	
Year? (1), Season? (1), Date? (1), Day of week? (1), Month? (1)	5	Ask the patient to say "no ifs, ands, or buts." (1 pt. if successful on first try)	1
Place Orientation		**Verbal Commands**	
State? (1), County? (1), Town? (1), Building? (1), Floor / room? (1)	5	Give patient a plain piece of paper and say: "Take this paper in your right hand, fold it in half, and put it on the floor." (1pt. for each correct action)	3
Register 3 Objects		**Written Commands**	
Name 3 objects slowly and clearly. Ask the patient to repeat them. (1 pt. for each item correctly repeated)	3	Show patient a piece of paper with "**CLOSE YOUR EYES**" printed on it. (1 pt. if the patient's eyes close)	1
Serial Sevens		**Writing**	
Ask patient to count backwards from 100 by 7 five times, OR ask to spell "world" backwards. (1 pt. for each correct answer or letter)	5	Ask patient to write a sentence. (1 pt. if sentence has a subject, a verb, and makes sense)	1
Recall 3 Objects		**Drawing**	
Ask patient to recall the objects mentioned above. (1 pt. for each item correctly remembered)	3	Ask patient to copy a pair of intersecting pentagons onto a piece of paper. (1 pt. for 10 corners and 2 intersecting lines)	1
Naming		**Scoring (max.)**	30
Point to your watch and ask the patient what it is. Repeat with a pencil.	2	24-30: within normal limits - ≤ 23: cognitive impairment (further formal testing recommended)	
mod. per Folstein			

C.3 Review of Systems

Proceed head to toe	
Head	Do you have any: headaches, dizziness, syncope?
Eyes	Vision changes, photophobia, dryness, discharge, pain?
Ears	Hearing changes, tinnitus, vertigo, history of ear infections?
Nose	Nose bleeds, sinus pain/tenderness, polyps, change in ability to smell?
Throat	Bleeding gums, oral lesions?
Respiratory	Chest pain or shortness of breath, coughing up blood, recent lung infections? When was your last PPD? What was the result?
Cardiovascular	Chest pain with exertion/at rest, orthopnea, paroxysmal nocturnal dyspnea, murmurs, claudication, peripheral edema, palpitations?
Gastrointestinal	Abdominal pain, nausea/vomiting, dysphagia, heartburn, hematemesis, constipation/diarrhea, melena, hematochezia?
Gynecologic	Number of pregnancies (G? P?), age at menarche/menopause, last menstrual period (frequency, duration, flow), dysmenorrheal, type of contraception, sexual history, STD's, sexual orientation?
GU	Urinary frequency, urgency, hesitancy, dysuria, hematuria, polyuria, nocturia, discharge, STD's, impotence, sexual history including high risk activity for HIV?
Musculoskeletal	Arthralgias, arthritis, trauma, joint swelling, back pain, gout, trauma?
Vascular/ Hematologic	Varicose veins, claudication, thrombophlebitis/thromboembolic disease, anemia, bleeding, easy bruising
Endocrine	Polyuria, polydypsia, polyphagia, temperature intolerance, hormonal supplements, changes in skin or hair?
Neuropsychiatric	Syncope, seizures, weakness, coordination problems, altered mood, memory sleep pattern, emotional disturbances, drug or alcohol problems?

C.4 SOAP Note - Daily Progress Note

Date, Time, PGY/MS Progress Note

Subjective: Events over night

Objective:

PE, Labs, Studies

Current Medications List:

PE: Vital signs
Gen:
HEENT:
Neck:
Lungs:
CV:
Abd:
Ext:
Labs:

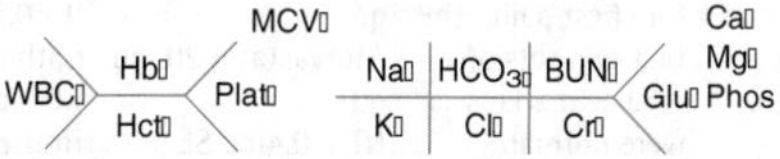

Culture results:
New radiographic findings:

Assessment:
Example: This is an 84 year old woman with pneumonia

Plan:
Organized by organ system:
Cardiovascular, Endo, GI, Hem/Onc, ID, Nephrology, Neurology; Pulm, F/E/N, Pain, DVT prophylaxis

Will discuss with Dr. X (the attending)

Your Name, pager#, year (PGY/MS)
Signature

C.5 Daily Signout Note

Date, Time, PGY/MS, Team, Resident, Attending (phone#)			
Patient Info	**Problem List**	**Medication List**	**To Do**
Patient Information Name Location MR# Allergies Code status Attending	Medical Status Specifics to watch for Recent changes	Medication with date of change or start date	Specific instructions for physician taking over patient's care.
Examples:			
Doe, John #1234567 12th floor South room 1234-1 NKDA Full Code Attending: Dr. House	55 yo man with HTN who was admitted for chest pain. The first two sets of cardiac markers were normal. Planning stress test in the AM	Aspirin 81mg po qd Atenolol 50 mg po qd Atorvastatin 20 mg qd NTG 0.4mg SL q5min	Please follow-up third Trop I at 10pm. If <0.1 there is nothing to do. If >0.1 please call Dr. House at home. The ph# is 123-4321
Smith, Jane #9876543 15th floor East room 1543 ALL: Penicillin DNR Attending: Dr. Shepherd	45 y.o woman with no PMH who was admitted with pyelonephritis and high temps. She was started on IV Ceftriaxaone on 2/12. If fevers persist > 72 hrs planning CT scan urology consult	Ceftriaxone 1g IV qd ½ NS @ 100/hr Reglan 10mg IV prn	Nothing to do overnight

C.6 Admission Orders, Transfer Orders

ADC-VAAN-DIML-HC **Physician Order Sheet**

Medications:	**Other Orders:**
Date: __/__/__ Time: ____am/pm All medications listed here: (hold parameters for BP meds) Common additions while hospitalized Tylenol 650mg PO q12 prn for HA Zolpidem 5mg PO qhs prn Heparin 5000 units SQ tid Name ______ Signature ______ pgr:__	Date: __/__/__ Time: ____am/pm **A**dmit:Floor,team,attending,resident, intern **D**iagnosis: primary diagnosis **C**ondition: stable/fair/guarded/ critical **V**itals: routine/q shift/q 4 **A**llergy: NKDA **N**ursing: wet to dry dressing changes, QD **D**iet: regular/1800 ADA (diabetic) Name ______ Signature ______ pgr:__
Date: __/__/__ Time: ____am/pm Name ______ Signature ______ pgr:__	Date: __/__/__ Time: ____am/pm **I**ns and Outs: strict I's and O's **M**onitors: on telemetry **L**abs: CBC, basic metabolic panel in AM **H**ouse Officer Calls: please notify house officer for BP > 180/110 Code Status: Patient is Full Code/DNR Name ______ Signature ______ pgr:__
Date: __/__/__ Time: ____am/pm Name ______ Signature ______ pgr:__	Date: __/__/__ Time: ____am/pm **Notes:** -If non-ambulatory and not on heparin SQ consider Venodynes -Be polite and always present/explain your orders to the nursing staff -Write legibly -If you are not sure...Ask for help! Name ______ Signature ______ pgr:__

C.7 On Service Note (Use SOAP format)

Date, Time, PGY/MS Progress Note
Admission Date:
Admission Diagnosis:
Hospital Course:
Subjective: Events over night
Objective:
PE, Labs, Studies

Current Medications List:

PE: Vital signs
Gen:
HEENT:
Neck:
Lungs:
CV:
Abd:
Ext:
Labs:

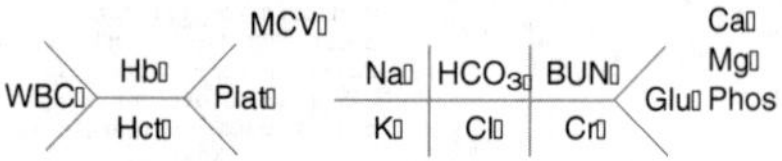

Culture results:
New radiographic findings:

Assessment:
Example: This is an 84 year old woman with pneumonia
Plan:
Organized by organ system:
Cardiovascular, Endo, GI, Hem/Onc, ID, Nephrology, Neurology, Pulm, F/E/N, Pain, DVT prophylaxis

Will discuss with Dr. X (the attending)

Your Name, pager#, year (PGY/MS)
Signature

C.8 Discharge Summary / Dictation Format

1. Date of Admission:
2. Date of Discharge:
3. Admitting Diagnosis:
4. Discharge Diagnosis:
5. Secondary Diagnoses:
6. Attending:
7. Ward team: Service, fellow, resident, intern
8. Procedures and tests: Radiology/lab-tests/other studies from this admission
9. Brief PMH:
10. Hospital Course:
11. Disposition: Where the patient will go following discharge
12. Discharge Medications:
13. Instructions/wound care:
14. Follow-up plans

Signed ______________ PGY________ Pager ______
Co-signed by attending________________________
(for dictations: "please send a copy to Dr. Organized")

C.9 PreOp Note

Date, Time, PGY/MS Pre-Operative Note

Pre-op diagnosis:
Procedure:
(E + 7C's):
EKG:
CBC:
Chem 7:
Coagulation:
Cross Match: Cross Match for 2 units PRBC's or Type and Screen in lab
Culture and Sensitivity (urine): U/A with C & S sent to lab
Chest X-ray:
Consent: Informed consent signed, in the front of the chart
Pre-op orders to consider:

- NPO after midnight for surgery
- Begin antibiotics (often Kefzol 1gm IV) on call to OR- then 1g IV q8h
- Anesthesia to see patient

C.10 Postoperative Note 4-6 Hrs Post-Op

Date, Time, PGY/MS Post-Operative Note
Procedure: Patient status post Appendectomy
S: Patient tolerated procedure. Pt alert and responsive, and without complaints. Pt reports pain is well controlled.
O: Vitals: Temp-current, T-max, BP, HR, RR, O2 sat, pain, Urine and drain output
PE: Brief
Meds:
Labs: New lab results since surgery
A: Assessment based on data above (15 year old male POD #0 s/p appendectomy, tolerated surgery well)
P: Encourage incentive spirometry, NPO, IV fluids, Meds (pain meds, antibiotics), consults, labs

C.11 Operative Note

Date, Time, PGY/MS Brief Op Note
Pre-Op diagnosis: Appendicitis
Post-Op diagnosis: Appendicitis
Procedure(s): Appendectomy
Surgeon: Attending, residents, and students present
Anesthesia: GETA (General Endotracheal Anesthesia), Spinal, or Local
Fluids: D5LR 2 L, 2 units of PRBC's
Estimated Blood Loss (EBL):Amount in ml
Drains: Foley, JP in RUQ
Specimens: Items sent to pathology
Complications: None or specify
Findings: Enflamed appendix with surrounding edema
Disposition: Patient to PACU, stable, extubated
Dictation: by Dr. Brilliant

Your name, pager#, year (PGY/MS)
Signature

C.12 Procedure Note

Date, Time, PGY/MS Procedure Note

Procedure: Right Internal Jugular TLC
Indication: Patient in septic shock for emergent IV access
Permission: Informed consent signed, in front of chart
Technique: Modified seldinger
Anesthesia: 2% lidocaine, local
Description:
(including complications/estimated blood loss/ and how pt tolerated procedure)

Example:
Anatomic landmarks identified. Area cleaned with betadine, sterile drape placed. Area anesthetized with 2% lidocaine. Left internal jugular vein cannulated and a TLC placed over wire using modified seldinger technique. There was good return in all three ports. The TLC was secured using 4 sutures and a sterile dressing was placed. The patient tolerated the procedure well. EBL ~30ml. Procedure was supervised by the Chief Resident on call, Dr. Bailey.

Resident/Fellow ____________________ Attending ________________

C.13 Delivery Note

Date, Time, PGY/MS Delivery Note

On (date and time) a (age) year-old delivered a healthy (male/female) infant weighing ______ with APGAR scores of (0-10) and (0-10) at 1 and 5 minutes. Delivery was (SVD-spontaneous vaginal delivery/LTCS-Low transverse C-section/ classical CS) over (intact perineum/mid-line episiotomy). The infant was (De Lee/ Bulb) suctioned. A nuchal cord was (easily reduced/not present). The cord was clamped, cut and the infant was (placed on maternal abdomen, handed to waiting nurse/pediatrician/neonatologist). The infant was noted to be spontaneously crying. Cord blood was obtained, and the placenta was delivered (spontaneously and intact/ with manual extraction). The placenta was grossly (normal/abnormal) and contained a three vessel cord. (Uterus/cervix/vagina/rectum) explored and a (___degree spontaneous laceration in the perineum was repaired with (2-0 chromic suture). EBL (estimated blood loss)= _____. Infant was sent to nursery and mother to recovery, both in stable condition.

Delivered by: Attending, resident, and student names

Things to consider prior to delivery:
- Consent for C-Section
- Blood consent form

If patient is on MgSO4, things you need to order:
- Pulse OX
- DTR's q2hrs
- Mg levels
- Fluid Restriction
- Ca Gluconate at bedside

Must d/c Pitocin (oxytocin) if:
- Non-reassuring tracings are found
- There is fetal distress.

Common pain meds:
- Demerol 50mg IM/IV x 1

C.14 Post-Partum Note (SOAP format)

Date, Time, PGY/MS Post-partum Note
Admission Date:
Delivery Date:
Complications:
Subjective: Events over night. Key questions: pain control, breast tenderness, vaginal bleeding, urination, flatus, bowel movements, lower extremity swelling, ambulation, nursing comments

Objective:
PE, Labs, Studies, Current Medications (list)
PE: Vital signs
Gen
HEENT:
Neck:
Lungs:
CV: Flow murmur may be normal
Abd: Bowel sounds present, fundal height/consistency
Pelvic: Incision/episiotomy condition
Ext: Lower extremity edema
Labs:

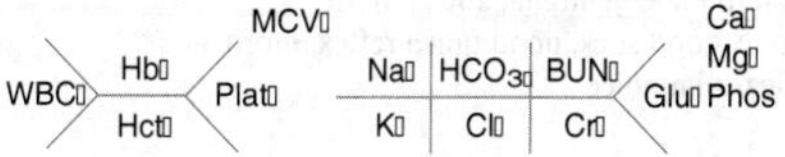

Rh status:
Culture results:
New radiographic findings:

Assessment: (eg, This is an 84 year old woman with pneumonia)
Plan:
Organized by organ system: OBGYN, Cardiovascular, Endo, GI, Hem/Onc, ID, Nephrology, Neurology, Pulm, F/E/N, Pain, DVT prophylaxis
Will discuss with Dr. X (the attending)

Your name, pager#, year (PGY/MS)
Signature

C.15 Newborn Nursery Admission Note

Date, Time, PGY/MS Newborn Nursery Note

Summary: This is a ___ week (female/male) AGA (appropriate for gestational age) born by NSVD (normal spontaneous vaginal delivery) to a __ y/o G_P_ mother (ABO+/-, HbsAg +/-, HIV +/-, Rubella immune, RPR +/non-reactive, GBS negative). The mother received adequate prenatal car. Maternal past medical history is significant for ______. No complications at delivery. Labor was around ___ hours.

Baby: Birth Date: ______Time:______, Child's Blood Type_____, RH:____

Apgars _______ @ 1 min, _____@ 5 min

Birth weight: _____g, length: _____cm, head circumference: ____cm

Objective: PE, Labs, Studies

PE: Baby is awake, alert, pink, NAD

Head: AFOF (anterior fontanelle open and flat), MMM (moist mucus membranes), normal facial features, red reflex present, no caput, no cleft lip or palate

Neck: Supple, no masses, clavicles intact

Lungs: Good air entry b/l, no wheezing, rales or ronchi

Heart: RRR, S1 S2 wnl, no murmurs, pulses strong and equal

Abdomen: Soft, NTND (non tender non-distended), no masses, no HSM (hepatosplenomegaly)

Ext: Full range of motion, brisk capillary refill

Hips: No clicks, no clunks, hips stable

GU: Normal male/female genitalia, anus patent

Neuro: Good tone, good suck, good grasp reflex, moro +

Skin: No significant jaundice

Labs/Studies:

Assessment: Day of life #, FT (full term) male/female well newborn feeding house formula exclusively, +voiding, +stooling

Plan: Routine well baby car, Anticipatory guidance

Your name, pager#, year (PGY/MS)

Signature

C.16 Apgar Score

Points	0	1	2
Appearance	entire body is blue	extremities are blue	entire body is pink
Pulse	absent	< 100 / min	> 100 / min
Grimace (response to suction)	no response	grimace	cough, sneeze, or cry
Activity (muscle tone)	atonic	decreased, some extremity flexion	active motion
Respiratory effort	absent	gasping or irregular	good
Scoring is done at 1 and 5 minutes after birth			
8 points: mild risk; 6-8 points: newborn is impaired; < 6 points: newborn's life is severely threatened, transfer immediately to NICU			

C.17 Writing a Prescription

The following information needs to be included as shown in the example below:

- Name of medication and dose in mg
- Number of pills to dispense
- Instructions

Authenticating Stamp

Patient Name: ______________ Date: __________
Address: __________________ Age: _____
City: _____________________ Sex: M / F
State, Zip: ________________

Name of medication and dose in mg: `Furosemide 20mg`
Number of pills to dispense: `Dispense #30`
Instructions: `sig: 1 tablet by mouth twice per day`

Refills ______ Signature ______________
Maximum daily dose ____ Printed Name ______________

C.18 How to Call a Consult

6) Write down the following key pieces of information (at least the first few times you call a consult)
- Patient's name
- Medical record number
- Room number, floor
- Attending name
- Age
- Primary diagnosis
- Why they came to the hospital- and when
- Few key facts - For example, if you are calling an endocrinology consult, know the blood sugars from the past few days and the hemoglobin A1c level.

7) Have the chart in front of you, with the most recent medication list
8) Provide a brief summary, not a full history
9) Speak confidently and concisely

On a good day, it might go something like this:

You: Hello, is this vascular surgery?

Them: Yes, this is Dr. Bigshot. I was paged to this number.

You: This is Dave from the medicine A team. We have a patient named Jon Doe, his medical record number is 327765, and he is in room 1402, on the 14th Floor East Wing. He is a 75 year old man with hypertension who was found to have an abdominal aortic aneurysm measuring 6 cm on a CT scan performed this morning. We would appreciate your input regarding surgery in this patient.

Them: Does he have any other medical problems?

You: Yes, besides hypertension, he has arthritis and GERD.

Them: How was the aneurysm diagnosed?

You: The patient was admitted for pneumonia last night. On physical exam he was found to have a pulsatile abdominal mass. A CT scan was ordered, and performed this morning.

Them: Why have you waited so long to consult vascular surgery?

You: We wanted to confirm our findings on CT scan

Them: We'll see him this morning

You: Thanks

Them: And who am I speaking to?

You: This is Dave Johnson. I'm a fourth-year medical student.

Them: Fine. From now on tell your resident to call her own consults.

C.19 Sample ICU patient tracker

Page 2. Patient Name__________________

Date							
pH							
pCO2							
pO2							
HCO3							
O2 Sat							
FIO2							
Ca							
Mg							
Phos							

Hx:

Test Results:

Consults:

To Do:

D Medical Abbreviations

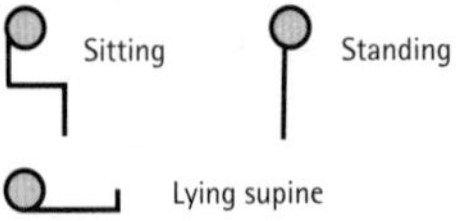

#	number; fracture; pounds
~	approximate; similar
@	at
+ve	positive
-ve	negative
↓ ; ↑	down, lowered; up, raised
f	steady, normal, unchanged
2x, 3x ...	twice, three times ...
AA	African-American; Alcoholics Anonymous
AAA	abdominal aortic aneurysm
Ab	antibody; abortion
ABC	airway, breathing, circulation
ABG	arterial blood gases
ac	before meals (Lat: ante cibum)
ACE(I)	angiotensin-convert. enzy. (inhibitors)
A(C)LS	advanced (cardiac) life support
ACU	ambulatory (acute) care unit
ADD	attention deficit disorder
ADL	activities of daily living
AF	acid-fast
AFB	acid-fast bacilli
Afib	atrial fibrillation
AI	aortic insufficiency
aka	also known as
ALC	alternative level of care
Alk Phos	alkaline phosphatase
ALL	acute lymphocytic leukemia
ALS	amyotrophic lateral sclerosis
ALT	alanine aminotransferase
AMA	against medical advice; antimitochondrial Ab
AMI	acute myocardial infarction
AML	acute myelogenous leukemia
ANA	antinuclear antibody
ANCA	antineutrophil cytoplasmic antibodies
ANP	atrial natriuretic peptide
A&O	alert and oriented
AOB	alcohol on breath
AP	anteroposterior
APC	atrial premature contraction
ARDS	adult respiratory distress syndrome
ARF	acute renal/respiratory failure; acute rheumatic fever
AS	aortic stenosis; arteriosclerosis
ASA	acetylsalicylic acid (aspirin)
ASAP	as soon as possible
ASD	atrial septal defect
ASHD	arteriosclerotic heart disease
AST	aspartate transaminase
ASVD	arteriosclerotic vascular disease
AV	arteriovenous; atrioventricular; aortic valve
AVM	arteriovenous malformation
AVR	aortic valve replacement
AVRT	atrioventr. reentrant tachycardia
AXR	abdominal x-ray
BAL	blood alcohol level; bronchoalveolar lavage

BBB	bundle branch block; blood-brain barrier
BC	blood culture; basal cell; birth control
BCG	bacillus Calmette-Guerin
BF	black female
bid	two times daily (Lat: bis in die)
biw	twice a week
BJ	biceps jerk; bone + joint
BJP	Bence Jones protein
BLS	basic life support
BM	black male; bowel movement; bone marrow
BMI	body mass index
BP	blood pressure; bullous pemphigoid
BPH	benign prostatic hypertrophy
BPM	beats/breaths per minute
BRBPR	bright red blood per rectum
BS	breath (or bowel) sounds; blood sugar
BUN	blood urea nitrogen
BW	black woman; birth weight
Bx	biopsy
c	with (Lat: cum)
C	Celsius; chlamydia; concentration; cyanosis
CA	cancer, carcinoma
CABG	coronary artery bypass graft (pron.: 'cabbage')
CAD	coronary artery disease
CAH	chronic active hepatitis
CAT	computed axial tomography
CBC	complete blood count
CBD	common bile duct
CC	chief complaint; creatinine clearance
CCB	calcium channel blocker
CCE	clubbing, cyanosis, edema
CCU	coronary (critical) care unit
CDC	Centers for Disease Control
CDH	congenital dislocation of hip
CEA	carcinoembryonic antigen
CF	complem. fixation; cystic fibrosis
CHD	congenital heart disease
CHF	congestive heart failure
CI	cardiac index; coronary insuff.
CIS	carcinoma in situ
CK(-MB)	creatine kinase (MB)
CLL	chronic lymphocytic leukemia
CMV	cytomegalovirus
CML	chronic myelogenous leukemia
CN	cranial nerve
CNS	central nervous system
CO	cardiac output
c/o	complains of
COPD	chronic obstructive pulmonary disease
CP	chest pain; cerebral palsy
CPAP	continuous positive airway pressure
CPK	creatinine phosphokinase
CPR	cardiopulmonary resuscitation
CRF	chronic renal failure
CRI	chronic renal insufficiency
CRP	C-reactive protein
C/S	Cesarean section
C&S	culture + sensitivity; conjunctiva + sclera
CSF	cerebrospinal fluid; colony-stimulating factor
CT	computed tomography
CV	cardiovascular; curriculum vitae

CVA	cerebral vascular accident, stroke; costovertebral angle
CVP	central venous pressure
CVS	cardiovascular system/surgery
c/w	consistent with
CXR	chest x-ray
d	days
DARF	dosage adjustment in renal failure
DAT	dementia of Alzheimer's type; diet as tolerated
D/C	discontinue; discharge
D&C	dilation and curettage
DD (Ddx)	differential diagnosis
D&E	dilation and evacuation
DHS	dynamic hip screw
DHx	drug history
DI	diabetes insipidus
DIC	disseminated intravascular coagulation
DJD	degenerative joint disease
DKA	diabetic ketoacidosis
DM	diabetes mellitus
DNKA	did not keep appointment
DNR	do not resuscitate
DO	disorder; Doctor of Osteopathy
DOA	date of admission; dead on arrival
DOB	date of birth
DOE	dyspnea on exertion
DPT	diphtheria, pertussis, tetanus
DSA	digital subtraction angiography
DSM	Diagnostic and Statistical Manual of Mental Disorders
DT	delirium tremens
DTR	deep tendon reflex
DU	duodenal ulcer; decubitus ulcer
DUB	dysfunctional uterine bleeding
D&V	diarrhea and vomiting
DVT	deep vein thrombosis
D5W	5% dextrose in water
Dx	diagnosis
EBL	estimated blood loss
EBV	Epstein-Barr virus
ECF	extracellular fluid
ECG	electrocardiogram
ECT	electroconvulsive therapy
ED	emergency department; epidural
ED50	median effective dose
EDC	estimated date of confinement
EDD	estimated delivery date
EEG	electroencephalogram
EF	ejection fraction
EGD	esophagogastroduodenoscopy
EKG	electrocardiogram
ELISA	enzyme-linked immunosorbent assay
EMD	electromechanical dissociation
EMG	electromyogram
EMS	emergency medical services
ENT	ear, nose and throat
EOM(I)	extraocular muscles (intact)
EOS	eosinophil(s)
ER	emergency room
ERCP	endoscopic retrograde cholangiopancreatography
ESR	erythrocyte sedimentation rate
ESRD	end stage renal disease
EtOH	ethanol
ETT	exercise tolerance test; endotrach. tube
F	father; female; Fahrenheit
FB	foreign body
FBS	fasting blood sugar
FD	Forceps delivery; fully dilated

FEV	forced expiratory volume
FFP	fresh frozen plasma
FH(x)	family history
FMP	first menstrual period
FNA	fine-needle aspiration
FOBT	fecal occult blood testing
FOC	father of child
FRC	functional residual capacity
FT	full-term
FTND	full-term normal delivery
FTT	failure to thrive
F/U	follow up
FUO	fever of unknown origin
FVC	forced vital capacity
Fx	fracture
G	gravida
GA	general anesthesia; gestational age
GB	gall bladder
GBS	Guillain-Barré syndrome
GCS	Glasgow Coma Scale
GDM	gestational diabetes mellitus
GERD	gastroesophageal reflux disease
GFR	glomerular filtration rate
GI(T)	gastrointestinal (tract)
GIFT	gamete intrafallopian transfer
gluc	glucose
GN	glomerulonephritis
G6PD	glucose-6-phosphate dehydrog.
GSW	gun shot wound
GTT	glucose tolerance test
gtt	drops, drip (Lat: guttae)
GU	gastric ulcer; genitourinary
HA	headache; hemolytic anemia
HAV	hepatitis A virus

Hb	hemoglobin
HBP	high blood pressure
HBV	hepatitis B virus
Hct	hematocrit
HCV	hepatitis C virus
HDL	high-density lipoprotein
HD	hemodialysis (high dependency) unit
HEENT	head, eyes, ears, nose and throat
HI	head injury; hepatic insufficiency
HIB	haemophilus influenzae type B
HIV	human immunodeficiency virus
HLA	human leukocyte antigen
HMO	health maintenance organization
h/o	history of
HOCM	hypertrophic obstructive cardiomyopathy (pron.: 'hocum')
H&P	history and physical examination
HPI	history of present illness
HPV	human papilloma virus
HR	heart rate
HS	heart sounds; herpes simplex
hs	at bedtime, hour of sleep (Lat: hora somni)
HSM	hepatosplenomegaly; holosystolic murmur
HSP	Henoch-Schönlein purpura
HSV	herpes simplex virus
HTN	hypertension
HUS	head ultrasound, hemolytic uremic syndrome
HVA	homovanillic acid
Hx	history; hospitalization
IA	intraarterial
IBD	inflammatory bowel disease
ICD-9	International Classification of Diseases, 9th Revision

ICH	intracerebral hemorrhage
ICP	intracranial pressure
ICS	intercostal space
ICU	intensive care unit
ID	infectious disease
I&D	incision and drainage
IDA	iron deficiency anemia
IDDM	insulin-dependent diabetes mell.
IFN	interferon
Ig	immunoglobulin
IHD	ischemic heart disease
IL	interleukin
IM	intramuscular
IMI	inferior myocardial infarction
imp	impression; important; improved
IMV	intermitt. mandatory ventilation
INR	international normalized ratio
I&O	intake and output
IP	inpatient
IPPB	intermitt. pos. pressure breathing
IRDS	infant resp. distress syndrome
ITP	idiopathic thrombocytopenic purpura
IUD	intrauterine contraceptive device
IUGR	intrauterine growth retardation
IUP	intrauterine pregnancy
IV	intravenous
IVC	inferior vena cava
IVCD	intraventr. conduction defect
IVDU	intravenous drug user
IVF	intravenous fluids; in vitro fertilization
IVH	intraventricular hemorrhage
IVIG	intravenous immunoglobulin
IVP	intravenous pyelogram/push
IVU	intravenous urogram

JOD (M)	juvenile onset diabetes mellitus
JPC	junctional premature contraction
JRA	juvenile rheumatoid arthritis
JVC	jugular venous catheter
JVD	jugular venous distension
JVP	jugular venous pulse/pressure
KJ	knee jerk
KS	Kaposi sarcoma; kidney stone
KUB	kidneys, ureters, bladder (x-ray)
;L	left
LA	left atrium; local anesthesia
Lab	laboratory
lac	laceration
LAD	left anterior descend. (coronary artery); left axis deviation
LAE	left atrial enlargement
LAFB	left anterior fascicular block
LAHB	left anterior hemiblock
LAP	leukocyte alkaline phosphatase; left atrial pressure
lap	laparoscopy
lapt	laparotomy
LBBB	left bundle branch block
LBP	lower back pain
LBW	low birth weight
LDH	lactate dehydrogenase
LDL	low-density lipoprotein
LE	lower extremity; lupus erythematosus
LFD	low fat diet
LFT	liver function test
LGA	large for gestational age
LGV	lymphogranuloma venerum
LKS	liver, kidney, spleen
LLE	left lower extremity

LLL	left lower lobe
LLQ	left lower quadrant
LMN	lower motor neuron
LMP	last menstrual period
LN	lymph node
LOC	loss (level) of consciousness
LP	lumbar puncture
LPFB	left posterior fascicular block
LPHB	left posterior hemiblock
LPN	licensed practical nurse
LSB	left sternal border
LUE	left upper extremity
LUL	left upper lobe
LUQ	left upper quadrant
LV	left ventricle
LVEDP	left ventric. end-diast. pressure
LVF	left ventricular failure
LVH	left ventricular hypertrophy
M	mother; male
m	murmur
MAE	moves all extremities
MAO (I)	monoamine oxidase (inhibitor)
MAP	mean arterial pressure
MAT	multifocal atrial tachycardia
MCH (C)	mean corpuscular hemoglobin (concentration)
MCL	midclavicular line
MCTD	mixed connective tissue disease
MCV	mean corpuscular volume
MDD	max. daily dose, manic-depr. DO
MDI	metered-dose inhaler
meds	medication
MEN	multiple endocrine neoplasia
MGF	maternal grandfather
MGM	maternal grandmother
MHC	major histocompatib. complex
MI	myocardial infarction; mental illness; mitral insufficiency
MIC	minimal inhibitory concentration
MLC	mixed lymphocyte culture
M&M	morbidity and mortality
MMFR	maximal midexpiratory flow rate
MMPI	Minnesota Multiphasic Personality Inventory
MMR	measles, mumps, rubella
MOS	mitral opening snap
MPGN	membranoproliferative glomerulonephritis
MR	mitral regurgitation; mental retardation
MRA	magnetic resonance angiogr.
MRDD	max. recommended daily dose
m/r/g	murmurs, rubs, gallops
MRI	magnetic resonance imaging
MRSA	methicillin-resistant Staphylococcus aureus
MRT	magnetic resonance tomography
MS	mitral stenosis; multiple sclerosis; mental status; medical student; morphine sulfate
MSE	mental status examination
MSO4	morphine sulfate
MV	mitral valve
MVA	motor vehicle accident
MVI	multivitamin
MVP	mitral valve prolapse
MVR	mitral valve replacement
MVV	maximum voluntary ventilation
N	nerve
N/A	not applicable
NAD	no acute distress

NAI	nonaccidental injury
NAS	no added salt
NBN	newborn nursery
NC	no change; nasal cannula; normocephalic
NC/AT	normocephalic, atraumatic
ND	not detected/diagnosed/done
NDI	nephrogenic diabetes insipidus
NE	norepinephrine
NEC	necrotizing enterocolitis
neg	negative
NG	nasogastric
NGT	nasogastric tube
NH	nursing home
NHL	non-Hodgkin's lymphoma
NIDDM	non-insulin-dependent DM
N/K	not known
NKDA	no known drug allergies
NL	normal limits
NM	neuromuscular
NMS	neuroleptic malignant syndrome
NOS	not otherwise specified
NP	nasopharyngeal, nurse practitioner
NPH	neutral protamine Hagedorn (regular insulin); normal pressure hydrocephalus
NPO	nothing by mouth (Lat: nihil per orem)
NQW MI	non-Q wave myocard. infarction
NS	normal saline; not specific
NSAID	nonsteroidal anti-inflamm. drug
NSR	normal sinus rhythm
NT	nasotracheal; not tested; not tender
NTD	nothing to do; neur. tube defect
NTT	nasotracheal tube
NTG	nitroglycerine
N&V	nausea and vomiting
NVD	nausea, vomiting, diarrhea
O	objective
OA	osteoarthritis; occiput anterior
OAF	osteoclast-activating factor
OB	obstetrics
OBS	organic brain syndrome
occ	occasionally
OCG	oral cholecystogram
OCR	oculocephalic reflex
OCT	oral contraceptive therapy
OD	overdose; once daily; right eye
OE	on examination
OF	open fracture
OGTT	oral glucose tolerance test
OM	otitis media
OOB	out of bed
OP	oropharynx; occiput posterior; opening pressure
O&P	ova and parasites
OPD	outpatient department
OPV	oral polio vaccine
OR	operating room
OREF	open reduction, external fixation
ORIF	open reduction, internal fixation
orth	orthopedic
OS	by mouth (Lat: os); left eye (Lat: oculus sinister); overall survival; opening snap (heart sound)
OSA	obstructive sleep apnea
osmo	osmolality
OT	occupational therapy
OTC	over the counter
OU	both eyes (Lat: oculus uterque)

P	after (post); parent; plan; pulse
P_2	second pulmonic heart sound
PA	patient; posteroanterior (x-ray); physician's assistant; pulmonary artery
PAC	premature atrial contraction
PAN	polyarteritis nodosa
PAP	pulmonary artery pressure
PAT	paroxysmal atrial tachycardia
PAWP	pulm. artery wedge pressure
PBC	primary biliary cirrhosis
PBP	penicillin-binding protein
PC	present complaint
pc	after meals (Lat: post cibum)
PCA	patient-controlled analgesia
PCB	postcoital bleeding
PCN	penicillin
PCOS	polycystic ovarian syndrome
PCP	pneumocystis carinii pneumonia; primary care physician
PCR	polymerase chain reaction
PCV	packed cell volume
PCW	pulmonary capillary wedge
PD	peritoneal dialysis; Paget's disease; Parkinson's disease
PDA	patent ductus arteriosus, personal digital assistant
PDR	Physician's Desk Reference
PE	pulmonary embolism; physical examination
PEEP	positive end-expiratory pressure
PEF(R)	peak expiratory flow (rate)
PEG	percutaneous endoscopic gastrostomy
PERRLA	pupils equal, round, react to light and accommodation
PET	positron emission tomography

PFT	pulmonary function test
PG(E)	prostaglandin (E)
PGF	paternal grandfather
PGM	paternal grandmother
PH	past history; pulmonary HTN
PI	present illness
PICC	peripherally inserted central catheter
PICU	pediatric intensive care unit
PID	pelvic inflammatory disease
PKD	polycystic kidney disease
PKU	phenylketonuria
PLT	platelets
PM	postmortem; postmenopausal
PMB	postmenopausal bleeding
PMH	past medical history
PMI	point of maximal impulse; past medical illness
PMN	polymorphonuclear leukocyte
PMR	polymyalgia rheumatica; phys. medicine and rehabilitation
PMS	premenstrual syndrome
PNA	pneumonia
PND	paroxysmal nocturnal dyspnea
PNH	paroxysmal nocturnal hemoglobinuria
PNS	peripheral nervous system
PO	by mouth (Lat: per os); postoper.
POC	postoperative care; product of conception
POD	postoperative day
POP	plaster of Paris
PPD	purified protein derivative; packs per day
PPH	postpartum hemorrhage
PPHN	persistent pulmon. hypertension
PPN	peripheral parenteral nutrition
PPP	peripheral pulses present

PPS	peripheral pulmonary stenosis; postpartum sterilization
PPTL	postpartum tubal ligation
PR	per rectum; pulse rate
PR(B)C	packed red (blood) cells
prn	as required (Lat: pro re nata)
PROM	premature rupture of membrane
PS	pulmonary stenosis
PSA	polysubstance abuse
PSH	past surgical history
PSS	progressive systemic sclerosis
PSVT	paroxysmal supraventricular tachycardia
PT	prothrombin time; paroxysmal tachycardia; physical therapy
pt	patient
PTA	prior to admission
PTC	percutaneous transhepatic cholangiogram
PTCA	percutaneous transluminal coronary angioplasty
PTE	pulmonary thromboembolism
PTL	preterm labor
PTSD	posttraumatic stress disorder
PTT	partial thromboplastin time
PTX	pneumothorax
PU	passed urine; peptic ulcer
PUD	peptic ulcer disease
PUO	pyrexia of unknown origin
PUPPP	pruritic urticarial papules and plaques of pregnancy
PV	examination per vagina; pemphigus vulgaris; polycythemia vera; portal vein
PVC	premature ventric. contraction
PVD	peripheral vascular disease

PVR	peripheral vascular resistance; pulse-volume recording
PVT	paroxysmal ventr. tachycardia
py	pack years (of cigarettes)
q	every, each (Lat: quaque)
qam	every morning
qd	every day, once a day (quaque die)
qh	every hour (Lat: quaque hora)
q2h	every two hours
qhs	every bedtime (Lat: hora somni)
qid	4 times daily (Lat: quater in die)
QNS	quantity not sufficient
qod	every other day
qpm	every evening
QS	as much as will suffice (Lat: quantum sufficit); quantity sufficient (Lat: quantum satis)
;R	right
RA	rheumatoid arthritis; right atrium; room air
RAD	reactive airway disease; right axis deviation
RAIU	radioactive iodine uptake
RAST	radioallergosorbent test
RBBB	right bundle branch block
RBC	red blood (cell) count
RCA	right coronary artery
RDI	recommended daily intake
RDS	respiratory distress syndrome
reg	regular(ly)
REM	rapid eye movement
RES	reticuloendothelial system
RF	rheumatic fever; rheumatoid factor; renal failure; risk factor
RHD	rheumatic heart disease; renal hypertensive disease

RIND	reversible ischemic neurol. deficit
RL	Ringer's lactate; right leg/lung
RLE	right lower extremity
RLL	right lower lobe
RLQ	right lower quadrant
RML	right middle lobe
RN	registered nurse
R/O	rule out
ROM	range of motion; rupture of membranes
ROS	review of systems/symptoms
RPF	renal plasma flow
RPGN	rapidly progressive glomerulonephritis
RPR	rapid plasma reagin (syphilis tx)
RR	respiratory rate
RRP	relative refractory period
RRR	regular rate and rhythm
RS	right side
RSB	right sternal border
RSV	respiratory syncytial virus
rt	right
RTA	renal tubular acidosis
RTC	return to clinic
RTS	Revised Trauma Score
RUE	right upper extremity
RUL	right upper lobe
RUQ	right upper quadrant
RV	right ventricle; residual volume
RVH	right ventricular hypertrophy
Rx	drug; treatment; prescription (Lat: recipe)
Rxn	reaction
s	without (Lat: sine)
S_1 ... S_4	heart sounds, 1st to 4th
SA	sinoatrial; salicylic acid; suicide attempt

SAB	spontaneous abortion
SAD	seasonal (schizo-) affective DO
SAH	subarachnoid hemorrhage
SBE	subacute bacterial endocarditis
SBO	small bowel obstruction
SBP	systolic blood pressure
SC	subcutaneous
SD	standard deviation
SDH	subdural hematoma
SEM	systolic ejection murmur
SEMI	subendocardial MI
SES	socioeconomic status
SGA	small for gestational age
SGOT	serum glutamic oxaloacetic transaminase (now called AST)
SGPT	serum glutamic pyruvic transaminase (now called ALT)
SHx	social history
SIADH	synd. of inappropriate ADH secr.
SICU	surgical intensive care unit
SIDS	sudden infant death syndrome
SK	streptokinase
SL	sublingual
SLE	systemic lupus erythematosus
SLR	straight leg raising (Lasègue)
SMA	sequential multiple analyzer
SNF	skilled nursing facility
SOB	shortness of breath
SP	suprapubic; systolic pressure
s/p	status post, no change
SPEP	serum protein electrophoresis
SQ	subcutaneous
SR	systems review; sustained release
SROM	spontaneous rupture of membrane
S&S	signs and symptoms
SSE	soapsuds enema

SSPE	subacute scleros. panencephalitis
SSS	sick sinus syndrome; scalded skin syndrome
ST	sinus tachycardia
stat	immediately (Lat: statim)
STD	sexually transmitted diseases
STS	serologic test for syphilis
SVC	superior vena cava
SVR	systemic vascular resistance
SVT	supraventricular tachycardia
SW	social worker
Sx	signs, symptoms
SZ	schizophrenia; seizure
T	temperature
T_3	triiodothyronine
T_4	thyroxine
T&A	tonsillectomy + adenoidectomy
tab	tablet
TAH	total abdominal hysterectomy
TAT	Thematic Apperception Test
TB	tuberculosis
T&C	type and cross-match (blood)
TCA	tricyclic antidepressant
TCI	to come in (hospital)
TD	tolerance dose
TEE	transesophageal echocardiogram
TEF	tracheoesophageal fistula
TFT	thyroid function test
TG	triglycerides
TGA	transient global amnesia
TGV	transposition of great vessels
T&H	type and hold
THC	transhepatic cholangiogram
THR	total hip replacement
TIA	transient ischemic attack
TIBC	total iron-binding capacity
tid	three times daily (Lat: ter in die)
TIPS	transjugular intrahepatic portosystemic shunt
tiw	three times a week
TLC	total lung capacity
TM	tympanic membrane
TMP	trimethoprim
TNM	tumor, node, metastasis
TOA	tubo-ovarian abscess
TOP	termination of pregnancy
TOS	thoracic outlet syndrome
TPA	tissue plasminogen activator
TPN	total parenteral nutrition
TPR	temperature, pulse, respirations; total peripheral resistance
TSH	thyroid-stimulating hormone
tsp	teaspoon
TSS	toxic shock syndrome
TT	tetanus toxoid; thrombin time
TTE	transthoracic echocardiogram
TTP	thrombotic thrombocytopenic purpura
TUR (P/BT)	transurethral resection (of prostate/bladder tumor)
TV	tidal volume
Tx	treatment
U	units
UA	urinalysis; uric acid
UC	ulcer. colitis; urinary catheter
UE	upper extremity
UGI	upper gastrointestinal (series)
UMN	upper motor neuron
UO	urinary output
unk	unknown
URI	upper respiratory infection
US	ultrasound

UTD	up to date
UTI	urinary tract infection
UV	ultraviolet
VA	Veterans Admin.; ventriculoatrial
VB	vaginal bleeding
VC	vital capacity
VCUG	voiding cystourethrogram
VD	venereal disease
VDRL	VD Research Lab (syphilis test)
VE	vaginal examination
VF	ventricular fibrillation
VH	vaginal hysterectomy
VIP	vasoactive intestinal peptide
VLDL	very low-density lipoprotein
VMA	vanillylmandelic acid
VNS	visiting nurse service
VO	verbal order
VPC	ventr. premature contraction
V/Q	ventilation-perfusion ratio
VS	vital signs
VSD	ventricular septal defect
VT	ventricular tachycardia
VZV	varicella-zoster virus
WB	whole blood
WBC	white blood (cell) count
WCC	white cell count
WD	ward; wound; well-developed

WF	white female
wk	week
WM	white male
WN	well-nourished
WNL	within normal limits
WPW	Wolff-Parkinson-White
wt	weight
X	times, except, cross
x/12	x number of months
x/24	x number of hours
x/40	x number of gestation weeks
x/52	x number of weeks
x/7	x number of days
XR	x-ray
XRT	(external) radiation therapy
y	year
yo	year(s) old
ZES	Zollinger-Ellison syndrome

E Medical Resources on the Web

Needle Sticks

CDC Emergency Needlestick Information Website:
http://www.cdc.gov/niosh/topics/bbp/emergnedl.html

National Clinicians Post-Exposure Prophylaxis Hotline (PEPLine): 888-448-4911

CDC, National Institute of Occupational Safety and Health Hotline (for reporting HIV seroconversions in health care workers with and without post-exposure prophylaxis): 800-893-0485

Bioterrorism information

CDC Bioterrorism Portal: www.cdc.gov or www.bt.cdc.gov/bioterrorism

Travel Medicine

CDC Travel Information Portal and Yellow Book: http://wwwnc.cdc.gov/travel/

Essential Online References

UpToDate: www.uptodateonline.com
New England Journal of Medicine: www.nejm.org
Medscape Emedicine Portal: emedicine.medscape.com
Google Scholar: scholar.google.com
National Guideline Clearinghouse: www.guideline.gov

Evidence Based Medicine

Cochrane database: www.cochrane.org
Pubmed: www.ncbi.nlm.nih.gov/entrez
Ovid: password required- ask your librarian!

Residency/Fellowship Information

Freida Online: ww.ama-assn.org/vapp/freida/srch/
National Residency Match: www.nrmp.org

Essential Downloads and Resources for Mobile Devices

iMedicalApps (medical app reviews): www.imedicalapps.com
Epocrates App Portal: apps.epocrates.com
Medscape Mobile: http://www.medscape.com/public/mobileapp
Cleaveland Clinic Mobile App Portal: my.clevelandclinic.org/mobile-apps/default.aspx
Borm Bruckmeier Publishing Medical Reference Mobile Apps: www.media4u.com

F Answers to Board Questions

1 Fluids, Electrolytes, Acid-Base

1) C - Caffeine
2) Increased Na^+ reabsorption, increased H^+ and K^+ secretion
3) A - an increase in plasma oncotic pressure
4) A,C - lack of antidiuretic hormone, nephrogenic diabetes insipidus
5) Low, High

2 Cardiology

1) β1 selective β-blockers
2) Atropine and possible pacemaker placement
3) Coronary catheterization; Stress testing is contraindicated in aortic stenosis.
4) Mitral stenosis
5) No prophylaxis is indicated

3 Endocrinology

1) The hypothyroidism should NOT be treated first as this may precipitate adrenal crisis, a medical emergency
2) D-autoimmune adrenalitis
3) Vitamin D3 (1,25-OH-vitamin D)
4) PTU
5) Kallman's syndrome, GnRH analogues via portable pump may be of value

4 Gastroenterology

1) Intestinal lymphoma as a complication of celiac disease
2) Scleroderma in a patient with decreased sphincter tone.
3) Gilbert's syndrome
4) Polyarteritis nodosa as a complication of Hepatitis B
5) VIPoma

5 Geriatrics

1) Treat restless leg syndrome with any of the following: pramipexole (Mirapex) or ropinirole (Requip), L-dopa/carbidopa (Sinemet), clonazepam, or gabapentin.
2) This patient with carotid sinus hypersensitivity should avoid triggers, such as tight collars. He may require cardiac pacing if cardio-inhibitory response is elicited.
3) Benadryl can cause delirium, confusion, constipation, and urinary retention and should not be used as a sleep aid.
4) Meperidine (Demerol) is metabolized to normeperidine an active metabolite with 2-3 times the CNS effects of meperidine, that can accumulate with decreased renal function.
5) Tetanus diphtheria booster every 10 years, Influenza vaccine every year, and Pneumococcal vaccine once after age 65.

6 Hematology

1) Hodgkin disease in a patient with a Reed-Sternberg cell.
2) Paroxysmal Nocturnal Hemoglobinuria (PNH)- where GPI (glycosyl-phosphatidyl-inosityl)-linked proteins are missing from the surface of PNH hematopoietic cells. The most specific test is analysis of RBCs for the absence of the GPI-anchored proteins CD55 (DAF) and CD59.
3) MRI of the hip to confirm avascular necrosis of the femoral head
4) Erythropoietin can cause hypertension, thrombosis in shunts, seizures, and hyperkalemia.
5) Rho(D) immune globulin (WinRho) may delay time to splenectomy in patients who are Rh+ with ITP.

7 HIV

1) Varicella, oral polio, MMR, and BCG (for tuberculosis).
2) HIV- associated lipodystrophy
3) H. capsulatum glycoprotein antigen can be detected in the urine of 90% of patient with disseminated histoplasmosis and 75% of those with diffuse acute pulmonary histoplasmosis. Serologic tests are another option, although the antibody levels may be lower in this immunosuppressed individual.
4) The patient should be treated for latent tuberculosis with INH (300mg QD or 900mg 2x/week) for nine months. Another acceptable regimen is rifampin (600mg daily or 2x/week) for 4 months
5) Patients are typically highly infectious during acute HIV due to a very high viral load in blood an genital secretions. They may continue to engage in risky sexual activities and expose others to HIV. An HIV viral load will confirm the diagnosis.

8 Infectious Diseases

1) Ceftriaxone 125mg IM + azithromycin 1 gram PO x 1 dose. As a note, doxycycline should be avoided in pregnancy.
2) The soon the person begins prophylaxis for HIV after a needle stick the better. They should not wait to finish their shift.
3) Vancomycin 1gm IV every 12 hours- Coverage for MRSA.
4) ELISA testing for Leptospirosis is rapid and widely available. The gold standard is the MAT (macroscopic agglutination test), although it requires live organisms, and is performed only by specialized laboratories like the CDC.
5) Empiric antifungal therapy with amphotericin B and surgical evaluation for possible mucormycosis (zygomycosis).

9 Internal Medicine

1) Esophagitis caused by bulimia. Eating habits should be discussed and the patient should be referred to a psychiatrist.
2) Stop the medication and check the CK level.
3) Don't give measles vaccine since it is a live vaccine. Give γ-globulin 0.25 mg/kg IM
4) Give steroids. Steroids should be given before a biopsy is performed in this case.

10 Womens'Health

1) Give HBIg + HepB vaccine to the child at the time of delivery
2) b
3) c
4) c
5) e

11 Nephrology

1) No
2) Multiple Myeloma with light chain production (Bence-Jones proteins) should be excluded in all patients with proximal RTA, unless another cause can be identified.
3) IgA nephropathy. Poststrepococcal nephropathy usually occurs 1-3 weeks after an infection.
4) Supportive care for Henoch-Schonlein purpura includes hydration, rest, and pain control. NSAIDS may be considered for abdominal pain Naproxen 10-20 mg/kg bid. For severe abdominal pain Prednisone 1-2 mg/kg/d may be considered although they do not shorten the disease course.
5) Serum assay for anti-Glomerular basement membrane antibodies along with the findings on immunofluoroscence are found in Goodpastures' Syndrome.

12 Neurology

1) Classic Migraine; Subcutaneous Imitrex +/- metoclopramide
2) Multiple sclerosis; MRI of the brain and cervical spine with gadolinium
3) Epidural abscess; MRI of the spine with gadolinium, and blood cultures
4) Left, Middle Cerebral Artery; CT is often normal within the first few hours of an ischemic stroke.
5) Tardive dyskinesia from long term antipsychotic medications. There is no treatment, however traditional antipsychotics (ie, Haldol) should be changed to atypicals (ie, Seroquel) when possible.

13 Oncology

1) Colonoscopy- there is an association between colonic neoplasia and S. bovis bacteremia.
2) Uterine cancer- tamoxifen is as risk factor for the development of uterine cancer. It also increases the risk of thromboembolic disease as well as vision changes. This patient should be referred for an endometrial biopsy.
3) Burkitt's lymphoma in Africa, non-Hodgkin's lymphoma, Hodgkin's disease, nasopharyngeal carcinoma, T-cell lymphoma (rare)
4) Chemotherapy and radiation
5) Prostate gland biopsy. Usually a TRUS-(transrectal ultrasound) guided prostate biopsy is the procedure of choice.

16 Psychiatry

1) c
2) b
3) b
4) a
5) e

17 Pulmonary and Critical Care

1) Exercise challenge test. Methacholine challenge may have equivocal results in these patients.
2) Prednisone 1-1/5 mg/kg/day x 4-8 weeks, then tapered to 0.5-1 mg/kg/day for the next 6 weeks.
3) Trimethoprim sulfamethoxazole (Bactrim) 2 double strength tablets PO every 8 hours for 21days with prednisone: 40 mg BID PO for 5 days, then 40 mg once daily PO for 5 days, and then 20 mg once daily PO for 11 days.

4) e: The current recommendations from the Centers for Disease Control state that the single most important test for Legionnaires' disease is isolation of the organism by culture. When the disease is suspected both a urinary antigen and respiratory specimen should be ordered. Since the urinary antigen is specific for L. pneumophilia serogroup 1 - accounting for 70% of Legionella infections- it may not be reliable for diagnosis of disease caused by non-serogroup 1 organisms.
5) Emergent intervention for tension pneumothorax: do not wait for cxr. Administer 100% oxygen. Locate anatomic landmarks and quickly prepare the area to be punctured with an iodine-based solution (eg, Betadine). Insert a large-bore (ie, 14-gauge or 16-gauge) needle with a catheter into the second intercostal space, just superior to the third rib at the midclavicular line, 1-2 cm from the sternal edge (ie, to avoid injury to the internal thoracic artery). Use a 3-6 cm long needle, and hold it perpendicular to the chest wall when inserting; however, note that some patients may have a chest wall thickness greater than 3 cm and failure for the symptoms to resolve may be attributed to inadequate needle length. Once the needle is in the pleural space, listen for the hissing sound of air escaping, and remove the needle while leaving the catheter in place. Secure the catheter in place, and install a flutter valve. Prepare the patient for tube thoracostomy.

18 Rheumatology

1) SLE. The findings of proteinuria would not be expected in a patient with RA. Atypical renal, cardiac, and endocrine complication have only been reported in a few cases of adult-onset Still's disease.
2) Thromboangiitis obliterans (Buerger's disease). The patient should be instructed to stop smoking cigarettes.
3) Ruptured popliteal cyst (Baker's cyst). However, an ultrasound should still be performed to rule out a deep vein thrombosis.
4) Hypothyroidism. Hypothyroidism, Diabetes, and acromegaly are all associated with carpal tunnel syndrome.
5) Felty's syndrome

July 2012

Tu	1	
We	2	
Th	3	
Fr	4	Independence Day
Sa	5	
Su	6	
Mo	7	
Tu	8	
We	9	
Th	10	
Fr	11	
Sa	12	
Su	13	
Mo	14	
Tu	15	
We	16	
Th	17	
Fr	18	
Sa	19	
Su	20	
Mo	21	
Tu	22	
We	23	
Th	24	
Fr	25	
Sa	26	
Su	27	
Mo	28	
Tu	29	
We	30	
Th	31	

August 2012

Fr	1	
Sa	2	
Su	3	
Mo	4	
Tu	5	
We	6	
Th	7	
Fr	8	
Sa	9	
Su	10	
Mo	11	
Tu	12	
We	13	
Th	14	
Fr	15	
Sa	16	
Su	17	
Mo	18	
Tu	19	
We	20	
Th	21	
Fr	22	
Sa	23	
Su	24	
Mo	25	
Tu	26	
We	27	
Th	28	
Fr	29	
Sa	30	
Su	31	

September 2012

Mo	1	Labor Day
Tu	2	
We	3	
Th	4	
Fr	5	
Sa	6	
Su	7	
Mo	8	
Tu	9	
We	10	
Th	11	
Fr	12	
Sa	13	
Su	14	
Mo	15	
Tu	16	
We	17	
Th	18	
Fr	19	
Sa	20	
Su	21	
Mo	22	
Tu	23	
We	24	
Th	25	
Fr	26	
Sa	27	
Su	28	
Mo	29	
Tu	30	

October 2012

We	1	
Th	2	
Fr	3	
Sa	4	
Su	5	
Mo	6	
Tu	7	
We	8	
Th	9	
Fr	10	
Sa	11	
Su	12	
Mo	13	Columbus Day
Tu	14	
We	15	
Th	16	
Fr	17	
Sa	18	
So	19	
Mo	20	
Tu	21	
We	22	
Th	23	
Fr	24	
Sa	25	
Su	26	
Mo	27	
Tu	28	
We	29	
Th	30	
Fr	31	Halloween

November 2012

Sa	1	
Su	2	
Mo	3	
Tu	4	
We	5	
Th	6	
Fr	7	
Sa	8	
Su	9	
Mo	10	
Tu	11	Veterans Day
We	12	
Th	13	
Fr	14	
Sa	15	
Su	16	
Mo	17	
Tu	18	
We	19	
Th	20	
Fr	21	
Sa	22	
Su	23	
Mo	24	
Tu	25	
We	26	
Th	27	Thanksgiving Day
Fr	28	
Sa	29	
Su	30	

December 2012

Mo	1	
Tu	2	
We	3	
Th	4	
Fr	5	
Sa	6	
Su	7	
Mo	8	
Tu	9	
We	10	
Th	11	
Fr	12	
Sa	13	
Su	14	
Mo	15	
Tu	16	
We	17	
Th	18	
Fr	19	
Sa	20	
Su	21	
Mo	22	
Tu	23	
We	24	Christmas Eve
Th	25	Christmas Day
Fr	26	
Sa	27	
Su	28	
Mo	29	
Tu	30	
We	31	New Year's Eve

January 2013

Th	1	New Year's Day
Fr	2	
Sa	3	
Su	4	
Mo	5	
Tu	6	
We	7	
Th	8	
Fr	9	
Sa	10	
Su	11	
Mo	12	
Tu	13	
We	14	
Th	15	
Fr	16	
Sa	17	
Su	18	
Mo	19	Martin Luther King Day
Tu	20	
We	21	
Th	22	
Fr	23	
Sa	24	
Su	25	
Mo	26	
Tu	27	
We	28	
Th	29	
Fr	30	
Sa	31	

February 2013

Su	1	
Mo	2	
Tu	3	
We	4	
Th	5	
Fr	6	
Sa	7	
Su	8	
Mo	9	
Tu	10	
We	11	
Th	12	
Fr	13	
Sa	14	Valentine's Day
Su	15	
Mo	16	Washington's Birthday
Tu	17	
We	18	
Th	19	
Fr	20	
Sa	21	
Su	22	
Mo	23	
Tu	24	
We	25	
Th	26	
Fr	27	
Sa	28	

March 2013

Su	1	
Mo	2	
Tu	3	
We	4	
Th	5	
Fr	6	
Sa	7	
Su	8	
Mo	9	
Tu	10	
We	11	
Th	12	
Fr	13	
Sa	14	
Su	15	
Mo	16	
Tu	17	
We	18	
Th	19	
Fr	20	
Sa	21	
Su	22	
Mo	23	
Tu	24	
We	25	
Th	26	
Fr	27	
Sa	28	
Su	29	
Mo	30	
Tu	31	

April 2013

We	1	
Th	2	
Fr	3	
Sa	4	
Su	5	
Mo	6	
Tu	7	
We	8	
Th	9	
Fr	10	
Sa	11	
Su	12	
Mo	13	
Tu	14	
We	15	
Th	16	
Fr	17	
Sa	18	
Su	19	
Mo	20	
Tu	21	
We	22	
Th	23	
Fr	24	
Sa	25	
Su	26	
Mo	27	
Tu	28	
We	29	
Th	30	

May 2013

Fr	1	
Sa	2	
Su	3	
Mo	4	
Tu	5	
We	6	
Th	7	
Fr	8	
Sa	9	
Su	10	
Mo	11	
Tu	12	
We	13	
Th	14	
Fr	15	
Sa	16	
Su	17	
Mo	18	
Tu	19	
We	20	
Th	21	
Fr	22	
Sa	23	
Su	24	
Mo	25	Memorial Day
Tu	26	
We	27	
Th	28	
Fr	29	
Sa	30	
Su	31	

June 2013

Mo	1	
Tu	2	
We	3	
Th	4	
Fr	5	
Sa	6	
Su	7	
Mo	8	
Tu	9	
We	10	
Th	11	
Fr	12	
Sa	13	
Su	14	
Mo	15	
Tu	16	
We	17	
Th	18	
Fr	19	
Sa	20	
Su	21	
Mo	22	
Tu	23	
We	24	
Th	25	
Fr	26	
Sa	27	
Su	28	
Mo	29	
Tu	30	

July 2013

We	1	
Th	2	
Fr	3	
Sa	4	Independence Day
Su	5	
Mo	6	
Tu	7	
We	8	
Th	9	
Fr	10	
Sa	11	
Su	12	
Mo	13	
Tu	14	
We	15	
Th	16	
Fr	17	
Sa	18	
Su	19	
Mo	20	
Tu	21	
We	22	
Th	23	
Fr	24	
Sa	25	
Su	26	
Mo	27	
Tu	28	
We	29	
Th	30	
Fr	31	

August 2013

Sa	1	
Su	2	
Mo	3	
Tu	4	
We	5	
Th	6	
Fr	7	
Sa	8	
Su	9	
Mo	10	
Tu	11	
We	12	
Th	13	
Fr	14	
Sa	15	
Su	16	
Mo	17	
Tu	18	
We	19	
Th	20	
Fr	21	
Sa	22	
Su	23	
Mo	24	
Tu	25	
We	26	
Th	27	
Fr	28	
Sa	29	
Su	30	
Mo	31	

September 2013

Tu	1	
We	2	
Th	3	
Fr	4	
Sa	5	
Su	6	
Mo	7	Labor Day
Tu	8	
We	9	
Th	10	
Fr	11	
Sa	12	
Su	13	
Mo	14	
Tu	15	
We	16	
Th	17	
Fr	18	
Sa	19	
Su	20	
Mo	21	
Tu	22	
We	23	
Th	24	
Fr	25	
Sa	26	
Su	27	
Mo	28	
Tu	29	
We	30	

October 2013

Th	1	
Fr	2	
Sa	3	
Su	4	
Mo	5	
Tu	6	
We	7	
Th	8	
Fr	9	
Sa	10	
Su	11	
Mo	12	Columbus Day
Tu	13	
We	14	
Th	15	
Fr	16	
Sa	17	
Su	18	
Mo	19	
Tu	20	
We	21	
Th	22	
Fr	23	
Sa	24	
Su	25	
Mo	26	
Tu	27	
We	28	
Th	29	
Fr	30	
Sa	31	Halloween

November 2013

Su	1	
Mo	2	
Tu	3	
We	4	
Th	5	
Fr	6	
Sa	7	
Su	8	
Mo	9	
Tu	10	
We	11	Veterans Day
Th	12	
Fr	13	
Sa	14	
Su	15	
Mo	16	
Tu	17	
We	18	
Th	19	
Fr	20	
Sa	21	
Su	22	
Mo	23	
Tu	24	
We	25	
Th	26	Thanksgiving Day
Fr	27	
Sa	28	
Su	29	
Mo	30	

December 2013

Tu	1	
We	2	
Th	3	
Fr	4	
Sa	5	
Su	6	
Mo	7	
Tu	8	
We	9	
Th	10	
Fr	11	
Sa	12	
Su	13	
Mo	14	
Tu	15	
We	16	
Th	17	
Fr	18	
Sa	19	
Su	20	
Mo	21	
Tu	22	
We	23	
Th	24	Christmas Eve
Fr	25	Christmas Day
Sa	26	
Su	27	
Mo	28	
Tu	29	
We	30	
Th	31	New Year's Eve

Key Telephone Numbers

	Telephone Number	
Emergency Call		
Wards		
–		
–		
–		
–		
–		
–		
–		
–		
–		
House Staff		
–		
–		
–		
–		
–		
–		
–		
–		
–		
–		

	Telephone Number	
Attending Staff		
–		
–		
–		
–		
–		
–		
–		
–		
–		
Department		
Admitting		
Anesthesia		
CCU		
ECG		
EEG		
ER		
ICU		
Laboratory		
– Chemistry		
– Hematology		
– Microbiology		
– Other		

	Telephone Number	
Nuclear Medicine		
OR		
Pathology		
Pharmacy		
Physical Therapy		
Pulmonary Function		
Imaging		
- CT		
- MRI		
- X-Ray		
Recovery Room		
Security		
Social Service		
Sonography		
Surgery		
-		
-		
-		
-		
-		
-		
-		
-		
-		

	Telephone Number	
Nursing Stations		
–		
–		
–		
–		
–		
–		
–		
–		
–		
–		
–		
–		
Call Pagers		
–		
–		
–		
–		
–		
–		
–		
–		
–		
–		

	Telephone Number	
Consults		
– Anesthesia		
– Cardiology		
– Gynecology/OB		
– Nephrology		
– Neurology		
– Pediatrics		
– Oncology		
– Pulmonary		
– Psychiatry		
– Radiology		
– Surgery		
–		
–		
–		
–		
–		
–		
Other Numbers		
– Police		
– Taxi		
–		
–		
–		

Numerics

A

B

Trade name = bold *Drug name = italic*

Trade name = bold *Drug name = italic*

Trade name = bold *Drug name = italic*

Trade name = bold *Drug name = italic*

Q

Trade name = bold *Drug name = italic*

Trade name = bold *Drug name = italic*

T

Trade name = bold *Drug name = italic*

U

Trade name = bold *Drug name = italic*

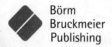

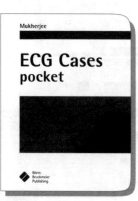